A Prehabilitation Guide for All Providers

Alexander Watson • Karen Barr
Editors

A Prehabilitation Guide for All Providers

Springer

Editors
Alexander Watson
University of Pittsburgh Medical Center
Pittsburgh, PA, USA

Karen Barr
University of Pittsburgh Medical Center
Pittsburgh, PA, USA

ISBN 978-3-031-72864-8 ISBN 978-3-031-72862-4 (eBook)
https://doi.org/10.1007/978-3-031-72862-4

This Springer imprint is published by the registered company Springer Nature Switzerland AG
The registered company address is: Gewerbestrasse 11, 6330 Cham, Switzerland

Contents

Introduction to Prehabilitation

Alexander Watson and Karen Barr

Pre-habilitation, prehabilitation, or "prehab" is the concept of using many traditional rehabilitation strategies to prepare for surgery or other major medical interventions such as chemotherapy. The premise is that by improving the individual's health and functional status prior to the physical stress, the individual will have greater resilience, resulting in better outcomes. Many prehabilitation plans set tangible goals such as improvements in holistic measurements of function such as the 6-minute walk test (6MWT), weight loss of a certain amount, normalization of abnormal lab values such as blood glucose or liver enzymes, or improvement in respiratory function. These changes are associated with improved surgical outcomes such as reduced complication rates, shorter length of stay, and lower rates of reoperation, depending on the intervention they precede. Many surgeries—particularly orthopedic—often have body mass index (BMI) maximums and will refer patients who exceed these cutoffs for evaluation by a weight loss specialist prior to surgery [1]. In some cases, surgery is contingent upon achieving certain goals.

Even if other specialists do not have absolute BMI or hemoglobin A1c maximums, interested patients and clinicians can pursue risk reductions for upcoming procedures by deliberately targeting specific high-yield metrics. As obesity-associated comorbidities span endocrinologic/metabolic, orthopedic, psychiatric, pulmonologic/sleep, and neurologic systems, healthcare providers must screen patients with obesity for distinct conditions prior to surgery, ensuring these individuals have optimal resilience and stamina to run the gauntlet and even persevere through the low [2, 3] but nonzero risks of complications. Notably, complication rates are relatively higher in the older adult population, with one meta-analysis

A. Watson (✉)
Admire Medical, Middletown, DE, USA
e-mail: Alexander@admiremedical.com

K. Barr
University of Pittsburgh, Pittsburgh, PA, USA
e-mail: barrkp@upmc.edu

A. Watson, K. Barr (eds.), *A Prehabilitation Guide for All Providers*,
https://doi.org/10.1007/978-3-031-72862-4_1

calculating a pooled rate of 14.7% for older adults undergoing bariatric surgery and attributing it to multiple factors including decreased cell proliferation, cell migration, growth factors, and extracellular matrix functioning [4]. Similarly, complication rates in joint replacement surgeries increase steadily with increasing age, and one review notes approximately 5% of patients over 80 years old experience at least one complication relative to 0.35% in patients <50 years old [5].

Prehabilitation practitioners can be integral partners in fostering this resilience through a multifaceted regimen—less about blindly screening and more related to targeted preparation, education, and patient empowerment. Moreover, while this framework and these principles are currently employed predominantly prior to cancer treatment and organ transplantation, a multimodal prehabilitation program should be the scaffolding on which most major surgical preparation is built.

As has already been introduced, the benefits of prehabilitation are intuitive, particularly if the patient is significantly deconditioned and/or has components of metabolic disease. Thorough medical weight loss plans involve many of the same principles as multimodal surgical preparation. Weight loss, decreased pain, and improved independent function restore the patient's quality of life. These multimodal programs in tandem with the newest pharmacotherapies are the most effective nonsurgical way to target obesity, given the many contributing factors including diet, genetics, environmental cues, activity level, and disability and the countless comorbidities associated with obesity.

There are other primary reasons for addressing the overlap of prehabilitation and obesity medicine early in this text. First, obesity is a well-established risk factor for most cancers [6, 7], osteoarthritis (OA) [8–10], and degenerative spinal disease [11, 12]. Treating obesity and metabolic disease aggressively at the root cause with nutritional modifications, exercise, and modern pharmacology will at least *slow* the progression of obesity-related comorbidities, if not halt or even reverse some. Further, as obesity is often accompanied by low-grade inflammation [13, 14], treating obesity has been shown to ease this inflammatory state in some cases [15, 16], which may also improve pain symptoms in painful musculoskeletal pathology [17, 18]. Although these improvements are unlikely to reverse the need for surgical intervention, they may extend the preoperative period and allow for further health optimization.

Moreover, clinicians with a bird's-eye view of the patient's health can extend screening beyond what is required for their impending intervention, as the obesity-related comorbidities do not "wait their turn" until their presenting condition is addressed. For example, the patient presenting with end-stage knee osteoarthritis anticipating a total knee arthroplasty (TKA) is also significantly more likely to have nonalcoholic fatty liver disease (NAFLD), which is now the leading cause of liver transplantation [19]. As such, the prehabilitation program for the first illness may function as treatment for or primary/secondary/tertiary prevention of other pathology. In fact, medications that are prescribed primarily for glycemic control in the outpatient setting like glucagon-like peptide-1 (GLP-1) receptor agonists [20, 21], sodium-glucose cotransporter-2 (SGLT2) inhibitors [22], and metformin [23, 24] are associated with end organ benefits beyond what would be expected by simply achieving optimal glucose control. Therefore, those utilizing these medications may have ancillary metabolic effects that patients would only previously achieve following significant weight loss.

Finally, metabolic syndrome may impact surgical recovery, and in some instances, chemotherapeutic agents may worsen insulin resistance. For reasons such as these, appropriate pre-procedural preparation can improve postoperative wound healing, reduce pain and complications, and mitigate the side effects of the intervention. For example, achieving glycemic control in the perioperative period is one critical step in minimizing surgical site infections [25] and may make maintaining appropriate blood glucose levels easier when other factors like chemotherapy may perturb homeostasis.

One meta-analysis [26] assessing the benefit of weight loss before bariatric surgery on the patient's success following surgery demonstrated an additional 5% greater weight loss postoperatively for participants who lost *any* weight preoperatively. They also determined that for bariatric procedures, preoperative weight loss decreases the time of the operation room by approximately 20 min although there were no other significant benefits identified in this meta-analysis like decreased complication rates despite the shorter operative time. Individual studies have had varying results comparing preoperative weight loss and operative length, however. The intent of this study was partly to ensure that the required preoperative weight loss at least was not *causing* harm, as theoretically, if this weight loss is accomplished through restrictive dieting to the point of developing nutritional deficiencies, this could theoretically lead to harm with poor tolerating of stress in the operating room and postoperative complications. As other research has shown that even "modest" weight loss of approximately 10% excess body weight could improve hypertension, diabetes, and obstructive sleep apnea symptoms (all of which worsen operative outcomes), a well-tailored, multimodal, prehabilitation plan could potentially result in better outcomes for bariatric and other kinds of surgery. Overall, programs should be multimodal with both a focus on functional improvements in endurance and exercise tolerance [28] and weight loss for patients with metabolic disease, particularly visceral/liver fat as this will be associated with decreases in blood pressure and blood glucose. Nutritional professionals should oversee dietary interventions to ensure intake of the appropriate amount of calories, protein, and micronutrients.

1 Exercise Is a Key Component of Prehabilitation

In one published review of prior studies of patients with obesity undergoing prehabilitation prior to both bariatric and non-bariatric surgeries [27], the authors identified an inverse relationship between fitness level and 30-day medical complications, particularly if providers referred patients to these programs due to the presence of comorbidities instead of simply elevated BMI—the latter being considered "metabolically healthy obesity." The more typical instances in which preoperative weight loss was associated with *worse* surgical outcomes occurred when individuals achieved this weight loss through bariatric surgery prior to orthopedic surgeries. In these cases, it is plausible that the malabsorptive state created by bariatric surgery contributed to insufficient nutrient absorption. In these cases, readmission and surgical revisions were higher in groups who had bariatric surgery before joint replacement. Not every study demonstrates improved surgical outcomes with exercise alone. In unsuccessful interventions, the outcomes were likely the result of insufficient intensity of the interventions. Some consisted only of counseling on exercise and diet or were impacted by poor adherence and high dropout rates. Alternatively, many studies showed significant positive benefits of preoperative weight loss—some more intensive programs such as weekly meetings with a physician, nutritionist, personal trainer, and psychologist showed improvements in length of stay, complications such as poor wound healing and infection, reoperation, and mortality. As outlined in the condition-specific chapters that follow, the combination of nutritional optimization, moving toward a healthy body weight, and exercise constitutes a potent framework to improve surgical outcomes.

Finally, these programs are only as effective as the participation level of the individuals. Therefore, great strides should be made to increase engagement and adherence to the program through frequent touchpoints with team members, reward systems/gamification, and other strategies [29].

Besides weight loss and optimization of metabolic parameters for patients with metabolic disease, the goals of a multimodal program include optimizing body composition. These improvements are effectively an investment into a figurative kind of functional health savings account—not the financial instrument offered by employers—from which the patient will withdraw post-procedurally during periods of inactive recovery, caloric deficit, or cachexia. While there are physiologic limits to fat loss and muscle mass/strength gains within a limited period, astute practitioners have tools at their disposal to prime the patient's physiology to be most receptive to making these changes.

2 Low Body Weight and Sarcopenia Also a Risk Factor for Poor Outcomes

Alternatively, treating other patient populations that often suffer from *low* BMI, frailty, and cachexia such as those with advanced cancer, pulmonary diseases like COPD and fibrosis, and cardiac/renal failure utilizes similar principles and pharmacology as treating patients with metabolic syndrome–associated comorbidities. The principles of optimizing nutrition, prescribing exercise modifications in the setting of barriers to participation, and treating mood disorders span across the BMI spectrum. Understanding which tenets are universally applicable versus those that must be personally tailored is a core competency of pre-procedural health optimization.

3 Other Key Components That Make Up Multimodal Prehabilitation

Mental health care and sleep optimization are critical components of a multimodal program, as poor sleep and nutrition potentiate catabolic processes and are frequently implicated in conditions such as cancer [30], metabolic disease, sarcopenia

[31], infertility [32], and vascular disease [33]. Similarly, depression and anxiety are often comorbid in these cases and contribute to poor sleep, low energy, lack of motivation, and pain that make participation in prehabilitation more difficult for the patient.

4 Patient Education

During the preoperative/preprocedural counseling period, patient education can have multiple benefits toward achieving a successful intervention. For example, in a meta-analysis of patients prior to cancer surgery, face-to-face education (vs written or audiovisual instruction) was most efficacious in improving patient satisfaction, knowledge, anxiety, and even potentially lower healthcare costs [34]. In other literature on patients prior to surgery for colorectal cancer, specifically, preoperative education improved patients' postoperative self-image, reduced length of stay, and enhanced the recovery of self-reported global health status [35]. Similar educational interventions before orthopedic surgery were equally effective when delivered in person or via telehealth [36].

As healthcare, in general, migrates toward a culture of shared decision-making, comprehensive education prior to invasive treatments is a crucial component of empowering patients to make informed decisions. The improvement in patient satisfaction is logical, partly attributable to the perceived extra effort involved in leading these discussions and the predictability of the medical course throughout the continuum of care [37]. By better understanding the rationale behind the treatment plans, patient adherence is improved, which may be a contributing factor to fewer complications and improved outcomes. Additionally, by being upfront about potential side effects and complications, physicians can foster the physician–patient relationship and maintain faith in the long-term plan during any short-term setbacks.

Innovative alternatives to improve patient education are emerging. Shared medical appointments (SMAs) function as a means of providing standardized information to a group of patients who are all undergoing a similar treatment course or share a common disease process. The setting allows practitioners to limit the repetitive nature of these standardized information sessions while facilitating patient understanding of the course as others may voice questions/concerns they had not considered or were unable to ask. Research suggests that these appointments also increase patient satisfaction [38] and can mitigate some of the rote aspects of a practitioner's job, thereby potentially mitigating one source of burnout [39]. Given the greater patient volumes clinicians can counsel and potentially treat, SMAs offer an opportunity to improve access to care and reduce health system expenditures [40]. The limited existing data also suggest a potential for improved clinical outcomes in chronic diseases like T2DM and hypertension [41].

One study published in the *Annals of Family Medicine* [38] compared case mix index-matched patients who attended shared medical appointments versus those who participated in usual care within the same multispecialty practice. Patients highlighted a few common themes, particularly significantly improved satisfaction with access to care, personal communication with the physician including "perceived time spent" and "personalized concern expressed" by the physician, and sensitivity to the patient's needs. These are important takeaways, as shifting from an individualized appointment structure to a shared appointment model inherently implies the physician's time and attention during the appointment are divided among all participants. These data counter that perception and propose both patient and provider benefits that may justify the added logistical complexity of coordinating these appointments.

5 Getting Started

Designing a prehabilitation plan and coordinating with all the involved specialists is not an easy role. The purpose of this text is to present the tools available to practitioners as well as the unique situations in which they may be used, grouped into several main cohorts: orthopedic and spine, oncologic, bariatric, solid organ transplant, and obstetrics and infertility. Each population has unique treatments and considerations when designing a personalized plan. While practitioners of physical medicine and rehabilitation are well-trained in coordinating care between multiple therapists (i.e., physical, occupational, and speech therapy) as well as managing most sequelae of metabolic disease, other medical specialties should feel comfortable using this resource to complement their own unique training in leading a prehabilitation team.

References

1. Ricciardi BF, Giori NJ, Fehring TK. Clinical faceoff: should orthopaedic surgeons have strict BMI cutoffs for performing primary TKA and THA? Clin Orthop Relat Res. 2019;477(12):2629–34.
2. Arafat M, Norain A, Burjonrappa S. Characterizing bariatric surgery utilization and complication rates in the adolescent population. J Pediatr Surg. 2019;54(2):288–92.
3. Chang S-H, Freeman NLB, Lee JA, Stoll CRT, Calhoun AJ, Eagon JC, et al. Early major complications after bariatric surgery in the USA, 2003–2014: a systematic review and meta-analysis. Obes Rev. 2018;19(4):529–37.
4. Giordano S, Victorzon M. Bariatric surgery in elderly patients: a systematic review. Clin Interv Aging. 2015;10:1627–35.
5. Fang M, Noiseux N, Linson E, Cram P. The effect of advancing age on total joint replacement outcomes. Geriatr Orthop Surg Rehabil. 2015;6(3):173–9.
6. García-Jiménez C, Gutiérrez-Salmerón M, Chocarro-Calvo A, García-Martinez JM, Castaño A, De la Vieja A. From obesity to diabetes and cancer: epidemiological links and role of therapies. Br J Cancer. 2016;114(7):716–22.
7. Steele CB, Thomas CC, Henley SJ, Massetti GM, Galuska DA, Agurs-Collins T, et al. Vital signs: trends in incidence of cancers associated with overweight and obesity—United States, 2005–2014. Morbid Mortal Weekly Rep. 2017;66(39):1052.
8. Lementowski PW, Zelicof SB. Obesity and osteoarthritis. Am J Orthop-Belle Mead. 2008;37(3):148.
9. Kulkarni K, Karssiens T, Kumar V, Pandit H. Obesity and osteoarthritis. Maturitas. 2016;89:22–8.
10. Francisco V, Pérez T, Pino J, López V, Franco E, Alonso A, et al. Biomechanics, obesity, and osteoarthritis. The role of adipokines: when the levee breaks. J Orthop Res. 2018;36(2):594–604.

11. Maas F, Arends S, van der Veer E, Wink F, Efde M, Bootsma H, et al. Obesity is common in axial spondyloarthritis and is associated with poor clinical outcome. J Rheumatol. 2016;43(2):383.
12. Bakirci S, Dabague J, Eder L, McGonagle D, Aydin SZ. The role of obesity on inflammation and damage in spondyloarthritis: a systematic literature review on body mass index and imaging. Clin Exp Rheumatol. 2020;38(1):144–8.
13. Visser M, Bouter LM, McQuillan GM, Wener MH, Harris TB. Elevated C-reactive protein levels in overweight and obese adults. JAMA. 1999;282(22):2131–5.
14. Timpson NJ, Nordestgaard BG, Harbord RM, Zacho J, Frayling TM, Tybjærg-Hansen A, et al. C-reactive protein levels and body mass index: elucidating direction of causation through reciprocal Mendelian randomization. Int J Obes (Lond). 2011;35(2):300–8.
15. Garvey WT, Batterham RL, Bhatta M, Buscemi S, Christensen LN, Frias JP, et al. Two-year effects of semaglutide in adults with overweight or obesity: the STEP 5 trial. Nat Med. 2022;28(10):2083–91.
16. Selvin E, Paynter NP, Erlinger TP. The effect of weight loss on C-reactive protein: a systematic review. Arch Intern Med. 2007;167(1):31–9.
17. Briggs MS, Givens DL, Schmitt LC, Taylor CA. Relations of C-reactive protein and obesity to the prevalence and the odds of reporting low back pain. Arch Phys Med Rehabil. 2013;94(4):745–52.
18. Macphail K. C-reactive protein, chronic low back pain and, diet and lifestyle. Int Musculoskelet Med. 2015;37(1):29–32.
19. Gill MG, Majumdar A. Metabolic associated fatty liver disease: addressing a new era in liver transplantation. World J Hepatol. 2020;12(12):1168.
20. Greco EV, Russo G, Giandalia A, Viazzi F, Pontremoli R, De Cosmo S. GLP-1 Receptor agonists and kidney protection. Medicina. 2019;55(6):233.
21. Nizari S, Basalay M, Chapman P, Korte N, Korsak A, Christie IN, et al. Glucagon-like peptide-1 (GLP-1) receptor activation dilates cerebral arterioles, increases cerebral blood flow, and mediates remote (pre)conditioning neuroprotection against ischaemic stroke. Basic Res Cardiol. 2021;116(1):32.
22. Panchapakesan U, Pollock C. Organ protection beyond glycaemic control with SGLT2 inhibitors. Nat Rev Nephrol. 2021;17(4):223–4.
23. Riksen NP, El Messaoudi S, Rongen GA. It takes more than one CAMERA to study cardiovascular protection by metformin. Lancet Diab Endocrinol. 2014;2(2):105–6.
24. Luo F, Das A, Chen J, Wu P, Li X, Fang Z. Metformin in patients with and without diabetes: a paradigm shift in cardiovascular disease management. Cardiovasc Diabetol. 2019;18(1):54.
25. Iqbal U, Green JB, Patel S, Tong Y, Zebrower M, Kaye AD, et al. Preoperative patient preparation in enhanced recovery pathways. J Anaesthesiol Clin Pharmacol. 2019;35(Suppl. 1):S14.
26. Livhits M, Mercado C, Yermilov I, Parikh JA, Dutson E, Mehran A, et al. Does weight loss immediately before bariatric surgery improve outcomes: a systematic review. Surg Obes Relat Dis. 2009;5(6):713–21.
27. Smith NA, Martin G, Marginson B. Preoperative assessment and prehabilitation in patients with obesity undergoing non-bariatric surgery: a systematic review. J Clin Anesth. 2022;78:110676.
28. García-Delgado Y, López-Madrazo-Hernández MJ, Alvarado-Martel D, Miranda-Calderín G, Ugarte-Lopetegui A, González-Medina RA, et al. Prehabilitation for bariatric surgery: a randomized, controlled trial protocol and pilot study. Nutrients. 2021;13(9):2903.
29. Tran S, Smith L, El-Den S, Carter S. The use of gamification and incentives in mobile health apps to improve medication adherence: scoping review. JMIR Mhealth Uhealth. 2022;10(2):e30671.
30. Huang B-H, Duncan MJ, Cistulli PA, Nassar N, Hamer M, Stamatakis E. Sleep and physical activity in relation to all-cause, cardiovascular disease and cancer mortality risk. Br J Sports Med. 2022;56(13):718–24.
31. Lucassen EA, De Mutsert R, Le Cessie S, Appelman-Dijkstra NM, Rosendaal FR, Van Heemst D, et al. Poor sleep quality and later sleep timing are risk factors for osteopenia and sarcopenia in middle-aged men and women: the NEO study. PLoS One. 2017;12(5):e0176685.

32. Palnitkar G, Phillips CL, Hoyos CM, Marren AJ, Bowman MC, Yee BJ. Linking sleep disturbance to idiopathic male infertility. Sleep Med Rev. 2018;42:149–59.
33. Cappuccio FP, Miller MA. Sleep and cardio-metabolic disease. Curr Cardiol Rep. 2017;19(11):110.
34. Waller A, Forshaw K, Bryant J, Carey M, Boyes A, Sanson-Fisher R. Preparatory education for cancer patients undergoing surgery: a systematic review of volume and quality of research output over time. Patient Educ Couns. 2015;98(12):1540–9.
35. Koet LL, Kraima A, Derksen I, Lamme B, Belt EJT, van Rosmalen J, et al. Effectiveness of preoperative group education for patients with colorectal cancer: managing expectations. Support Care Cancer. 2021;29(9):5263–71.
36. Buvanendran A, Sremac AC, Merriman PA, Della Valle CJ, Burns JW, McCarthy RJ. Preoperative cognitive–behavioral therapy for reducing pain catastrophizing and improving pain outcomes after total knee replacement: a randomized clinical trial. Reg Anesth Pain Med. 2021;46(4):313–21.
37. Yeh M-Y, Wu S-C, Tung T-H. The relation between patient education, patient empowerment and patient satisfaction: a cross-sectional-comparison study. Appl Nurs Res. 2018;39:11–7.
38. Heyworth L, Rozenblum R, Burgess JF, Baker E, Meterko M, Prescott D, et al. Influence of shared medical appointments on patient satisfaction: a retrospective 3-year study. Ann Fam Med. 2014;12(4):324–30.
39. Lacagnina S, Tips J, Pauly K, Cara K, Karlsen M. Lifestyle medicine shared medical appointments. Am J Lifestyle Med. 2021;15(1):23–7.
40. Mahajan UV, Sharma N, Maynard M, Kang L, Labak CM, Raghavan A, et al. Inpatient virtual shared medical appointments to improve health literacy, increase patient self-efficacy, and reduce provider burnout in acute cerebrovascular pathology patients and their caregivers: a pilot study. Neurosurg Focus. 2022;52(6):E12.
41. Edelman D, McDuffie JR, Oddone E, Gierisch JM, Nagi A, Williams JW Jr. Shared medical appointments for chronic medical conditions: a systematic review. Washington (DC): Department of Veterans Affairs (US); 2012.

Basic Prehabilitation Pillars

Alexander Watson and Jason Bitterman

The tenets of prehabilitation are reversing risk factors that predispose individuals to worse outcomes when the body is stressed and anticipating the surgery's impact on postoperative function to best mitigate the negative consequences of surgery. Further, practitioners should address medical issues such as components of metabolic syndrome that may negatively impact the response to and recovery from various surgeries and cancer therapies. Prehabilitation ultimately aims to improve outcomes, prevent disease recurrence, and maintain function.

This chapter aims to educate practitioners on foundational concepts of prehabilitation, including why it is critical for certain populations, the benefits of various exercise regimens, nutritional considerations, and dietary/supplement strategies. These described populations often fall into two broad phenotypes such as individuals with multiple comorbidities of metabolic disease like obesity, diabetes mellitus, and metabolic associated fatty liver disease/elevated visceral fat burden and those with sarcopenia and frailty. Exercise regimens and nutritional considerations describe strategies for building/maintaining skeletal muscle and, where appropriate, different approaches for caloric restriction to reverse elements of metabolic disease.

1 Considerations for Program Design: Encouraging Provider Investment

Comprehensive *re*habilitation begins with a multimodal *pre*habilitation program. Increasingly, best practices call for prior to surgery, prehabilitation can reduce recovery time, reduce complication rates, and augment the response to the

A. Watson (✉)
Admire Medical, Middletown, DE, USA
e-mail: alexander@admiremedical.com

J. Bitterman
Hartford Healthcare Medical Group, Hartford, CT, USA

A. Watson, K. Barr (eds.), *A Prehabilitation Guide for All Providers*,
https://doi.org/10.1007/978-3-031-72862-4_2

intervention [1]. Even in nonelective operations, such as tumor resection, many surgeons recognize that a therapeutic delay of surgery to allow for prehabilitation (in appropriate patients) can result in better outcomes. For example, an overwhelming majority of cardiothoracic surgeons in one study were willing to delay surgical resection of lung cancer beyond the current average 20-day waiting period to allow patients to participate in prehabilitation [2].

The "Enhanced Recovery After Surgery (ERAS®) guidelines generally refer to evidence-based, multidisciplinary methods of reducing patients' stress response to surgery, facilitating recovery, and optimizing physiologic function and recommend best practices for specific surgical procedures [3]. The 2019 update for lung surgical procedures [1], ERAS, and the European Society of Thoracic Surgeons (ESTS) recommended prehabilitation for high-risk patients as well as other components of a multimodal program pretreatment, such as nutritional screening and smoking cessation. The 2021 ERAS update for bariatric surgery presented similar recommendations [4].

2 Considerations for Program Design: Participation

To do the work involved in a prehabilitation program, most patients will need to understand why they are necessary. The chapters in this book delve into disease-specific evidence of the efficacy of prehabilitation to improve surgical outcomes, and communicating this information to patients is often helpful. In addition to improving immediate surgical outcomes such as decreasing surgical morbidity and mortality and decreasing hospital length of stay, prehabilitation can decrease some of the challenges of posttreatment rehabilitation caused by disease symptoms, side effects of treatments, and decline in health status [5]. Clinicians should emphasize prehabilitation as a means of maintaining the current function, improving surgical outcomes, and enhancing posttreatment function and quality of life.

Despite best intentions and a desire to participate in prehabilitation, there are many factors that can interfere with adherence. Patients are often burdened by many medical appointments during pre-procedural planning, the psychological burden of their disease, and the symptoms of their disease. In the Perioperative Rehabilitation in Operable Lung Cancer Patients (PROLUCA) study [6], patients attributed difficulty adhering to a home-based exercise program due to the number of appointments required within the abbreviated 8-day average preoperative window. In terms of *initiating* a prehabilitation program, one study [2] listed access to professionals, comorbidities, and transportation as top barriers. One innovative means of improving access to care is to mirror/expand upon the approach taken by cancer and transplant centers, in which interdisciplinary appointments or sequential appointments allow patients to visit their specialists batched together. Coordinating elements of prehabilitation with other appointments would limit transportation time and cost and may be more favorable to patients or caregivers who must request time off work.

Even with programs solely targeting nutritional goals, convenience can have a significant impact on improving preoperative health status. Since almost 15% of patients in one Dutch hospital setting were already malnourished at admission for elective surgeries, researchers assessed the impact of a high-protein meal delivery service in improving nutrition and outcomes. For the 3 weeks prior to surgery, the service delivered six high-protein meals/snacks per day. Participants in the intervention group averaged about 93% of the target protein goal (1.2 g/kg of body weight), whereas participants in the control group averaged only 78% of the target. Additionally, patients in the intervention group were significantly more satisfied with meal preparation and presentation. Another prospective study recruited patients newly diagnosed with non-small cell lung cancer (NSCLC) and high-performance status (PS = 0 or 1) to assess the feasibility of adhering to a structured exercise program prior to and during treatment initiation [7]. Of all consented patients, the completion rate for the 16-session program was 44%; the most cited reasons for nonadherence were physical deterioration and feeling unwell. These findings suggest preoperative programs should prioritize medical team buy-in to manage symptoms as able to facilitate prehabilitation.

The psychological burdens the patients face also need to be recognized. A new cancer or other serious diagnosis often involves a grieving process [8]. A patient's mood may impact participation during a crucial pretreatment window, where each day participating in therapeutic interventions could tangibly reduce the risk of complications, improve resilience for withstanding treatment, and benefit long-term outcomes. Practitioners should be mindful of this and support patients as appropriate. Programs that focus on patient convenience and the individualization of treatments to accommodate patients' symptoms and psychological state are the most likely to be successful [9].

The content and length of the program are other essential features that determine the likelihood of success. Typical features of successful programs are those that are multimodal in nature (i.e., attend to nutrition, exercise, and mental health), are of sufficient length and intensity, and include sufficient supervision/attention to adherence. Prehabilitation programs that fail to significantly improve perioperative/periprocedural metrics (such as complication rate, length of stay, or physical functioning) often share common design flaws such as being too short in duration to allow for meaningful improvement. Likewise, providing photocopied handouts of standard exercises and healthy food choices without direct instruction is also unlikely to make a clinically meaningful change in a patient with other health concerns. Thoughtful and personalized design of prehabilitation programs is required to maximize benefits in the typically short pre-procedural period. Moreover, the practitioner's skillset must include the ability to motivate patients to participate as completely as they are able, given the integral nature of each component in the plan.

3 Motivational Interviewing for Change

Throughout the prehabilitation process, motivational interviewing is a crucial skill for understanding patients' willingness, readiness, and motivation for implementing behavioral change. For habits that are particularly psychologically and biochemically engrained, such as tobacco use, these skills are especially prudent. A patient-centered approach to counseling begins by qualifying the patient's readiness and support for change as a stage along a continuum, proceeding through pre-contemplation, contemplation, preparation, action, maintenance, and (potentially) relapse [9]. To elicit these details, practitioners should employ the "core skills" of motivational interviewing based on the mnemonic "OARS": *open-ended questions*, *affirmations* (of positive insights), *reflections* (i.e., reflective listening), and *summarization* (to promote continued introspection) [10].

Another mnemonic, RULE, is critical to controlling (*resisting*) one's own impulse to immediately insert suggestions for improvement into the conversation. Instead, *understand* the motivation by *listening* with empathy before *empowering* the patient through targeted feedback. Empowerment should illustrate to patients that they are responsible for their decisions and the subsequent outcomes of those decisions.

The "5 A's" is one final commonly used framework when determining readiness for change and providing support. These different approaches are not used linearly but instead complement each other during the motivational interviewing process. With the 5 As, the *ask*, *assess*, *advise*, *agree*, and *arrange/assist* steps may be peppered throughout OARS, RULE, and Feedback, Responsibility, Advice, Menu Options, Empathy and Self-Efficacy (FRAMES), as *ask* signals the interviewer to inquire about the patient's understanding of health risks and their current habits around their behavior before *assess*ing his/her readiness for change [11]. Provide detailed, unambiguous, and solicited advice (*advise)*, ideally as a menu of choices from which both parties may *agree* on the best solution for the patient. *Assist* them in implementing the change whether it be, for example, through nicotine replacement therapy (NRT) or resources on group therapy sessions for smoking cessation or substance abuse recovery, respectively. Also, prescheduling follow-up sessions for ongoing support demonstrates the provider's understanding of the patient's difficult journey ahead and establishes regular check-ins for supporting adherence while motivation is highest.

Practitioners should not strictly follow every step of each framework, particularly since these frameworks overlap at different points. Instead, structuring conversations with these in mind may help drive progress through what may be a ruminative process while simultaneously ensuring the patient is in the appropriate mindset for implementing the ultimate changes.

4 External Limitations to Prehabilitation

Some of the most significant barriers to prehabilitation are patient and surgeon buy-in, symptoms related to the patient's illness or other comorbidities limiting participation, and the psychological burdens patients may be facing. A new cancer diagnosis often involves a grieving process like other life-altering events [8]. A patient's mood may dramatically diminish motivation during a crucial pretreatment window, where each day participating in therapeutic interventions could tangibly reduce the risk of complications, improve resilience for withstanding treatment, and benefit long-term outcomes. Practitioners should be mindful of this and other barriers to prehabilitation.

5 Exercise Intervention

Screening

Per the 2014 ACSM guidelines, the number of people who require screening before initiating an exercise regimen is fewer than previously recommended. This change reflects the overly sensitive previous guidelines (95% of individuals over 40 met the criteria for requiring a screening) despite the low *absolute* risk of a cardiovascular event. The new algorithm recommends that individuals who do not currently participate in regular exercise undergo pre-exercise "clearance" if they have known signs/symptoms of renal, metabolic, or cardiovascular disease [12]. Following this evaluation, they should begin with light–moderate intensity exercise before progressing gradually to vigorous exercise. Among individuals who are currently participating in regular exercise, those with known disease should be cleared prior to escalating to vigorous intensity if asymptomatic. If these individuals have any signs/symptoms during exercise, such as chest pain, shortness of breath out of proportion to the activity, feeling faint or dizzy, nausea, atypical pain, or other concerning symptoms, they should discontinue exercise and undergo a medical evaluation. The most suggestive signs/symptoms of disease encompass broadly suggestive symptoms such as chest, jaw, neck, or arm pain (particularly on exertion); unusual shortness of breath or fatigue with mild exertion, usual activities, or at rest; syncope or dizziness; lower extremity edema; tachycardia; palpitations; paroxysmal nocturnal dyspnea; or orthopnea.

Traditional Exercise Programs

One of the main objectives of prehabilitation is to improve baseline cardiopulmonary function, particularly when considering the effects certain surgeries may have on pulmonary function (e.g., lobectomy [13]), the impact of comorbid pulmonary disease that is prevalent in patients with obesity or a smoking history, or effects of deconditioning after even brief posttreatment immobility [14]. Aerobic conditioning is critical to optimize cardiopulmonary function.

Building lean muscle mass is also crucial for *any* individual, but intuitively, it is of even greater importance for individuals preparing for a battle with cancer or anticipating rapid weight loss following bariatric surgery. One prospective study found nearly 70% of patients with advanced lung cancer experienced cachexia and almost 50% experienced sarcopenia [15]. In a 2022 meta-analysis of outcomes following bariatric surgery, researchers identified an average lean body mass decrease of over 8 kg in the first year with over 3 kg specifically from skeletal muscle. Worse, the majority of this occurs in the first 3 months following surgery [16]. Given the important contribution of skeletal muscle mass to resilience and longevity, exercise is the foundation of prehabilitation, with the *best* type of exercise being "whatever exercise the patient will complete."

An ideal starting exercise prescription should include a mix of resistance and aerobic training. Depending on the lead time before surgery/treatment, prescribers should vary the intensity, frequency, and volume to maximize participation. This should be balanced with not overtraining the patient, as too high an intensity or frequency of exercise could risk injury or potentiate muscle mass loss when paired with caloric restriction and inadequate protein consumption. Practitioners can personalize a patient's exercise plan by adjusting the balance of resistance and aerobic training based on preexisting deficits and the anticipated effects of their impending intervention. One must also consider medications and baseline health status, which can both impact a patient's risk for injury and rate of recovery from exercise. Training styles are broadly categorized as shown in Table 1.

Aquatherapy is a good modality for individuals with typical musculoskeletal disorders, as it is low impact and thermoconductive (provoking less physical discomfort during exertion), maintains a social component for better adherence, and can combine aerobic and resistance training in one setting. In one review and meta-analysis of studies assessing the benefits of exercise in patients with obesity and low back pain [17], researchers compared the effects of Pilates/yoga, aerobic exercise, resistance exercise, and aquatic-based exercise on multiple metrics. Overall, *all* forms of exercise substantially improved perceived disability, with aquatic having the best overall profile. In this analysis, aquatic therapy most meaningfully improved pain severity (on par with resistance and Pilates/yoga), quality of life, and functionality (on par with Pilates/yoga). Of note, this paper also found benefits specific to resistance training. Resistance training decreased body fat percentage while increasing skeletal muscle, whereas the included studies on aerobic training and yoga/Pilates did not report changes in body composition. Resistance training produced greater improvements in fear avoidance and pain catastrophizing than aerobic training.

Based on these data, interested and untrained patients can initiate an exercise plan starting at a mild–moderate intensity to establish a baseline level of fitness and

Table 1 Differentiating between typical aerobic versus resistance training exercises

Training	Description
Aerobic	Activities involving dynamic work with large muscle groups, e.g., walking, cycling, running. These in turn may be divided into two subcategories: • Continuous (isokinetic) training: Long-duration sessions performed at a continuous pace without rest • Interval training: Short (e.g., 4 min), high-intensity bouts interspersed with active recovery (e.g., 3 min) at a lower intensity. This cycle is typically repeated 3–4 times/session
Resistance	The use of (typically isotonic) resistance to muscular contraction to build strength and size of skeletal muscles using different tools: elastic bands, free weights, machines, or body weight exercises

build a tolerance to exertional discomfort. As their conditioning improves, dedicated land-based resistance training may produce greater benefits for mitigating pain and isolating focal areas of dysfunction, for example, by targeting scapular dyskinesis or lumbopelvic core stabilization.

Blood Flow Restriction Training

Blood flow restriction (BFR) or *kaatsu* is a technique whereby the user performs the exercise, often resistance training, while a tourniquet cuff is applied as proximal as possible to the working muscle(s). The pressure applied by the tourniquet is adjusted until it occludes venous outflow and only partly occludes arterial inflow. By obstructing outflow, metabolic by-products accumulate more quickly in the working muscles. According to current research, these by-products appear to be the metabolic impetus for satellite cell proliferation, myostatin inhibition, and ultimately muscle hypertrophy [18]. As a result, individuals can elicit a greater recovery response in muscles using lower loads, which makes it particularly suitable for rehabilitation after an injury with resultant weight-bearing limitations or prehabilitation for individuals with baseline deconditioning and musculoskeletal disease.

For example, for a patient who was previously physically active with a relatively limited lower extremity weight limit (such as in advanced osteoarthritis), this weight limit may render “typical” resistance training nearly meaningless. However, if a tourniquet cuff were applied to the proximal thigh, a circuit of lightweight knee extension, lying leg curls, and standing calf raises can potentially target the major muscles of the leg with an adequate stimulus for hypertrophic benefit. Similarly, this individual could benefit from BFR to overcome similar weight-bearing restrictions in the upper extremity such as in chronic elbow tendinopathy.

There are three settings in which BFR may be used: resistance exercise (BFR-RE), aerobic exercise (BFR-AE), and passively without an exercise component (P-BFR) [19]. To begin using the equipment, practitioners must appropriately measure the arterial occlusive pressure (AOP) with the size/length of the cuff they will ultimately prescribe, as the size of the cuff and patient characteristics will affect these values [20]. As such, BFR requires some training since off-the-shelf cuffs that do not require calibration are currently not widely available. Additionally, the cuff must be removed in between sets, both to achieve the intended effect and to minimize risks of complications due to prolonged occlusion [19].

Overall, BFR training is generally safe, effective, and easy to perform with the guidance of trained rehabilitation professionals although there are potential risks and contraindications. In untrained individuals with diminished recovery capacity (e.g., patients with cachexia), practitioners should start BFR training with very low resistance to reduce the risk of overtraining-related injury. There are case reports of rhabdomyolysis following overtraining with BFR [21]. Realistically, untrained individuals are at higher risk of rhabdomyolysis when initiating *any* training program, but instances published in the literature describe a high-intensity level not typical in guided prehabilitation [22]. In fact, a systematic review published in the *American*

Journal of Sports Medicine found that in populations with chronic musculoskeletal disorders such as inflammatory myopathies, thoracic outlet syndrome, and knee osteoarthritis, rates of adverse events were not significantly different when comparing BFR-RE and exercise alone [18].

It is important to note that individuals undergoing prehabilitation for advanced chronic diseases like heart failure or COPD are less likely to have been included in the majority of studies assessing the efficacy and safety of BFR, and therefore, the bulk of literature is likely underrepresenting individuals with comorbid cardiovascular, neuromuscular, or pulmonary disease. However, isolated studies *have* demonstrated safety and efficacy within populations. First, in studies of patients with obesity [23], BFR resulted in higher metabolic demand, as evidenced by significantly higher HR, VCO_2/VO_2, and a 20.5% and 11% increase in energy expenditure in male subjects and female subjects, respectively, despite low perceived exertion. This study population did not exhibit higher rates of adverse events, thus suggesting individuals who are at risk for developing chronic disease due to obesity may likely safely employ BFR as a means of course correction.

The volume of literature within specific high-risk populations is limited but also suggests a likely favorable benefit/risk profile. For example, in one small study ($n = 36$) of individuals with congestive heart failure, BFR using low load resistance training significantly improved quality of life, isometric strength, and mitochondrial respiratory function when compared with control, while the alternative intervention (remote ischemic conditioning) provided no benefit beyond control [24]. A subsequent systematic review of BFR in patients with heart disease and chronic heart failure included the prior study and corroborated the results with similar data and expanded the potential benefits to include improvements in left ventricular function, systemic inflammation, and symptoms of dyspnea and fatigue without any significant increase in adverse events [25].

With regard to COPD, one pilot study demonstrated low load BFR with resistance training was equal to high load resistance training for increasing isometric muscle strength, and BFR was superior for improving functional exercise capacity and physical activity with lower perceived dyspnea [26]. Another pilot study showed comparable improvements over a two-week period between low load BFR-RE and high load resistance training without any acute muscular or cardiac events in either population [27]. For patients with chronic kidney disease, low load BFR-RE similarly reproduces the benefits of higher load resistance training without an increase in adverse events [28]. BFR-AE achieves comparable outcomes when compared with standard aerobic training in patients on dialysis, as well [29].

In summary, while the data for specific use cases of BFR in populations with different chronic diseases are not yet comprehensive, available data suggest comparable benefits and safety profiles as BFR studies in healthy populations. As such, patients who are unable to participate in any form of standard exercise due to load intolerance may benefit from BFR as a means of incorporating some element of structured, progressive overload-focused physical activity. However, it is presently imprudent to provide clear, standardizable guidance for incorporating BFR training with particularly high-risk individuals.

Exercise Tailored to Reverse Metabolic Disease

Exercise and dietary interventions have additional benefits beyond improving weight, blood pressure, lipids, and diabetes. These lifestyle interventions can incite a positive feedback loop in improving health outcomes. For example, in individuals with very high BMIs, weight loss does not have to be substantial to significantly improve obesity-related comorbidities. A "mere" 5% reduction in body weight leads to significant improvements in blood pressure, osteoarthritis symptoms [30], polycystic ovarian syndrome (PCOS) [31], GERD in women (men need 10% weight loss reduction) [32], and dyslipidemia [33]. A greater than 7% reduction in body weight is necessary for reducing the risk of developing type 2 diabetes [34], and a 10% reduction in body weight can improve obstructive sleep apnea (OSA) symptoms [35] and reduce the risk of nonalcoholic fatty liver disease (NAFLD)/metabolic-associated fatty liver disease (MAFLD).

As we better understand the pathophysiology of insulin resistance and MAFLD, more deliberately targeted lifestyle therapies can facilitate insulin sensitization without requiring as high a degree of weight loss as listed earlier [36]. Resistance and aerobic training affect different changes in muscle energy metabolism. Recall that skeletal muscle is the predominant reservoir for glucose storage in the body, and at rest, insulin binding to the insulin receptor promotes skeletal muscle uptake of glucose using GLUT4 transporters [37]. Aerobic exercise, however, has the capacity to promote GLUT4 transporter uptake of glucose without requiring insulin [38, 39], a clinically relevant feature when intending to acutely improve blood glucose levels in patients with insulin resistance.

Muscle biopsies of patients with insulin resistance and diabetes demonstrate mitochondria with limited capability to oxidize fatty acids for energy, as should occur during aerobic exercise or prolonged fasting in healthy individuals. Insulin resistance instead promotes the deposition of lipids (fatty acids) within muscle [40]. This becomes self-reinforcing as research has identified the accumulation of diacylglycerol (a by-product of triglyceride metabolism) as one indirect mediator of insulin resistance, ultimately reducing insulin-dependent GLUT4 activity in skeletal muscle. Hyperinsulinemia develops to overcome this resistance and, in tandem with elevated circulating free fatty acids, contributes to MAFLD development [41].

Exercise strategies to address this must clear intramuscular fat while reducing the hyperinsulinemia needed to maintain glucose homeostasis. Fortunately, research supports targeting these two mechanisms with the synergy of aerobic exercise to immediately improve insulin sensitivity and resistance training for both acute and chronic improvement, the latter likely by increasing the glucose storage capacity acutely (via glycolytic pathways) and chronically by hypertrophy [39, 42].

Specifically, current research supports a strategy of aerobic training with intensity of at least 40–60% of VO_2 max although, higher intensity may be more favorable over lower intensity at a higher volume [43], provided the patient can safely participate in this intensity. By evenly dividing these sessions to allow participation in aerobic activity at least every 48 h, the acute insulin-sensitizing effects are sustained while the chronic effects accumulate. Presuming "leisure" time availability as the limiting factor for exercise participation, this higher intensity/lower volume would free other available time for incorporating resistance training. To maximize the metabolic benefit of resistance training, individuals should strive to engage the greatest number of muscle groups via 5–10 exercises, incorporating working sets to near-failure in the range of 8–15 reps per exercise set [38]. In a tailored exercise approach such as this, individuals may potentially achieve improvements in insulin sensitivity (i.e., lower risk of developing type 2 diabetes) with potentially as little weight loss as 3% instead of the conventional 7–10% [36].

Prescribing Exercise

Exercise prescriptions should follow a common structure, such as the FITTE (frequency, intensity, time spent, type, and enjoyment) framework [44]. This ensures thoughtful consideration of the patient's fitness level and preferred exercise modalities. Practitioners should first consider activities the patient most enjoys like walking, biking, swimming, and hiking and consider fitness barriers they may face based on their health status and baseline conditioning. Exercise prescriptions should also specify precautions, such as weight-bearing restrictions, maximum target heart rate (if known), or case-specific precautions due to advanced musculoskeletal pathology, such as requiring a thoracolumbosacral orthotic (TLSO) or avoiding concurrent bending/twisting maneuvers due to vertebral compression fractures.

Additionally, prescriptions should set realistic goals based on a shared decision-making process with the patient. This is particularly important if the prescription will be provided to a physical or occupational therapist. These goals can be a certain level of cardiovascular exercise such as jogging for 30 min or a specific activity a patient enjoys such as playing tennis. These goals will serve as therapy endpoints and help guide patients and therapists during their exercise training course. Finally, counsel the patient on what constitutes true "stop signals" for exercise, such as exertional chest pain, nausea, feeling faint, or severe pain. Patients should also be counseled on "caution" signals, such as excessive breathlessness, that signal to dial down the intensity.

6 Lifestyle Interventions

There are many other "lifestyle" interventions patients can incorporate beyond exercise during prehabilitation to improve health outcomes. These include smoking cessation, alcohol reduction/abstinence, and weight loss.

Arguably, smoking cessation is the highest-yield lifestyle intervention for any patient intending to increase their short-term intervention outcomes and long-term health status. Smokers may experience worsening respiratory function 1–2 weeks immediately following smoking cessation [45], so practitioners should recommend smoking cessation well before any significant medical intervention. One study related to preparation before cancer treatment used a 4-week cessation period prior to initiating chemotherapy without related adverse effects [46]. Similarly, an ERAS protocol prior to bariatric surgery recommends at least 4 weeks of cessation prior to surgery [4]. Practitioners should also provide supportive resources like nicotine replacement therapy or symptomatic management for increased mucus production to allow for adequate symptom resolution prior to their procedure.

Nutritional Considerations

Optimizing a patient's nutrition can have synergistic benefits with exercise prescriptions in improving metabolic parameters like hemoglobin A1C, healing from surgery/illness, and greater resilience to neurological trauma [45].

A full review of available literature on the "best" diet for short- and long-term wellness is beyond the scope of this text. In addition, nutritional research often has confounders that impact the broader applicability of findings. However, a few nutritional concepts may serve as guidelines for prehabilitation. However, a few nutritional heuristics may ease the complexity of identifying healthy food choices. Minimizing fructose consumption by avoiding high fructose corn syrup or added sucrose (an oligosaccharide of fructose + glucose) will have outsized returns relative to the required effort.

Fructose

First, bench and clinical researchers are increasingly identifying fructose as a significant contributor to metabolic disease. Ingested fructose over 3–4 g in one sitting [47] exceeds the ability of the intestine to convert it to glucose; however, this effect is reduced when fructose comes from a high dietary fiber source, such as with fruit. Fructose is readily absorbed by the intestine and sent to the liver via the portal circulation, where it has multiple negative effects on insulin sensitivity, energy storage, and other metabolic comorbidities like gout.

Studies have demonstrated that consuming a diet rich in fructose is associated with significantly longer intestinal villi [48], the component of the gut enterocytes responsible for absorbing nutrients. This response effectively increases the absorptive surface area of the intestine, thereby promoting greater absorption of consumed calories. Fructose also stimulates appetite due to the high ATP investment during its intracellular uptake and breakdown [49]. Health professionals have long known that high fructose consumption is a risk factor for elevated uric acid and subsequent gout attacks, but recent studies have implicated uric acid in mitochondrial dysfunction [50], elevated blood pressure [51], and kidney disease [52], as well.

Fructose also directly stimulates lipogenesis even in the absence of caloric surplus [53]. It is also one of many signals to upregulate the enzyme aldose reductase, leading to the in vivo conversion of glucose to fructose [54]. While hibernating mammals take advantage of these effects to rapidly store energy in adipose tissue, modern humans in a nutrient-abundant environment must exercise significant restraint against the biological drive to accumulate fat stores.

Nutritional takeaways for patients should be concise and explicit. To this end, recommend avoiding any sugar-sweetened beverages and fruit juices and substituting high-sugar/low-fiber fruits such as grapes, mangos, and figs with relatively lower fructose fruits such as citrus, berries, and kiwi. Similarly, making the behavioral nudge to swap sugar-sweetened beverages to artificially sweetened beverages may drastically reduce an individual's sugar intake. With regard to safety, research is confirming that artificial sweeteners alter the microbiota in rodents [55], with new data even suggesting subtle secondary impacts on insulin sensitivity particularly by the sweeteners saccharin and sucralose [56]. Regardless, transitioning sugar to artificial sweeteners is a harm reduction technique because, if the alternative was high fructose corn syrup or sucrose, then nonnutritive sweeteners are still a positive substitute [57].

Nutritional Supplements

Another potentially high-yield lifestyle intervention is nutritional supplementation for certain patient populations. Clinicians should examine patients for signs/symptoms of malnutrition and replete deficiencies through dietary counseling, oral supplementation, or parenteral nutrition when warranted and in accordance with the patient's wishes [58]. This examination should include a thorough inquiry about sensory disturbances (which may be indicative of neuropathy), fatigue/pallor (which could indicate an underlying anemia), and any restrictive eating patterns (which cause various nutritional deficiencies). In individuals pursuing bariatric surgery, these history questions or more formal screening with a panel of serum tests are typically standard, as any baseline deficiencies are likely to worsen in a postoperative malabsorptive state [59].

Creatine

Even for individuals without any identified deficiency, certain targeted supplements may accelerate recovery from exercise (and ultimately surgery), build lean mass, and even improve resilience to physical trauma. One such supplement is creatine, often consumed as creatine monohydrate. Athletes have used creatine for decades to increase muscle mass and physical performance. During this time, it has become one of the most extensively studied supplements. Meat products are a main dietary source of creatine, which is also produced de novo by the liver and kidneys. Biochemically, creatine functions as a source of energy as a phosphate donor (creatine phosphate) primarily in muscle cells, but it is also utilized in other metabolically active tissues, including the central nervous system [60]. Creatine may benefit patients undergoing a prehabilitation program. Unfortunately, although widely studied in healthy patients, studies of patients with significant medical illness are more limited, but in the available literature, "creatine supplementation appears safe and well tolerated in virtually all medical patient populations" [61].

One of the most pervasive concerns related to creatine is whether it contributes to water retention. This would be of particular concern in individuals with preexisting kidney or heart disease, as they are more sensitive to changes in fluid balance. Studies show that when an individual first starts creatine supplementation, his or her fluid status may increase (this effect is not universal), particularly if the creatine is "loaded" with several days of extremely high doses to facilitate faster uptake by skeletal muscle [62]. Over time, the fluid redistributes, mitigating the risk of pathologic fluid overload. This risk mitigation is evident, as studies of creatine administration and exercise therapy in patients with chronic heart failure demonstrate improvements in inflammation and endothelial dysfunction [63] without adverse effects, and plasma brain-derived natriuretic peptide (BNP) is inversely correlated with myocardial phosphocreatine/ATP ratio [64].

Similarly, despite concerns to the contrary, creatine does not cause or worsen kidney disease. This misconception is likely the result of measuring kidney function based on changes in serum creatinine [65]. By monitoring creatinine as a proxy for kidney function, any external cause of creatinine fluctuation may falsely suggest changes in renal function. All else held equal, healthcare professionals interpret rising creatinine levels with worsening kidney function. However, as *creatine* levels increase via supplementation, so does the metabolism of creatine into the creatinine by-product. Increases in skeletal muscle also correlate with higher creatinine levels. Increased serum creatinine levels are an anticipated result of creatine supplementation and do not necessarily represent an acute kidney injury. However, this can obfuscate the medical picture when following labs to evaluate for side effects of medications, for example. Overall, a 2023 narrative review addressing the specific concept of "creatinesupplementation-induced kidney failure" reiterated that available randomized controlled trials cumulatively show creatine does *not* induce kidney failure though concerned healthcare providers may find it prudent to monitor kidney function in older patients or those at risk of worsening kidney function due to the incomplete body of evidence [66].

Researchers had previously hypothesized that creatine-induced fluid shifts in the body could provoke muscle cramping, especially in hot/humid environments. When studying this presumption, the opposite was found to be true [67]. Users of creatine supplements had significantly less heat illnesses, dehydration, muscle tightness, and cramping. In fact, athletes supplementing creatine had fewer sports-related injuries, again, particularly when training in heat [67, 68]. This finding may be due to the hydrating effect of creatine, drawing water intracellularly into skeletal muscle via the osmotic gradient. Applying this to chronic disease, one study demonstrated a 60% reduction in muscle cramping during dialysis for patients who received intravenous pretreatment with a creatine monohydrate solution [69].

Considering its purported benefits, creatine supplementation may play a role in certain patients undergoing prehabilitation. When combined with resistance training, creatine allows for greater strength increases and hypertrophy with decreased pain from exercise. Without an exercise stimulus, creatine alone has minimal effect on muscle growth. Studies conflict on whether it can mitigate atrophy due to short-term inactivity such as when recovering from injury, illness, or surgery [70].

Creatine may also benefit individuals with metabolic disease. In individuals with central obesity and metabolic disease, physicians are seeing a rapid rise in cases of metabolic-associated fatty liver disease (MAFLD). Likely mediated through creatine's relationship with choline [71], studies have demonstrated improvements in

MAFLD with creatine supplementation [72]. Through uncertain mechanisms in the brain, creatine has been shown to have antidepressant effects in certain individuals, as well [73, 74]. One caveat is that individuals initiating creatine supplementation are also typically increasing their fitness participation, and exercise has well-documented psychiatric and metabolic benefits.

Protein Supplementation

Healthcare practitioners commonly recommend high-protein diets for patients interested in weight loss, as high-protein foods can be a good substitute for carbohydrate-rich foods. This substitution often promotes satiety while lowering calorie consumption. Protein also has the greatest thermic effect of all the macronutrients, which effectively reduces the net calories available for storage if in a calorie surplus.

The current recommended dietary allowance for protein is 0.8 grams per kilogram of body weight daily [61]. For an individual weighing 165 pounds, this is about 60 grams of protein per day. The recommendation was not intended to serve as an upper limit for protein consumption but instead represents the amount of protein required for maintaining "nitrogen balance," essentially the amount of protein required to avoid a physiologic state of muscle catabolism. A total of 0.8 grams of protein per kilogram is a relatively low bar to clear for the average individual. However, this target may be inadequate for many patients in a prehabilitation program.

Cancer, surgery, and above-average physical activity increase an individual's metabolic demands. In order to maintain energy and promote healing, situations like these may require higher protein intake in order to be in a stable or anabolic state. Furthermore, the bioavailability of consumed protein decreases with age. Thus, higher amounts of protein are required in older adults when factoring in this inefficiency [75]. Finally, some plant protein sources have lower efficacy for meeting metabolic demand compared to animal sources due to fiber-reducing protein bioavailability and lower concentration of crucial amino acids for skeletal muscle anabolism. Legumes, for example, lack cysteine and methionine; seeds, grains, and nuts contain phytates, enzyme inhibitors, and tannins that affect protein utilization from the diet through different mechanisms [76].

Based on the above, current research suggests the target protein intake should be at *least* 1.2–1.6 grams of protein per kilogram of body weight for these groups [77]. Nutritionally, greater than 1.5 g/kg a day is considered a high-protein diet, which for a 165-pound individual is approximately 112 g of protein per day. Some research even suggests intake as high as 2 g/kg a day to ensure adequate stimulation of the cellular growth regulator mTOR [78] in both older adults (due to "anabolic resistance" associated with aging) and in individuals with significantly elevated protein requirements such as postsurgically or during cancer treatment. However, consuming this amount would likely be very challenging without supplementation. Recent research [79] suggests individuals may overcome anabolic resistance with a lower *total* protein amount by maximizing protein intake from sources like animal proteins that are rich in the amino acids leucine, lysine, and methionine.

Additionally, protein *timing* is crucial to reverse the natural catabolism that occurs during the overnight fast and immediately after exercise. In individuals who are athletically "untrained," protein consumption within 2 h of exercise maximizes the muscle-building benefits of resistance training. This window is less critical for trained athletes. Promoting anabolism is crucial, as bed rest (which is common following surgery) can lead to rapid strength declines, muscle mass loss, and worsened anabolic resistance. Older adults are particularly susceptible to the deleterious consequences of bed rest [80].

Leucine-rich sources may have direct benefits for insulin sensitivity. Leucine directly activates mTOR for muscle anabolism and PPAR gamma/delta for mitochondrial biogenesis and GLUT4 expression [81]. Therefore, leucine indirectly supports insulin sensitivity by increasing glucose uptake by skeletal muscle (GLUT4) and increasing skeletal muscle mass as a depot for glycogen storage. Leucine-rich food sources include beans, chicken, certain fish (e.g., salmon, tuna), certain cheeses (e.g., cottage cheese, Swiss cheese, provolone), and eggs.

Patients with cirrhosis and chronic kidney disease are two special populations who have historically been advised to moderate protein consumption. In cirrhosis, practitioners had empirically given this recommendation to minimize the risk of elevated ammonia, a by-product of protein metabolism, which can increase the risk of hepatic encephalopathy. However, these patients are also at higher risk of sarcopenia and frailty, which predispose them to other serious complications. Protein diets are one critical tool in treating sarcopenia. With more literature supporting the long-term benefits of high-protein diets in patients with cirrhosis [82], the evolving recommendation is for these individuals to gradually increase their daily protein intake to 1.2 grams/kg of body weight per day [83]. This gradual increase allows time for the upregulation of enzymes involved in the urea cycle to manage the greater nitrogen load and minimize the risk of acutely provoking hepatic encephalopathy.

Published research is still divided on whether high-protein diets negatively affect kidneys in vulnerable populations. In fact, research that studied high dietary protein intake in patients with obesity typically failed to find any negative impact on kidney function in the absence of preexisting kidney disease although some report "hyperfiltration," which is considered a precursor to kidney disease [84–86]. In the minority of studies that suggest a negative impact on kidney function from increased dietary protein intake, there are a few recurring confounders. First, the study participants were predisposed to accelerated kidney function decline due to other illnesses such as recent heart attacks, high blood pressure, and diabetes, and the researchers presumed that the high dietary protein load simply intensified these negative effects. Also, the few negative associations were between *animal* protein sources and kidney disease [87]. In these studies, however, there is a strong likelihood of confounders that contributed to worsening kidney function since people with increased animal protein intake relative to other protein sources are also more likely to smoke, have high blood pressure and diabetes, and be less active.

In patients with established, advanced chronic kidney disease, there is a likely relationship between high protein intake and negative health consequences. Protein digestion/metabolism increases the acidity of blood and phosphate levels, which healthy kidneys normally regulate. In advanced kidney disease, the kidneys may be unable to regulate these and other electrolytes, which have myriad other negative health consequences, including worsening of kidney disease. Purine-rich protein sources increase uric acid levels, which also negatively impacts kidney function. In patients with more mild disease or at risk for kidney disease, the evidence is not as clear. In those without kidney disease, high protein intake is unlikely to meaningfully impact kidney function, especially within the prehabilitation period.

For the individual without significant kidney disease who is consuming a high-protein diet in the context of exercise, smoking cessation, and an otherwise balanced diet high in vegetables and lower-glycemic fruits, high-protein intake is a low-risk, critical tool to maintain muscle mass while losing weight [88]. Moreover, any individual can offset residual concern by limiting the protein derived from red meat/pork and instead consuming protein from poultry, dairy (and whey protein isolate), and vegetable sources [87, 89].

Fasting Strategies

It is fairly well established that improving skeletal muscle quality (i.e., increasing mitochondrial density and reducing intramuscular fat deposition) [90] and regular exercise can improve blood sugar control in type 2 diabetes [91]. Interestingly, medically supervised fasting programs may also be a method of insulin sensitization [92].

Intermittent fasting (IF) and time-restricted feeding (TRF) are two strategies to increase the time a patient is in a fasted state and reduce weekly caloric intake. IF programs rely on planned fasting days (>24 h) either grouped together (e.g. 5–2, for 5 fed and 2 fasting days paired) or an alternate day fast (alternating fed days and fasting days). TRF programs (sometimes erroneously also referred to as intermittent fasting) involve a narrow "eating window" each day. Common TRF regimens may be 16 fasting hours and 8 eating hours or 20 fasting hours and 4 eating hours. Some proponents of these programs attribute weight loss and health benefits of fasting to direct changes in insulin sensitivity and adipose tissue catabolism during fasted periods driven by mTOR inhibition/AMPK activation although the bulk of the literature suggests the primary mechanism of weight loss is simply the result of an overall caloric deficit [93]. In the latter explanation, TRF/IF does not have any unique benefit that standard "dieting" practices of caloric restriction at each meal are not also providing. It is also critical for healthcare providers to recognize that fasting may carry significant risks, such as hypoglycemia for patients on insulin/insulin-related medications and gallstones during multiday fasting [94].

As with choosing an exercise program, the best nutritional program is the one a patient can maintain. In the case of diets designed to restrict calories, some patients may find it easier to maintain an average calorie deficit through TRF or IF with ad libitum intake during the eating window instead of a simple daily caloric restriction diet. By scheduling their feeding window/day on days that they may be socially pressured to eat (such as work engagements, celebrations, or family meals), patients may be able to better maintain a feeling of "normalcy" while still meeting nutritional goals. Patients should maintain a high protein intake while in caloric deficit to minimize lean mass loss; however, some decrease in muscle mass may be unavoidable. As skeletal muscle mass maintenance or gain is a core presurgical goal, patients must minimize the effects of muscle catabolism during the extended fasting period. Weak data suggest no increased risk of perioperative surgical complications in TRF immediately before bariatric surgery [95]. The benefits of TRF may plausibly be potentiated in the presurgical population with resistance training and a high-protein diet to maximize the anabolic stimulus. Further research is necessary to determine an optimal strategy for different populations.

Medically Supervised Fasting in Patients with Diabetes

Objective assessments of muscle cell mitochondrial function and flexibility reside along a spectrum. On one end, highly trained athletes demonstrate capacity for high-output ATP production from various fuel sources like fatty acids, ketones, glucose, and lactate, for example [96]. On the other end of the spectrum, individuals with metabolic disease possess a lower density of mitochondria within myocytes with less capacity to oxidize fat for ATP production. The ability to utilize either glucose or fat for energy is the concept of "metabolic flexibility." This fat utilization refers to both dietary fat as well as fat that is mobilized from adipocytes and transported to the liver and muscles. Just as exercise retrains the body to use fat for energy, decreasing the amount of carbohydrates in the diet results in a similar adaptation.

Since fat oxidation requires greater oxygen utilization by the mitochondria than carbohydrates, clinicians can infer the ratio of carbohydrates to fat burned during different conditions by measuring oxygen uptake/CO_2 production, a figure known as the respiratory quotient (RQ). The higher the RQ, the greater the dependence on glucose for metabolism. Research has demonstrated a significantly *higher* respiratory quotient in patients with diabetes utilizing exogenous insulin for glycemic control [97], confirming the impaired uptake of fatty acids for fuel and suggesting an etiology for the weight gain seen in patients with insulin-dependent type 2 diabetes mellitus.

Insulin and insulin-related medications like sulfonylureas carry an inherent risk of hypoglycemia (low blood sugar) in patients who abruptly restrict carbohydrates, a risk that antidiabetic medications such as sodium–glucose cotransporter 2 (SGLT-2) inhibitors, glucagon-like peptide 1 (GLP-1) receptor agonists, and metformin typically do not have in isolation. As a result, individuals on insulin/insulin-related medications should only attempt significant dietary changes under medical supervision, as requirements may change quickly. This reduction in insulin/insulin-related medication requirements suggests an opportunity for patients to therapeutically restrict carbohydrates to lower their RQ, increase fat burning, and support weight loss.

After reducing carbohydrates and remaining on a stable diabetic medication regimen, it is feasible to trial medically supervised fasts in motivated patients to increase endogenous insulin sensitivity and reduce their daily exogenous insulin requirements. Because much of the glucose that these medications manage is from food consumption, it is difficult to wean these medications gradually, and the patient and their doctor must permit slightly elevated blood sugars while starting a medically supervised fasting program. Ultimately, the goal is to meet this lowered insulin target as the body becomes more sensitized to insulin.

Modern management of type 2 diabetes often starts with medications that increase the body's sensitivity to insulin and decrease the amount of glucose the body produces or retains. This is done by altering liver and intestinal glucose management (metformin); altering the metabolic functions of the pancreas, stomach, and brain (GLP-1 receptor agonists and other incretin analogues); and altering how the kidneys dispose of glucose (SGLT-2 inhibitors). As these medications become inadequate to maintain glucose homeostasis, the body requires more insulin, either provided directly via injection or indirectly by medications that increase the pancreas' secretion of insulin (sulfonylureas).

Prolonged fasting theoretically has an indirect effect on glucose management, like non-insulin medications. By not consuming *any* calories, the body utilizes glycogen in the liver and skeletal muscle for fuel. By depleting these reserves, the body effectively has available glucose storage capacity the next time the individual eats carbohydrates or protein that is converted to glucose. Therefore, immediately in a fasting program, insulin requirements will decrease as mealtime insulin must be held because there are no meals on fasting days. Eventually, the "basal" (long-acting) insulin requirements will decrease since the normal, small amounts of insulin the pancreas steadily releases throughout the day will become sufficient to keep glucose levels within a normal range during non-mealtimes.

Fasting's indirect effect on glucose management has not yet been demonstrated in large scale, randomized controlled trials (RCTs) though it has been documented in case reports. One such article summarized the experiences of three patients with long-standing diabetes who underwent medically supervised fasting programs [98]. The patients fasted for 3–4 days per week for 7–11 months. All three patients required daily insulin prior to starting their fasts, and all three were off exogenous insulin within the first month of their fasting program, with one of the patients weaned off insulin in only 5 days. Moreover, these patients all reported *feeling* subjectively better and reported more energy.

Reports like these must be considered with caution. These patients were all supervised by a specialized medical team. This level of close oversight may have had an impact on the results (the "Hawthorne Effect"). Likely, though, these patients were able to wean from exogenous insulin through lifestyle interventions like exercise and a low carbohydrate diet in combination with their fasting program; the fasting diet alone was likely not the reason for such noteworthy outcomes. Fasting is a no-cost intervention and helps halt the forward momentum of diabetes progression and escalating insulin requirements. Therefore, therapeutic fasting programs may be a complementary tool in special populations with insulin resistance and diabetes who are not finding success with diet and exercise alone. However, data are presently very limited, and therefore, providers should exercise caution in applying this strategy.

Other Nutritional Weight Loss Strategies

Other nutritional strategies for weight loss involve changing an individual's dietary composition, such as basic low carbohydrate (ketogenic) diets, low fat diets, or "themed" diets such as the Paleolithic ("Paleo") and Mediterranean diets. The literature supporting one specific diet over others is often contradicting [99].The relative effectiveness of each of these diets is likely a function of how willing an individual is to commit to the diet. There is also variability from person to person in how they physiologically respond to each of these diets. For example, some individuals experience greater satiety when eating a ketogenic diet [100], which allows them to maintain a caloric deficit. However, others do not experience this satiety effect and are less likely to commit to a ketogenic diet.

Ultimately, the efficacy for a particular diet on *weight loss* alone predominantly hinges on the total caloric deficit, with nuanced benefits based on the body's net utilization of calories consumed—for example, high-fiber foods are incompletely absorbed, and high-protein foods require greater energy expenditure to digest [101]. Moreover, both high-fiber and high-protein foods take longer to digest and may promote greater satiation [102].

7 Neuropsychiatric Pillar Interventions

Mood

The need for mental health consultation is not always indicated in patients undergoing a prehabilitation program. However, it should be considered for many patients, as the diseases and disorders they are managing may be causing a significant psychological burden. For example, the journey through cancer treatment is arduous. This along with the cancer diagnosis, itself, may burden patients so heavily that psychiatric support is a crucial, early component of prehabilitation. Similarly, most bariatric surgery centers require psychiatric screening due to the stress of surgery and recovery, as well as the increased risk of new/worsening addiction—typically to alcohol [103]. As a counter example, patients pursuing elective joint replacements are less likely to need empiric psychiatric consultation; however, screening is still warranted since living with chronic pain may promote maladaptive behaviors. Preexisting mood disorders can also substantially affect pain perception, and treating the former may lead to improvements in the latter.

As noted earlier, discussion of obesity-related comorbidities is appropriate in contexts outside of bariatric surgery as obesity is a risk factor for osteoarthritis, degenerative disc disease, cirrhosis, multiple cancers, and other prehabilitation-relevant diagnoses. The association between obesity and depression is bidirectional, with a stronger link in women [104]. This bidirectionality may not simply be due to the effects of mood on appetite. Obesity and psychiatric illness may also share neuroimmunologic etiologies or hypothalamic pituitary-axis abnormalities like thyroid disease or growth hormone deficiency [105, 106] and result in similar changes in the autonomic nervous system [107]. Treating depression can improve a patient's willingness to change. The eventual weight loss may also improve depressive symptoms. Bariatric surgery often improves depression and binge eating disorders but may increase the risk of new/recurrent disorders such as substance abuse, restrictive eating disorders, and suicidality [108].

Stress Management

Besides exercise and psychiatric consultation, individuals may pursue massage therapy and saunas as means of stress reduction. Research suggests that for some individuals, these modalities may be worthwhile components of a comprehensive prehabilitation program.

The data for massage therapy to promote recovery after exercise activities are mixed [109]. However, there may be potential benefits, such as decreased fatigue, improved perceived recovery, faster lactate clearance, improved performance time, and decreased soreness/tenderness 48 h after eccentric exercise. Although studies do not show clear improvements in sport performance or injury prevention, reductions in postexercise soreness and improved perceived recovery among nonathletes may encourage continued engagement. Moreover, decreased inflammatory markers and cortisol levels are objective measures of improved stress and may mediate metabolic benefits demonstrated in the available research [110, 111]. While the data supporting these effects are not robust, the limited risk of massage therapy suggests a likely favorable reward/risk ratio for interested patients.

Heat therapy has a long history of use for sore, tight muscles. Research has elucidated the mechanisms of these and additional benefits [112]. For example, sauna, which applies heat systemically, is effective in facilitating muscle relaxation after resistance training [113]. Hot water immersion has been shown to enhance recovery after anaerobic training and improve fast-twitch muscle function, as evidenced by increased jump height and faster recovery post-training [114]. However, serum values of plasma creatine kinase, often used as a proxy for muscle damage, are inconsistently reduced by warm/hot water immersion following exercise [115, 116].

The potential mechanisms of benefits from sauna and hot water immersion include upregulation of heat shock proteins (HSPs) and mTOR activation. HSPs prevent protein denaturing and pathologic protein aggregation while stimulating homeostatic mechanisms such as cell chaperoning and others to protect the cell from different stressors [117, 118]. mTOR is a master growth regulator in pathways stimulated by insulin, growth hormone (GH) [119], and leptin [120]. As introduced previously, exercise and branched chain amino acids such as leucine potently stimulate mTOR in skeletal muscle [119, 121].

Addressing Stigma

Certain individuals may be subjected to stigma, such as those with obesity or those diagnosed with cancers associated with unhealthy behaviors. Patients with lung cancer possess the greatest levels of psychological distress of all cancers, largely the result of the potential stigma of personal actions causing their disease [122]. This shame is associated with anxiety and depression [123], leading to worse survival and quality of life. This stigma may be seen regardless of whether the patient actually smoked [124].

Individuals with obesity have long been stereotyped of exhibiting slovenly or gluttonous behavior despite the medical insights into the neurobiologic basis of obesity as a disease. Often, individuals with obesity have experienced a lifetime of judgment and ridicule. This stigma even manifests in bariatric surgery being considered "the easy way out" [125].

To mitigate stigma, healthcare professionals should communicate clearly, openly, and inclusively. A nonjudgmental tone is crucial to earning a patients trust. Patients with lung cancer, obesity, and other "lifestyle-associated" diseases may be reluctant to discuss aspects of their life and their values, particularly when these are tied to behaviors perceived to be related to their pathology. In some cases, the goal with high-risk behaviors is harm-reducing behavioral modifications instead of adhering to puritanical, all or nothing recommendations. For example, eliminating sugar-sweetened beverages from an unhealthy diet is a better starting point than prescribing three square meals of lean meats and egg whites with a glass of water. Similarly, for patients who smoke cigarettes and have struggled to quit in the past, vaporizing (vaping) nicotine may be a better initial recommendation than immediate smoking abstinence [126] though the efficacy of vaping as a harm reduction tool is debated. Certainly, the ultimate goal is to guide the patient to the healthiest habits, but incremental progress toward that goal is often necessary.

Sleep Optimization

Sleep is an underappreciated pillar of health. There is a large amount of data documenting the benefits of at least 7 h of uninterrupted sleep per night [127]. Sleep is crucial for restoration and management of various bodily functions. This includes clearing accumulated waste products in the brain, recycling damaged proteins in the body, and reconstituting muscle fibers damaged by exercise. Sleep is also important for adequate recovery following exercise [128].

On the other hand, sleep *deprivation* has many negative effects. It impairs the body's ability to dispose of glucose into a storable form (glycogen) within muscles, which is necessary for performance in subsequent bouts of exercise. This inability to efficiently store glucose also contributes to the elevations in fasting blood sugar seen with sleep deprivation. Additionally, poor sleep also impairs muscle anabolism, slowing recovery and predisposing individuals to injury. Poor sleep also increases the release of the "hunger hormone" ghrelin, increases the release of cortisol, and decreases levels of the "satiety hormone" leptin. Altogether, these result in increased hunger eating larger portions and more processed foods like cookies, chocolate, and potato [129, 130]. Finally, short sleep is associated with higher BMI, likely as a function of multiple interacting effects [131].

In some clinical scenarios, a patient may be exhibiting excessive daytime sleepiness despite sufficient sleep quantity. Obstructive sleep apnea (OSA) or another sleep disorder may be blunting the restorative benefits of sleep and can contribute to weight gain and metabolic dysfunction [132]. OSA becomes a self-perpetuating cycle of poor sleep promoting weight gain, which then further worsens sleep quality. A good prehabilitation program should screen for OSA, as it is often a missed diagnosis with significant health consequences.

The effects of sleep apnea extend beyond decreased total sleep time due to frequent awakenings [133]. During apneic (absent breathing) or hypopneic (decreased breath volume) periods, carotid chemoreceptors detect hypercapnia and hypoxemia that causes an increase in sympathetic nervous system activity, which acutely raises blood pressure and contributes to the arousal from sleep. These apneic/hypopneic episodes have a dose-dependent association with hypertension severity. Moderate or severe OSA is also associated with elevated incident stroke risk. Similarly, severe OSA is associated with coronary artery disease, and apneic episodes can provoke acute cardiac syndrome and arrhythmias [134]. Additionally, apneic episodes raise pulmonary arterial pressure, which can ultimately result in vascular remodeling and permanent pulmonary hypertension.

Healthcare providers should screen patients for sleep disorders when they report typical signs/symptoms of poor sleep, such as excessive daytime sleepiness and loud snoring. They should also consider sleep disorders when patients report in poor concentration and mood issues. Specific diagnostic testing and treatment modalities for sleep disorders are explained in more detail in later chapters.

Pain Management

Chronic pain is a major feature of many chronic illnesses, particularly disorders that may require joint replacement, spine surgery, and limb amputation. Addressing pain within a comprehensive prehabilitation program is critical to maximize engagement in the other aspects of the treatment plan. Chronic pain can also be linked to mood, sleep quality, and social engagement—improving pain will hopefully improve those as well.

Not all pain is purely due to anatomic/biologic pathology that can be easily fixed with a single, straightforward medication, injection, or surgery. Chronic pain is linked to psychosocial elements as well. Chronic pain is also frequently complicated by fear and anxiety, leading patients to avoid activities which may exacerbate their pain, even if the activity is not causing actual damage to the patient.

Treatment of chronic pain often begins with appropriate goal setting. Often this requires initially setting functional goals (e.g., "being able to walk in a park for 20 minutes") for patients rather than purely pain-focused goals (e.g. achieving "zero out of ten pain"). Providers should use various treatment methods to guide patients to more tolerable pain levels and guide them toward resuming activities they may be avoiding due to their pain. These treatment methods may include physical therapy, occupational therapy, aquatic therapy, medications, bracing, injections, mental health management, and adjunctive treatments (such as massage or acupuncture).

Patients who have lived with chronic pain for years may have gradually accumulated maladaptive behaviors and thought processes that cannot be immediately unwound. A multidisciplinary approach is sometimes critical, but at minimum, healthcare providers should take a holistic approach in managing pain. In complex cases of chronic pain in which the patient is severely debilitated and consumed by their pain, pharmacologic interventions (discussed in later chapters) will have greater efficacy when integrated with counseling from a pain psychologist or other pain-specialized mental health professional. As a component of this psychological intervention, some prehabilitation research suggests benefits in a "neuroscience education" program. This included preoperative sessions with a physical therapist and take-home literature to help patients not associate their pain with tissue damage [4]. In these studies, patient satisfaction with the surgical procedure was higher, and in some cases, postoperative pain was lower [135].

Given the likelihood of post-interventional pain after surgery, chemotherapy, or childbirth, achieving pain control during the prehabilitation period can be crucial. This window allows the healthcare team time to determine which treatments are most effective for the individual patient, determine how a patient tolerates different pain medication classes and how to manage potential side effects, and build resilience prior to adding posttreatment pain to their baseline chronic pain. Of note, one study examining patients before cancer surgery incorporated a holistic and opioid-sparing approach to pain management during the preoperative period; interestingly, this was associated with reduced postoperative opioid utilization and the rate of cancer recurrence [136].

Action Points

1. Few interventions, including cancer treatment, require emergent enough treatment that precludes the ability to do a proper prehabilitation program. Convincing patients and other providers to intentionally delay treatment will require a comprehensive discussion of treatment goals, risks, and benefits.
2. Patients are often burdened by many medical appointments during the prehabilitation period. Providers should minimize this burden by consolidating appointments on the same day and (ideally) location as other specialist visits. Programs such as meal delivery services can streamline patients' care and help patients achieve health optimization goals with minimal cognitive burden.
3. Personalized exercise prescriptions begin with prescreening patients for signs and symptoms of cardiopulmonary, metabolic, or renal disease. Providers should prescribe exercise based on patient preferences and comorbid diseases. The best exercise regimen is the one to which a person will remain adherent. For patients without preferred activities, a combined resistance and aerobic training program may maximize benefit in a limited period and accelerate improvement of metabolic disease.
4. Consider alternative exercise modalities such as aquatic therapy and blood flow restriction training in patients with weight-bearing limitations due to pain or medical comorbidities.

5. Nutritional "nudges" can affect behavioral change with less resistance. Eliminating sugar-sweetened beverages and increasing protein consumption can have synergistic benefits, especially in patients with insulin resistance. Well-designed and gradually introduced high-protein diets may be safely prescribed even in patients with cirrhosis and chronic kidney disease during the prehabilitation window. Vegetable and low-purine animal sources such as whey protein isolate may mitigate any residual risk.
6. Medically supervised fasting programs like intermittent fasting and time restricted feeding are methods to reduce calorie consumption without constant calorie restriction. Periodic, prolonged fasting programs can also accelerate insulin sensitization and improve metabolic flexibility.
7. Treating pain, mood disorders, and sleep disturbances may improve quality of life, outcomes of treatment, and improve the efficacy of other prehabilitation interventions.

References

1. Batchelor TJ, Rasburn NJ, Abdelnour-Berchtold E, Brunelli A, Cerfolio RJ, Gonzalez M, et al. Guidelines for enhanced recovery after lung surgery: recommendations of the Enhanced Recovery After Surgery (ERAS®) Society and the European Society of Thoracic Surgeons (ESTS). Eur J Cardiothorac Surg. 2019;55(1):91–115.
2. Shukla A, Granger CL, Wright GM, Edbrooke L, Denehy L. Attitudes and perceptions to prehabilitation in lung cancer. Integr Cancer Ther. 2020;19:1534735420924466.
3. Ljungqvist O, Scott M, Fearon KC. Enhanced recovery after surgery: a review. JAMA Surg. 2017;152(3):292–8.
4. Stenberg E, dos Reis Falcao LF, O'Kane M, Liem R, Pournaras DJ, Salminen P, et al. Guidelines for perioperative care in bariatric surgery: Enhanced Recovery After Surgery (ERAS) Society recommendations: a 2021 update. World J Surg. 2022:1–23.
5. Missel M, Pedersen JH, Hendriksen C, Tewes M, Adamsen L. Exercise intervention for patients diagnosed with operable non-small cell lung cancer: a qualitative longitudinal feasibility study. Support Care Cancer. 2015;23(8):2311–8.
6. Sommer MS, Trier K, Vibe-Petersen J, Missel M, Christensen M, Larsen KR, et al. Perioperative Rehabilitation in Operable Lung Cancer Patients (PROLUCA) a feasibility study. Integr Cancer Ther. 2016;15(4):455–66.
7. Temel JS, Greer JA, Goldberg S, Vogel PD, Sullivan M, Pirl WF, et al. A structured exercise program for patients with advanced non-small cell lung cancer. J Thorac Oncol. 2009;4(5):595–601.
8. Gökler-Danışman I, Yalçınay-İnan M, Yiğit İ. Experience of grief by patients with cancer in relation to perceptions of illness: the mediating roles of identity centrality, stigma-induced discrimination, and hopefulness. J Psychosoc Oncol. 2017;35(6):776–96.
9. Norcross JC, Krebs PM, Prochaska JO. Stages of change. J Clin Psychol. 2011;67(2):143–54.
10. Haque SF, D'Souza A. Motivational interviewing: the RULES, PACE, and OARS. Curr Psychiatr Ther. 2019;18(1):27–9.
11. Sherson EA, Yakes Jimenez E, Katalanos N. A review of the use of the 5 A's model for weight loss counselling: differences between physician practice and patient demand. Fam Pract. 2014;31(4):389–98.

12. Riebe D, Franklin BA, Thompson PD, Garber CE, Whitfield GP, Magal M, et al. Updating ACSM's recommendations for exercise preparticipation health screening. Med Sci Sports Exerc. 2015;47(11):2473–9.
13. Bobbio A, Chetta A, Carbognani P, Internullo E, Verduri A, Sansebastiano G, et al. Changes in pulmonary function test and cardio-pulmonary exercise capacity in COPD patients after lobar pulmonary resection. Eur J Cardiothorac Surg. 2005;28(5):754–8.
14. Knight J, Nigam Y, Jones A. Effects of bedrest 1: cardiovascular, respiratory and haematological systems. Nurs Times. 2009;105(21):16–20.
15. Srdic D, Plestina S, Sverko-Peternac A, Nikolac N, Simundic A-M, Samarzija M. Cancer cachexia, sarcopenia and biochemical markers in patients with advanced non-small cell lung cancer—chemotherapy toxicity and prognostic value. Support Care Cancer. 2016;24(11):4495–502.
16. Nuijten MA, Eijsvogels TM, Monpellier VM, Janssen IM, Hazebroek EJ, Hopman MT. The magnitude and progress of lean body mass, fat-free mass, and skeletal muscle mass loss following bariatric surgery: a systematic review and meta-analysis. Obes Rev. 2022;23(1):e13370.
17. Wasser JG, Vasilopoulos T, Zdziarski LA, Vincent HK. Exercise benefits for chronic low back pain in overweight and obese individuals. PM&R. 2017;9(2):181–92.
18. Minniti MC, Statkevich AP, Kelly RL, Rigsby VP, Exline MM, Rhon DI, et al. The safety of blood flow restriction training as a therapeutic intervention for patients with musculoskeletal disorders: a systematic review. Am J Sports Med. 2020;48(7):1773–85.
19. Patterson SD, Hughes L, Warmington S, Burr J, Scott BR, Owens J, et al. Blood flow restriction exercise: considerations of methodology, application, and safety. Front Physiol. 2019;10:533.
20. Loenneke JP, Allen KM, Mouser JG, Thiebaud RS, Kim D, Abe T, et al. Blood flow restriction in the upper and lower limbs is predicted by limb circumference and systolic blood pressure. Eur J Appl Physiol. 2015;115(2):397–405.
21. Thompson KM, Slysz JT, Burr JF. Risks of exertional rhabdomyolysis with blood flow–restricted training: beyond the case report. LWW. 2018;28(6):491–2.
22. Carneiro A, Viana-Gomes D, Macedo-da-Silva J, Lima GHO, Mitri S, Alves SR, et al. Risk factors and future directions for preventing and diagnosing exertional rhabdomyolysis. Neuromuscul Disord. 2021;31(7):583–95.
23. Karabulut M, Garcia SD. Hemodynamic responses and energy expenditure during blood flow restriction exercise in obese population. Clin Physiol Funct Imaging. 2017;37(1):1–7.
24. Groennebaek T, Sieljacks P, Nielsen R, Pryds K, Jespersen NR, Wang J, et al. Effect of blood flow restricted resistance exercise and remote ischemic conditioning on functional capacity and myocellular adaptations in patients with heart failure. Circulation: Heart Failure. 2019;12(12):e006427.
25. Cahalin LP, Formiga MF, Owens J, Anderson B, Hughes L. Beneficial role of blood flow restriction exercise in heart disease and heart failure using the muscle hypothesis of chronic heart failure and a growing literature. Front Physiol. 2022;13:924557.
26. Kohlbrenner D, Kuhn M, Manettas A, Aregger C, Peterer M, Greco N, et al. Low-load blood flow restriction strength training in patients with COPD: a randomised single-blind pilot study. Thorax. 2024;79(4):340–8.
27. Lau CW, Leung SY, Wah SH, Yip CW, Wong WY, Chan KS. Effect on muscle strength after blood flow restriction resistance exercise in early in-patient rehabilitation of post-chronic obstructive pulmonary disease acute exacerbation, a single blinded, randomized controlled study. Chron Respir Dis. 2023;20:14799731231211845.
28. Rolnick N, de Sousa Neto IV, da Fonseca EF, Neves RVP, dos Santos RT, da Cunha ND. Potential implications of blood flow restriction exercise on patients with chronic kidney disease: a brief review. J Exerc Rehab. 2022;18(2):81.
29. Clarkson MJ, Brumby C, Fraser SF, McMahon LP, Bennett PN, Warmington SA. Hemodynamic and perceptual responses to blood flow-restricted exercise among patients undergoing dialysis. Am J Physiol Renal Physiol. 2020;318(3):F843–50.

30. Christensen R, Bartels EM, Astrup A, Bliddal H. Effect of weight reduction in obese patients diagnosed with knee osteoarthritis: a systematic review and meta-analysis. Ann Rheum Dis. 2007;66(4):433–9.
31. Graff SK, Mario FM, Ziegelmann P, Spritzer PM. Effects of orlistat vs. metformin on weight loss-related clinical variables in women with PCOS: systematic review and meta-analysis. Int J Clin Pract. 2016;70(6):450–61.
32. De Bortoli N, Guidi G, Martinucci I, Savarino E, Imam H, Bertani L, et al. Voluntary and controlled weight loss can reduce symptoms and proton pump inhibitor use and dosage in patients with gastroesophageal reflux disease: a comparative study. Dis Esophagus. 2016;29(2):197–204.
33. Brown JD, Buscemi J, Milsom V, Malcolm R, O'Neil PM. Effects on cardiovascular risk factors of weight losses limited to 5–10%. Transl Behav Med. 2016;6(3):339–46.
34. Aaboe J, Bliddal H, Messier S, Alkjaer T, Henriksen M. Effects of an intensive weight loss program on knee joint loading in obese adults with knee osteoarthritis. Osteoarthr Cartil. 2011;19(7):822–8.
35. Hudgel DW, Patel SR, Ahasic AM, Bartlett SJ, Bessesen DH, Coaker MA, et al. The role of weight management in the treatment of adult obstructive sleep apnea. An official American Thoracic Society clinical practice guideline. Am J Respir Crit Care Med. 2018;198(6):e70–87.
36. Swift DL, Houmard JA, Slentz CA, Kraus WE. Effects of aerobic training with and without weight loss on insulin sensitivity and lipids. PLoS One. 2018;13(5):e0196637.
37. Erion DM, Shulman GI. Diacylglycerol-mediated insulin resistance. Nat Med. 2010;16(4):400–2.
38. Colberg SR, Sigal RJ, Fernhall B, Regensteiner JG, Blissmer BJ, Rubin RR, et al. Exercise and type 2 diabetes: the American College of Sports Medicine and the American Diabetes Association: joint position statement executive summary. Diabetes Care. 2010;33(12):2692–6.
39. Mann S, Beedie C, Balducci S, Zanuso S, Allgrove J, Bertiato F, et al. Changes in insulin sensitivity in response to different modalities of exercise: a review of the evidence. Diabetes Metab Res Rev. 2014;30(4):257–68.
40. Simoneau J-A, Kelley DE. Altered glycolytic and oxidative capacities of skeletal muscle contribute to insulin resistance in NIDDM. J Appl Physiol. 1997;83(1):166–71.
41. Petta S, Gastaldelli A, Rebelos E, Bugianesi E, Messa P, Miele L, et al. Pathophysiology of non alcoholic fatty liver disease. Int J Mol Sci. 2016;17(12):2082.
42. Bweir S, Al-Jarrah M, Almalty A-M, Maayah M, Smirnova IV, Novikova L, et al. Resistance exercise training lowers HbA1c more than aerobic training in adults with type 2 diabetes. Diabetol Metab Syndr. 2009;1(1):1–7.
43. Boulé NG, Kenny GP, Haddad E, Wells GA, Sigal RJ. Meta-analysis of the effect of structured exercise training on cardiorespiratory fitness in Type 2 diabetes mellitus. Diabetologia. 2003;46(8):1071–81.
44. Katsukawa F. FITT principle of exercise in the management of lifestyle-related diseases. Clin Calcium. 2016;26(3):447–51.
45. Ussher M, West R, Steptoe A, McEwen A. Increase in common cold symptoms and mouth ulcers following smoking cessation. Tob Control. 2003;12(1):86–8.
46. Tarumi S, Yokomise H, Gotoh M, Kasai Y, Matsuura N, Chang SS, et al. Pulmonary rehabilitation during induction chemoradiotherapy for lung cancer improves pulmonary function. J Thorac Cardiovasc Surg. 2015;149(2):569–73.
47. Jang C, Hui S, Lu W, Cowan AJ, Morscher RJ, Lee G, et al. The small intestine converts dietary fructose into glucose and organic acids. Cell Metab. 2018;27(2):351–61. e3
48. Taylor SR, Ramsamooj S, Liang RJ, Katti A, Pozovskiy R, Vasan N, et al. Dietary fructose improves intestinal cell survival and nutrient absorption. Nature. 2021;597(7875):263–7.
49. Johnson RJ, Wilson WL, Bland ST, Lanaspa MA. Fructose and uric acid as drivers of a hyperactive foraging response: a clue to behavioral disorders associated with impulsivity or mania? Evol Hum Behav. 2021;42(3):194–203.
50. Sánchez-Lozada LG, Lanaspa MA, Cristóbal-García M, García-Arroyo F, Soto V, Cruz-Robles D, et al. Uric acid-induced endothelial dysfunction is associated with

mitochondrial alterations and decreased intracellular ATP concentrations. Nephron Exp Nephrol. 2013;121(3–4):e71–e8.
51. Lanaspa MA, Andres-Hernando A, Kuwabara M. Uric acid and hypertension. Hypertens Res. 2020;43(8):832–4.
52. Johnson RJ, Nakagawa T, Jalal D, Sánchez-Lozada LG, Kang D-H, Ritz E. Uric acid and chronic kidney disease: which is chasing which? Nephrol Dial Transplant. 2013;28(9):2221–8.
53. Softic S, Cohen DE, Kahn CR. Role of dietary fructose and hepatic de novo lipogenesis in fatty liver disease. Dig Dis Sci. 2016;61:1282–93.
54. Johnson R, Stenvinkel P, Andrews P, Sánchez-Lozada L, Nakagawa T, Gaucher E, et al. Fructose metabolism as a common evolutionary pathway of survival associated with climate change, food shortage and droughts. J Intern Med. 2020;287(3):252–62.
55. Suez J, Korem T, Zeevi D, Zilberman-Schapira G, Thaiss CA, Maza O, et al. Artificial sweeteners induce glucose intolerance by altering the gut microbiota. Nature. 2014;514(7521):181–6.
56. Suez J, Cohen Y, Valdés-Mas R, Mor U, Dori-Bachash M, Federici S, et al. Personalized microbiome-driven effects of non-nutritive sweeteners on human glucose tolerance. Cell. 2022;185(18):3307–28.e19.
57. Nadolsky KZ. Counterpoint: Artificial sweeteners for obesity—better than sugary alternatives; potentially a solution. Endocr Pract. 2021;27(10):1056–61.
58. Arends J, Bachmann P, Baracos V, Barthelemy N, Bertz H, Bozzetti F, et al. ESPEN guidelines on nutrition in cancer patients. Clin Nutr. 2017;36(1):11–48.
59. Peterson LA, Zeng X, Caufield-Noll CP, Schweitzer MA, Magnuson TH, Steele KE. Vitamin D status and supplementation before and after bariatric surgery: a comprehensive literature review. Surg Obes Relat Dis. 2016;12(3):693–702.
60. Andres RH, Ducray AD, Schlattner U, Wallimann T, Widmer HR. Functions and effects of creatine in the central nervous system. Brain Res Bull. 2008;76(4):329–43.
61. Harmon KK, Stout JR, Fukuda DH, Pabian PS, Rawson ES, Stock MS. The application of creatine supplementation in medical rehabilitation. Nutrients. 2021;13(6):1825.
62. Lopez RM, Casa DJ, McDermott BP, Ganio MS, Armstrong LE, Maresh CM. Does creatine supplementation hinder exercise heat tolerance or hydration status? A systematic review with meta-analyses. J Athl Train. 2009;44(2):215–23.
63. Hemati F, Rahmani A, Asadollahi K, Soleimannejad K, Khalighi Z. Effects of complementary creatine monohydrate and physical training on inflammatory and endothelial dysfunction markers among heart failure patients. Asian. J Sports Med. 2016;7(1):e28578.
64. Chida K, Otani H, Kohzuki M, Saito H, Kagaya Y, Takai Y, et al. The relationship between plasma BNP level and the myocardial phosphocreatine/adenosine triphosphate ratio determined by phosphorus-31 magnetic resonance spectroscopy in patients with dilated cardiomyopathy. Cardiology. 2006;106(3):132–6.
65. Willis J, Jones R, Nwokolo N, Levy J. Protein and creatine supplements and misdiagnosis of kidney disease. BMJ. 2010;340:b5027.
66. Longobardi I, Gualano B, Seguro AC, Roschel H. Is it time for a requiem for creatine supplementation-induced kidney failure? A narrative review. Nutrients. 2023;15(6):1466.
67. Dalbo VJ, Roberts MD, Stout JR, Kerksick CM. Putting to rest the myth of creatine supplementation leading to muscle cramps and dehydration. Br J Sports Med. 2008;42(7):567–73.
68. Greenwood M, Kreider RB, Greenwood L, Byars A. Cramping and injury incidence in collegiate football players are reduced by creatine supplementation. J Athl Train. 2003;38(3):216–9.
69. Chang CT, Wu CH, Yang CW, Huang JY, Wu MS. Creatine monohydrate treatment alleviates muscle cramps associated with haemodialysis. Nephrol Dial Transplant. 2002;17(11):1978–81.
70. Kreider RB, Stout JR. Creatine in health and disease. Nutrients. 2021;13(2):447.
71. Deminice R, de Castro GSF, Francisco LV, da Silva LECM, Cardoso JFR, Frajacomo FTT, et al. Creatine supplementation prevents fatty liver in rats fed choline-deficient diet: a burden of one-carbon and fatty acid metabolism. J Nutr Biochem. 2015;26(4):391–7.

72. Marinello PC, Cella PS, Testa MT, Guirro PB, da Silva Brito WA, Padilha CS, et al. Creatine supplementation protects against diet-induced non-alcoholic fatty liver but exacerbates alcoholic fatty liver. Life Sci. 2022;310:121064.
73. Candow DG, Forbes SC, Ostojic SM, Prokopidis K, Stock MS, Harmon KK, et al. "Heads Up" for creatine supplementation and its potential applications for brain health and function. Sports Med. 2023;53(1):49–65.
74. Bakian AV, Huber RS, Scholl L, Renshaw PF, Kondo D. Dietary creatine intake and depression risk among U.S. adults. Transl Psychiatry. 2020;10(1):52.
75. Traylor DA, Gorissen SHM, Phillips SM. Perspective: protein requirements and optimal intakes in aging: are we ready to recommend more than the recommended daily allowance? Adv Nutr. 2018;9(3):171–82.
76. Shaghaghian S, McClements DJ, Khalesi M, Garcia-Vaquero M, Mirzapour-Kouhdasht A. Digestibility and bioavailability of plant-based proteins intended for use in meat analogues: a review. Trends Food Sci Technol. 2022;129:646–56.
77. Phillips SM, Chevalier S, Leidy HJ. Protein "requirements" beyond the RDA: implications for optimizing health. Appl Physiol Nutr Metab. 2016;41(5):565–72.
78. Beck AM, Holst M. Nutritional requirements in geriatrics. interdisciplinary nutritional management and care for older adults. Cham: Springer; 2021. p. 19–30.
79. Layman DK, Anthony TG, Rasmussen BB, Adams SH, Lynch CJ, Brinkworth GD, et al. Defining meal requirements for protein to optimize metabolic roles of amino acids. Am J Clin Nutr. 2015;101(6):1330S–8S.
80. Biolo G, Pišot R, Mazzucco S, Di Girolamo FG, Situlin R, Lazzer S, et al. Anabolic resistance assessed by oral stable isotope ingestion following bed rest in young and older adult volunteers: relationships with changes in muscle mass. Clin Nutr. 2017;36(5):1420–6.
81. Schnuck JK, Sunderland KL, Gannon NP, Kuennen MR, Vaughan RA. Leucine stimulates PPARβ/δ-dependent mitochondrial biogenesis and oxidative metabolism with enhanced GLUT4 content and glucose uptake in myotubes. Biochimie. 2016;128:1–7.
82. Dhaliwal A, Armstrong MJ. Sarcopenia in cirrhosis: a practical overview. Clin Med (Lond). 2020;20(5):489–92.
83. Lizardi-Cervera J, Almeda P, Guevara L, Uribe M. Hepatic encephalopathy: a review. Ann Hepatol. 2003;2(3):122–30.
84. Rosenvinge Skov A, Toubro S, Bülow J, Krabbe K, Parving HH, Astrup A. Changes in renal function during weight loss induced by high vs low-protein low-fat diets in overweight subjects. Int J Obes. 1999;23(11):1170–7.
85. Cuenca-Sánchez M, Navas-Carrillo D, Orenes-Piñero E. Controversies surrounding high-protein diet intake: satiating effect and kidney and bone health. Adv Nutr. 2015;6(3):260–6.
86. Clifton P. Effects of a high protein diet on body weight and comorbidities associated with obesity. Br J Nutr. 2012;108(S2):S122–S9.
87. Ko G-J, Rhee CM, Kalantar-Zadeh K, Joshi S. The effects of high-protein diets on kidney health and longevity. J Am Soc Nephrol. 2020;31(8):1667–79.
88. Friedman AN, Ogden LG, Foster GD, Klein S, Stein R, Miller B, et al. Comparative effects of low-carbohydrate high-protein versus low-fat diets on the kidney. Clin J Am Soc Nephrol. 2012;7(7):1103–11.
89. Vasconcelos QDJS, Alves APNN, de Souza ACH, de Moraes MEA, Aragão GF. Impact of chronic use of whey protein isolate in two doses using an experimental model. Biointerface Res Appl Chem. 2023;13(2):116.
90. Lee S, Kim Y, White D, Kuk J, Arslanian S. Relationships between insulin sensitivity, skeletal muscle mass and muscle quality in obese adolescent boys. Eur J Clin Nutr. 2012;66(12):1366–8.
91. Sigal RJ, Kenny GP, Boulé NG, Wells GA, Prud'homme D, Fortier M, et al. Effects of aerobic training, resistance training, or both on glycemic control in type 2 diabetes: a randomized trial. Ann Intern Med. 2007;147(6):357–69.
92. Stange R, Pflugbeil C, Michalsen A, Uehleke B. Therapeutic fasting in patients with metabolic syndrome and impaired insulin resistance. Complement Med Res. 2013;20(6):421–6.

93. Liu D, Huang Y, Huang C, Yang S, Wei X, Zhang P, et al. Calorie restriction with or without time-restricted eating in weight loss. N Engl J Med. 2022;386(16):1495–504.
94. Stokes CS, Lammert F. Excess body weight and gallstone disease. Visceral Med. 2021;37(4):254–60.
95. Tat C, Barajas-Gamboa JS, Del Gobbo GD, Klingler M, Abdallah M, Raza J, et al. The effect of fasting during ramadan on outcomes after bariatric surgery at an Academic Medical Center in the Middle East. Obes Surg. 2020;30(11):4446–51.
96. Yang W-H, Park J-H, Park S-Y, Park Y. Energetic contributions including gender differences and metabolic flexibility in the general population and athletes. Meta. 2022;12(10):965.
97. Nakaya Y, Ohnaka M, Sakamoto S, Niwa Y, Okada K, Nomura M, et al. Respiratory quotient in patients with non-insulin-dependent diabetes mellitus treated with insulin and oral hypoglycemic agents. Ann Nutr Metab. 1998;42(6):333–40.
98. Furmli S, Elmasry R, Ramos M, Fung J. Therapeutic use of intermittent fasting for people with type 2 diabetes as an alternative to insulin. Case Rep. 2018;2018:bcr-2017-221854.
99. Kim JY. Optimal diet strategies for weight loss and weight loss maintenance. J Obes Metab Syndr. 2021;30(1):20–31.
100. Gibson AA, Seimon RV, Lee CMY, Ayre J, Franklin J, Markovic TP, et al. Do ketogenic diets really suppress appetite? A systematic review and meta-analysis. Obes Rev. 2015;16(1):64–76.
101. Sutton EF, Bray GA, Burton JH, Smith SR, Redman LM. No evidence for metabolic adaptation in thermic effect of food by dietary protein. Obesity. 2016;24(8):1639–42.
102. Halton TL, Hu FB. The effects of high protein diets on thermogenesis, satiety and weight loss: a critical review. J Am Coll Nutr. 2004;23(5):373–85.
103. Steffen KJ, Engel SG, Wonderlich JA, Pollert GA, Sondag C. Alcohol and other addictive disorders following bariatric surgery: prevalence, risk factors and possible etiologies. Eur Eat Disord Rev. 2015;23(6):442–50.
104. Jantaratnotai N, Mosikanon K, Lee Y, McIntyre RS. The interface of depression and obesity. Obes Res Clin Pract. 2017;11(1):1–10.
105. Chen X, Xiao Z, Cai Y, Huang L, Chen C. Hypothalamic mechanisms of obesity-associated disturbance of hypothalamic–pituitary–ovarian axis. Trends Endocrinol Metab. 2022;33(3):206–17.
106. Hauger RL, Saelzler UG, Pagadala MS, Panizzon MS. The role of testosterone, the androgen receptor, and hypothalamic-pituitary–gonadal axis in depression in ageing Men. Rev Endocr Metab Disord. 2022;23(6):1259–73.
107. Wilson JB, Ma E, Lopez B, Brown AK, Lutfy K, Friedman TC. The role of neurochemicals, stress hormones and immune system in the positive feedback loops between diabetes, obesity and depression. Front Endocrinol. 2023;14:1224612.
108. Becerra AZ, Khalid SI, Morgenstern AS, Rembert EA, Carroll MM, Omotosho PA, et al. The association between bariatric surgery and psychiatric disorders: a national cohort study. Obes Surg. 2022;32(4):1110–8.
109. Weerapong P, Hume PA, Kolt GS. The Mechanisms of massage and effects on performance, muscle recovery and injury prevention. Sports Med. 2005;35(3):235–56.
110. Wändell P, Ärnlöv J, Andreasson AN, Andersson K, Törnkvist L, Carlsson A. Effects of tactile massage on metabolic biomarkers in patients with type 2 diabetes. Diabet Metab. 2013;39(5):411–7.
111. Moraska A, Pollini RA, Boulanger K, Brooks MZ, Teitlebaum L. Physiological adjustments to stress measures following massage therapy: a review of the literature. Evid Based Complement Alternat Med. 2010;7:409–18.
112. McGorm H, Roberts LA, Coombes JS, Peake JM. Turning up the heat: an evaluation of the evidence for heating to promote exercise recovery, muscle rehabilitation and adaptation. Sports Med. 2018;48(6):1311–28.
113. Iguchi M, Shields RK. Prior heat stress effects fatigue recovery of the elbow flexor muscles. Muscle Nerve. 2011;44(1):115–25.

114. Skurvydas A, Kamandulis S, Stanislovaitis A, Streckis V, Mamkus G, Drazdauskas A. Leg immersion in warm water, stretch-shortening exercise, and exercise-induced muscle damage. J Athl Train. 2008;43(6):592–9.
115. Pournot H, Bieuzen F, Duffield R, Lepretre P-M, Cozzolino C, Hausswirth C. Short term effects of various water immersions on recovery from exhaustive intermittent exercise. Eur J Appl Physiol. 2011;111(7):1287–95.
116. Vaile J, Halson S, Gill N, Dawson B. Effect of hydrotherapy on the signs and symptoms of delayed onset muscle soreness. Eur J Appl Physiol. 2008;102(4):447–55.
117. Brinkmeier H, Ohlendieck K. Chaperoning heat shock proteins: proteomic analysis and relevance for normal and dystrophin-deficient muscle. Proteomics Clin Appl. 2014;8(11–12):875–95.
118. Noble EG, Milne KJ, Melling CJ. Heat shock proteins and exercise: a primer. Appl Physiol Nutr Metab. 2008;33(5):1050–75.
119. Deldicque L, Theisen D, Francaux M. Regulation of mTOR by amino acids and resistance exercise in skeletal muscle. Eur J Appl Physiol. 2005;94(1):1–10.
120. Maya-Monteiro C, Bozza P. Leptin and mTOR: partners in metabolism and inflammation. Cell Cycle. 2008;7(12):1713–7.
121. Moberg M, Apró W, Ekblom B, Gv H, Holmberg H-C, Blomstrand E. Activation of mTORC1 by leucine is potentiated by branched-chain amino acids and even more so by essential amino acids following resistance exercise. Am J Physiol Cell Physiol. 2016;310(11):C874–C84.
122. Cataldo JK, Slaughter R, Jahan TM, Pongquan VL, Hwang WJ. Measuring stigma in people with lung cancer: psychometric testing of the cataldo lung cancer stigma scale. Oncol Nurs Forum. 2011;38(1):E46–54. NIH Public Access
123. Brown Johnson CG, Brodsky JL, Cataldo JK. Lung cancer stigma, anxiety, depression, and quality of life. J Psychosoc Oncol. 2014;32(1):59–73.
124. Chapple A, Ziebland S, McPherson A. Stigma, shame, and blame experienced by patients with lung cancer: qualitative study. BMJ. 2004;328(7454):1470.
125. Vartanian LR, Fardouly J. Reducing the stigma of bariatric surgery: benefits of providing information about necessary lifestyle changes. Obesity. 2014;22(5):1233–7.
126. Glynn TJ, Hays JT, Kemper K. E-cigarettes, harm reduction, and tobacco control: a path forward? Mayo Clin Proc. 2021;96(4):856–62. Elsevier
127. Liew SC, Aung T. Sleep deprivation and its association with diseases—a review. Sleep Med. 2021;77:192–204.
128. Vitale KC, Owens R, Hopkins SR, Malhotra A. Sleep hygiene for optimizing recovery in athletes: review and recommendations. Int J Sports Med. 2019;40(08):535–43.
129. Yang C-L, Schnepp J, Tucker RM. Increased hunger, food cravings, food reward, and portion size selection after sleep curtailment in women without obesity. Nutrients. 2019;11(3):663.
130. Akhlaghi M, Kohanmoo A. Sleep deprivation in development of obesity, effects on appetite regulation, energy metabolism, and dietary choices. Nutr Res Rev. 2023:1–64.
131. Liu S, Wang X, Zheng Q, Gao L, Sun Q. Sleep deprivation and central appetite regulation. Nutrients. 2022;14(24):5196.
132. Gileles-Hillel A, Kheirandish-Gozal L, Gozal D. Biological plausibility linking sleep apnoea and metabolic dysfunction. Nat Rev Endocrinol. 2016;12(5):290–8.
133. Dempsey JA, Veasey SC, Morgan BJ, O'Donnell CP. Pathophysiology of sleep apnea. Physiol Rev. 2010;90(1):47–112.
134. Zapater A, Sánchez-de-la-Torre M, Benítez ID, Targa A, Bertran S, Torres G, et al. The effect of sleep apnea on cardiovascular events in different acute coronary syndrome phenotypes. Am J Respir Crit Care Med. 2020;202(12):1698–706.
135. Waller A, Forshaw K, Bryant J, Carey M, Boyes A, Sanson-Fisher R. Preparatory education for cancer patients undergoing surgery: a systematic review of volume and quality of research output over time. Patient Educ Counsel. 2015;98(12):1540–9.
136. Dawson S, Koneti KK. The role of pain management in cancer prehabilitation. In: Chakraborty A, Balakrishnan A, editors. Prehabilitation for cancer surgery. Singapore: Springer Nature Singapore; 2022. p. 217–47.

Relevant Pharmacology and Interventions

Alexander Watson and Sydney Hand

The medications available to prehabilitation practitioners broadly address myriad functions and may fall into the same pillar categories as the other components of pre-procedural preparation. The agents included within this chapter do not completely encompass all those available to prescribers and all those from which a patient may benefit during a multimodal prehabilitation program. Similarly, an ideally complete description of the medications and interventions included is beyond the scope of this text, as it would require volumes to adequately convey the nuances between agents within a certain class (i.e., corticosteroids), between patient characteristics in an algorithmic decision tree, and of the practical prescribing considerations for those operating within different models of healthcare delivery.

Instead, the following chapter intends to highlight how these medications, many of which are well-known to practicing healthcare professionals, uniquely intersect with the prehabilitation population. Further, few belong neatly within one category. Many, for example, will improve exercise performance, recovery, and mood and significantly assist in weight loss efforts which speak to the pleiotropic nature of these interventions. Finally, some classes of medications are within the research pipeline and are not commercially available at the time of this writing; these are included if data suggests that approval is likely and efficacy is potentially substantial.

A. Watson (✉)
Admire Medical, Middletown, DE, USA
e-mail: alexander@admiremedical.com

S. Hand
Admire Medical, Middletown, DE, USA

UPMC Mercy Hospital, Pittsburgh, PA, USA

A. Watson, K. Barr (eds.), *A Prehabilitation Guide for All Providers*,
https://doi.org/10.1007/978-3-031-72862-4_3

1 Exercise Performance and Recovery

Oxandrolone

Oxandrolone is a synthetic anabolic steroid with clinical uses in cases of extreme catabolism such as for patients with extensive burns. By reversing the negative nitrogen balance in a hypermetabolic state, oxandrolone prevents the catabolism of skeletal muscle for the short-term recovery benefit at the expense of long-term muscle. In trials of oxandrolone for frailty, the use is not restricted to male patients as oxandrolone has a high anabolic to androgenic ratio; this results in favorable anabolic potential without substantial risk of virilizing effects in women. Even in these cases, while lean mass significantly benefits from treatment, frailty/physical functioning does not consistently improve [1, 2].

However, off-label practitioners also use oxandrolone for its effect on sex-hormone-binding globulin (SHBG) [3]. Normally, sex hormones like testosterone and estrogen are mostly bound to SHBG, and physiologic activity is conveyed by the residual unbound steroid. Oxandrolone at low doses increases free testosterone by reducing SHBG [4]. Further, as oral synthetic steroids can provoke transaminitis—suggestive of low-grade liver injury—prescribers can theoretically offset this effect by administering oxandrolone sublingually to bypass the portal circulation; however, presently there are no supporting studies to confirm this. Regardless, periodic serum AST/ALT evaluation can identify acute liver injury in real time and prompt transitioning to a different agent.

Hormone Replacement Therapy (Estrogen ± Progesterone Analogues)

For several decades, prescribers widely prescribed hormone replacement therapy (HRT) for women in menopause. Replacing the hormones progesterone (when necessary) and estrogen relieves symptoms such as hot flashes, sleep disturbance, poor concentration/memory, and mood disorders for millions of women. For unclear reasons, these symptoms are absent/mild in some while severely debilitating in others. For the latter group, replacing these hormones provides substantial benefits and can restore a normal quality of life, previously without a clear understanding of the long-term effects of health and longevity. The Women's Health Initiative, the largest study ever designed at that time, attempted to clarify the risks and benefits of HRT. Following the publication of the results of this research, prescription of HRT decreased from nearly one-quarter of women in menopause to only about 5%.

The remarkable decline in prescriptions is largely the result of published findings of the study that initially described a 26% higher risk of breast cancer among women who had received estrogen and progesterone as part of their HRT program [5]. Later analysis of the study design showed glaring errors and even some effects opposite to the original findings. First, the increased risk of breast cancer was an uncertain finding [6]. This was further bolstered by the fact that when looking only at the group of women who had *never* been on HRT prior to being included in the research, there was definitively no link between getting hormones and breast cancer risk.

Beyond the subjective benefits for quality of life and the questionable impact on breast health, HRT has other systemic impacts to consider that extend beyond the prehabilitation timeline. Although beyond the scope of this text, these are considerations when weighing the risks and benefits of initiating HRT, a decision that patients may be making to begin optimizing wellness prior to making more effortful lifestyle changes during an early prehabilitation program.

Finally, HRT undoubtedly is the most effective pharmacologic preventative treatment for bone health/bone density in postmenopausal women [7]. Currently, bisphosphonates are a class of medications for preventing bone fractures in women with osteoporosis, but they have short-term GI side effects and long-term (>5 years) risk of atypical bone fractures. Estrogen does not carry either risk.

Some patients may benefit from also supplementing testosterone, which similarly declines rapidly after menopause. As long as the dose is physiologic, that is, adequate to boost testosterone to approximately the level prior to menopause, patients should not experience virilization effects such as acne, increased body hair, voice changes, and so on. The potential benefits, however, complement those of HRT well and include maintenance of muscle mass, bone health, libido, cognitive function, and energy level [8–10].

Literature is increasingly demonstrating that like testosterone, estrogen has beneficial effects for supporting muscle recovery through multiple mechanisms. In addition to estrogen supporting skeletal muscle mass maintenance, exercise may augment the effect of estrogen in maintaining/building muscle mass and strength, as well as enhancing the injury response for repair [11].

Testosterone Replacement Therapy

Testosterone is the primary sex hormone in men, and it is also present in women. It is anabolic to muscle and catabolic to fat and stimulates libido among other effects. Men naturally have a gradual decrease in testosterone levels as they age, whereas women will typically have a sudden decline of testosterone at menopause when all sex hormones decrease. These decreases in testosterone are a contributing factor toward many related conditions such as sarcopenic obesity, frailty, and "anabolic resistance." In some instances, testosterone levels may be lower than is normal for a given age, which may warrant supplementation to restore good health.

Understanding appropriate testosterone repletion requires recalling the hypothalamic–pituitary–gonadal axis. In brief, the hypothalamus senses gonadal hormonal levels in the body and, if low, will release gonadotropin-releasing hormone (GnRH) to induce the pituitary gland to release luteinizing hormone (LH). Then, in men, rising LH instructs the testes to increase testosterone production. Therefore, with testosterone deficiency, the etiology is typically categorized as either primary (the testes are no longer responding to LH appropriately) or secondary (the brain is not releasing enough LH). These designations are important because they will help guide treatment.

For cases of secondary testosterone deficiency, the brain is releasing inadequate LH to tell the testes to produce appropriate amounts of testosterone. This may occur for many reasons including poor sleep or other hormone abnormalities such as insulin resistance or hypercortisolemia. If LH and testosterone remain low after correcting poor diet, sleep, and insulin resistance, then practitioners can reasonably trial a medication to function like LH such as HCG. HCG is structurally like LH, but it is more stable and lasts longer in circulation, thereby requiring less frequent doses. HCG then tells the testes to produce more testosterone and can also improve other functions in the testes necessary for fertility as well.

Alternatively, if lab tests demonstrate low testosterone but abnormally high levels of LH, this implies that the brain's calls are going unanswered. In these situations, adding more LH (HCG) will not have a meaningful effect. Instead, supplementing testosterone directly would be indicated if the individual was having symptoms of low testosterone as well.

Patients and some practitioners unfamiliar with the literature on this topic may be concerned about reports of heart disease risk and increases in cholesterol from testosterone replacement. Studies are mixed on this topic, but the prevailing wisdom is that an increased risk of heart disease only occurs with supra-therapeutic levels of testosterone. The TRAVERSE trial concluded in 2022 after a 4-year trial period of repleting testosterone in men with hypogonadism. While the data suggested an increased risk of pulmonary embolism in men in the intervention group, overall major adverse cardiac events were not significantly different in the control and intervention groups. In earlier research, when compared with individuals who do not replete low testosterone, individuals (particularly men with obesity) who supplement testosterone have less heart disease as well as many other benefits to overall health [12]. The TRAVERSE trial also demonstrated no change in blood pressure among men receiving testosterone repletion.

The primary benefit of supplementing testosterone for prehabilitation goals is an increase in lean body mass while simultaneously losing fat mass. Metabolic parameters improve such as insulin sensitivity may also improve through multiple mechanisms, including simply having more muscle mass, which increases the space to store glucose. These benefits in isolation ideally translate to improvements in more holistic measurements such as function, independence, and overall quality of life. By increasing exercise tolerance, individuals can then make fundamental changes to activity and alter their health permanently. This is particularly relevant for patients with sarcopenic obesity (addressed elsewhere) or frailty.

Frailty is a syndrome seen in older individuals that involves metabolic dysfunction, loss of bone density and muscle mass, and slowed cognitive functioning. This syndrome is a risk factor for falls, fractures, and worse health outcomes from other chronic diseases such as heart failure, cancer, and diabetes among others. Individuals with low testosterone for their age are more likely to develop frailty, and restoring testosterone to normal levels in conjunction with physical therapy and dietary interventions has the potential to substantially increase longevity and quality of life.

In determining who is appropriate for TRT, identify signs/symptoms and lab values such as testosterone levels below the 50th percentile. Then, consider whether the etiology is primary or secondary based on LH levels [13]. At this time, evaluate the prolactin level that, if elevated, can suppress LH levels, and screening for diabetes is appropriate as well. Consider nonhormonal impacts on testosterone such as poor sleep, diet, and stress. After initiating repletion, evaluate the patient's subjective improvements every 6 months with discussions of when to stop—typically, the recommendation is <2 years due to the risk of testicular atrophy and impaired fertility. If the patient is not concerned with maintaining fertility, then practitioners can extend the treatment duration longer.

2 Lifestyle-Pillar-Related Medications and Supplements: Weight Loss, Nutrition, and Substance Use Cessation

Gut Peptide Hormone Analogues

The field of obesity and metabolic medicine is becoming increasingly more exciting as new pharmacologic agents are leading to substantial weight loss with additional benefits of end-organ protection from complications of metabolic disease. Analogues of gut peptide hormones such as the glucagon-like peptide 1 (GLP-1) receptor agonists (RA) and dual agonists of the GLP-1R and gastric inhibitory protein (GIP) receptor are facilitating 20+% total body weight loss, far beyond what could be achieved with prior medications. Leading the fanfare are the medications semaglutide (GLP-1RA) and tirzepatide (GLP-1RA & GIP RA) and related to prior medications like liraglutide, exenatide, dulaglutide, and lixisenatide, which had demonstrated weight loss [14], albeit less substantial than semaglutide [15]. These medications are FDA-approved to treat type 2 diabetes mellitus, with semaglutide 1 mg reducing hemoglobin A1c by approximately 1.55% over 30 weeks [16] and tirzepatide 15 mg achieving as much as 2.58% reduction in 52 weeks in the SURPASS-4 trial [17]. For weight loss, at the time of this writing, only liraglutide, semaglutide, and tirzepatide are FDA-approved for obesity. Other promising dual (combinations of two analogues of GLP, GIP, or glucagon receptor agonists) and triple agonists (analogues of GLP, GIP, and glucagon) trials are ongoing with the potential for greater weight loss and improvements in comorbidities of metabolic disease.

When looking at the data from prior trials, however, researchers noticed additional benefits being demonstrated. Specifically, in addition to their effect in controlling diabetes, this class of medication was found to reduce cardiovascular disease [18], strokes, and all causes of death overall in the agents tested for these outcomes. In fact, the benefits spanned multiple body systems beyond the brain and heart as patients treated also had protection against the progression of chronic kidney disease [19].

Bupropion/Naltrexone

Bupropion, when prescribed alone, is often used as an atypical antidepressant due to its activity as a dopamine-norepinephrine reuptake inhibitor or as a smoking cessation agent for its affinity for the nicotinic receptors. However, when coupled with the mu-receptor antagonist naltrexone, the combination capitalizes on bupropion's hypothalamic activity of suppressing appetite via the pro-opiomelanocortin (POMC)/cocaine-amphetamine-related transcript (CART) pathways. Naltrexone synergizes with bupropion by decreasing the autoinhibition of POMC/CART synergy [20]. Expected weight loss varies by the study, but in the meta-analysis, participants lost 8.07 kg over 56 weeks [21]. Moreover, this synergy does not decrease bupropion's individual properties, so practitioners can address comorbid depression while also treating various substance use disorders through the effects of naltrexone. When considering different pathologic eating behaviors, early literature spearheaded by the Mayo Clinic [22] suggests this combination may be most effective for hedonic eating phenotype and, in this subpopulation, can assist in approximately total body weight loss of approximately 10%. Given the risk of lower seizure threshold in susceptible individuals, bupropion (alone or in combination with naltrexone) is contraindicated for individuals with bulimia, known seizure disorders, alcohol use disorder/binge drinking, or those at risk of abrupt cessation of benzodiazepines/barbiturates or antiepileptic drugs. Anorexia nervosa is a relative contraindication,

Phentermine and Other Substituted Amphetamines ± Topiramate

Phentermine and related compounds like diethylpropion, phendimetrazine, and benzphetamine are some of the oldest compounds approved as anti-obesity medications. Like bupropion, these function through appetite suppression via the POMC/CART hypothalamic appetite control pathway, but these compounds add modest peripheral lipolysis activity via beta-adrenergic receptor agonism [23]. For added benefit, providers may prescribe phentermine in combination with topiramate; however, the mechanism for the synergistic benefit is unclear. Unless prescribed as the branded form of phentermine/topiramate, phentermine and related agents are typically the least expensive of the anti-obesity medications with the longest history of use. These medications do not have the same risk of dependence as amphetamine salts/methamphetamine due to primarily noradrenergic activity with minimal dopaminergic activity [24], but these are contraindicated in patients with cardiac disease, insomnia, anxiety, and other sensitivity to stimulant medications such as individuals with palpitations and hyperhidrosis. When in combination with topiramate, patients may experience additional side effects of dysgeusia (abnormal taste), mild cognitive slowing/word-finding difficulty, and irritability. Further, topiramate has known teratogenic effects and should be strictly avoided in patients who may become pregnant.

Orlistat

Orlistat is the only anti-obesity agent that functions through the mechanism of inhibiting pancreatic lipase, thus impairing the absorption of dietary fat. This decreases the total calories absorbed from the diet. The primary side effects of gastrointestinal distress like diarrhea or flatulence essentially provide negative feedback to minimize dietary indiscretions. Impaired fat absorption may secondarily limit absorption of the fat-soluble vitamins A, D, E, and K and some medications such as amiodarone. The modest weight loss of ~2.12 kg in meta-analysis [25], coupled with the prominent side effect profile, limits the use of orlistat clinically.

3 Off-Label Therapeutics for Metabolic Health

Sodium–Glucose Cotransporter 2 (SGLT2) Inhibitors

Sodium–glucose cotransporter 2 (SGLT2) inhibitors comprise one of the newest medication classes for managing diabetes, with later additional indications for slowing the progression of chronic heart and kidney disease. Inhibiting this cotransporter of sodium and glucose leads to wasting instead of reclaiming glucose in the urine. Due to this mechanism, the drugs in this class have a mild diuretic and antihypertensive effect as well [26] from the osmotic effect of glucose. Prescribers must be mindful of a unique adverse event profile that includes Fournier's gangrene and euglycemic ketoacidosis. These medications make for an effective adjunctive medication for diabetes and metabolic health; however, in select patients, SGLT2 inhibitors may raise serum low-density lipoprotein cholesterol (LDLc) and triglycerides (TAGs), possibly from the increased mobilization of TAGs for beta-oxidation [27]. Some patients report increased cravings for simple carbohydrate-rich foods [28], which may be minimized by co-prescribing GLP-1RAs or metformin.

Mirabegron

At approved doses, mirabegron functions as a selective beta-3-adrenergic receptor agonist. As the beta-3 receptor promotes smooth muscle relaxation and the bladder is studded with beta-3 receptors, mirabegron is FDA-approved to promote bladder relaxation for overactive bladder. When prescribing doses higher than the 25–50 mg used for reducing bladder tone, mirabegron is effective in stimulating the beta-3 receptor sufficiently to promote the "browning" of white adipose tissue, essentially increasing the expression of mitochondria for fatty acid metabolism. In doing so, mirabegron may significantly increase HDL cholesterol and improve insulin sensitivity [29]; however, absolute/relative excess body weight loss is limited. At doses higher than 100 mg, the medication loses relative selectivity for the beta-3 receptor and may raise blood pressure and heart rate due to beta-1-adrenergic receptor stimulation, and it may even core body temperature, likely through multiple mechanisms

[30]. Researchers are exploring this and other beta-3 agonists for metabolic health and potential weight loss benefits. Note that dose reduction is necessary in patients with eGFR 15-30, and it is contraindicated in individuals with eGFR <15.

Metformin

Metformin is one of the most widely prescribed medications in the world and is typically the first-line medication used to treat type 2 diabetes through unique mechanisms not shared by any other medication on the market. By reviewing large population-based studies, researchers identified lower rates of many age-related diseases and even reductions in all-cause mortality in patients both with and without diabetes who are taking metformin [31]. Metformin also mitigates fatty liver disease through multiple mechanisms, and some studies suggest protection against the development of certain cancers [13], cognitive decline [32], and Alzheimer's disease in patients with diabetes [33].

Broadly, metformin works through three primary mechanisms for treating diabetes. It decreases hepatic gluconeogenesis and glucose absorption by the gut, increases insulin sensitivity in skeletal muscle and the liver, and modulates insulin release by the pancreas. At the cellular level, metformin triggers many of the same pathways induced during periods of caloric deficit via AMP kinase activation, particularly those in the mitochondria. Predominantly through the downstream effects as a stimulator of AMP kinase, metformin inhibits lipogenesis/stimulates lipolysis, stimulates cellular autophagy, decreases cholesterol synthesis, and increases glycolysis. On top of this, it stimulates mitochondrial biogenesis in tissues including brown adipose tissue [34], which then increases heat production through glucose/fat oxidation by the cell.

Metformin is remarkably well-tolerated relative to many other diabetes medications, particularly in that it does not increase the risk of hypoglycemia in isolation. However, many patients will experience gastrointestinal distress upon starting the medication or with dose increases, which some suspect is related to changes in gut cellular metabolism as well as changes in the gut microbiome. This typically passes within 1–2 weeks of starting the medication or dose increases, and utilizing an XR formulation may lessen this side effect. The most concerning side effect is the potential for severe lactic acidosis in individuals who already have impaired lactate clearance such as individuals with liver and kidney disease. Since metformin is excreted by the kidneys, those with kidney disease are at higher risk of impaired clearance and supra-therapeutic levels.

For individuals with limited time and a rigorous exercise plan, metformin may impair the beneficial adaptions to exercise [35]. Practically, this will be apparent in delayed recovery following strenuous exertion and, over the longer term, attenuating the aerobic and muscle hypertrophy benefits. As such, its place within a multimodal preprocedural optimization program hinges on where the patient's deficits predominate; if the patient demonstrates metabolic syndrome without obvious sarcopenia or major functional impairments, then the benefits may outweigh the risks for metformin. Further, for patients already on metformin who are about to increase their resistance training, metformin may decrease the risk of tendinopathy, with the most notable published benefit demonstrating significant protective benefit against rotator cuff tendinopathy [36]. Alternatively, if the patient's personalized program involves a schedule heavy with physical therapy, aerobic training, and resistance training to address multiple impairments in strength and aerobic conditioning, alternative medications may have a greater risk/benefit profile. Unfortunately, literature has not yet identified a modified dosing schedule to effectively mitigate impairment of exercise adaptation by separating dosing times from exercise sessions.

Taurine

Taurine is an amino acid most ingested in animal products and is also a common ingredient in energy drinks due to its integral role in exercise physiology [37]. In a meta-analysis, taurine ingestion of at least 1 gram prior to exercise significantly increased time to exhaustion and power output in endurance performance [38]. Although they share no structural relation, like the amino acid agmatine, taurine has many neurologic functions including regulating neurotransmission, anti-inflammatory actions, and neuroprotection from excitotoxicity [39, 40]. Taurine may also help improve insulin sensitivity as well as the downstream effects of diabetes in promoting microangiopathy as well as diabetic nephropathy [41], in some part acting as a glycation inhibitor. Supplementing taurine is also associated with significant improvements in blood pressure (both SBP and DBP), serum triglycerides, and serum total cholesterol (although no significant association with HDL-C or LDL-C, alone) in meta-analysis [42]. In this study, taurine was not found to impact fasting blood glucose, conflicting with other literature. Another meta-analysis of studies assessing the relationship of taurine and inflammation found the ability to significantly decrease c-reactive protein (CRP) by an average of 1.95 [43]; however, it did not have any significant impact on other inflammatory markers like TNF-alpha or IL-6.

4 Neuropsychology, Sleep, and Pain

Sleep Medications

As introduced in earlier chapters, sleep is a critical but often sacrificed element of self-care. Short-changing adequate quality and quantity of sleep is associated with increased levels of cortisol and ghrelin, decreased leptin and testosterone, and worsened insulin resistance. Through these effects and elevated catecholamines, poor sleep elevates blood pressure and increases the risk for major adverse cardiovascular events and accidental trauma like motor vehicle accidents.

For many, shortened sleep quantity is not deliberate but instead secondary to insomnia. While the modern sleeping environment with blue light and cognitive stimulation from cell phones, computers, and televisions is arguably the worst it has ever been, drug developers have been working in vain to develop medications that decrease sleep latency (the time to fall asleep) and increase sleep duration for over half of a century. Early medications like barbiturates, quaaludes, and benzodiazepines (BZDs) bound to different components of GABA receptors to promote sedation and sleep. Besides their high dependence liability limiting their practicality for chronic use, polysomnography suggested these medications blunt REM and deep sleep, which are crucial restorative phases of sleep [44]. Now, BZDs and barbiturates have utility in treating other conditions like anxiety and acute withdrawal symptoms, and quaaludes are no longer sold/manufactured due to risk of harm.

Newer generations of GABA-ergic medications like zolpidem, zaleplon, and eszopiclone are more selective for GABA receptor subunits for a better risk profile. While manufacturers market these medications as the best agents for managing insomnia for short durations, those afflicted often take them chronically resulting in trading one etiology of insomnia for substantial rebound insomnia should they discontinue treatment [45]. Moreover, these agents carry short-term risks of parasomnia behaviors such as eating, shopping, and even driving with potentially catastrophic consequences; long-term studies suggest higher rates of cancer and all-cause mortality, with some speculating this is the result of inadequate slow-wave sleep [46]. Per Beers criteria, benzodiazepines and non-benzodiazepine "z-drugs" are contraindicated for treating insomnia in older adults due to increased risk of adverse events.

Alternatively, trazodone is an atypical antidepressant that offers the elusive benefit of sleep induction/maintenance with polysomnography-proven restoration of normal sleep architecture [47]. Initially, drug developers identified trazodone as an alternative antidepressant to tricyclic antidepressants (TCAs), but the primary side effect of sleepiness limited its use for this indication. Unlike other non-GABA sleep-inducing drugs like first-generation antihistamines (diphenhydramine and doxylamine), trazodone's mechanism of promoting sleep does not include anticholinergic activity and, therefore, likely will not carry the same relative risk of cognitive impairment later in life and delirium in older adults.

Mirtazapine has similar activity to trazodone in promoting sleep through its antihistaminic and alpha-2-adrenergic activity, but due to stronger antagonism of $5HT_2$ and $5HT_3$ receptors, it is also a potent antiemetic/appetite stimulant. For this reason, it may be highly useful in patients with anorexia but likely should be avoided for patients with obesity. As it is a non-serotonergic antidepressant, mirtazapine may be an effective adjunct to selective serotonin reuptake inhibitors (SSRI)/serotonin and norepinephrine reuptake inhibitor (SNRI) medications for discrete symptoms such as insomnia [48].

TCAs, SSRIs, and SNRIs

Serotonin-norepinephrine-reuptake inhibitors (SNRIs) describe a class of medications developed for similar indications to the predecessor selective serotonin reuptake inhibitors (SSRIs) and tricyclic antidepressants (TCAs). Drug developers designed these medications in consideration with the "monoamine hypothesis" in mind, a theory that deficiency of available monoamines like serotonin, norepinephrine, and/or dopamine in the synapse contributes or is causal to illnesses like depression and anxiety. Although efficacy of these medications and further research suggest a more complex relationship between neurotransmitters and mood, these medications are effective for some in managing mood disorder symptoms [49].

Besides managing depressive and anxiety disorders, these antidepressants have additional applications for treating neuropathic pain and migraines. Although they are among the older class of antidepressants, TCAs may be one of the most effective in also treating pain for the same reason they are not typically the first-line agent [50, 51]. The effects of modulating each of these monoamines occur in different places; for example, norepinephrine reuptake increases the stimulation of alpha-2-adrenergic receptors on presynaptic neurons. This leads to decreased sympathetic output and analgesic benefit [52]. TCAs, however, are "dirty drugs" in that they have off-target effects that may include N-methyl-D-aspartate antagonism that modulates the centralization component of neuropathic/chronic pain as well [53]. The "dirtiness" of TCAs extends to common acute anticholinergic effects like somnolence, constipation, and urinary retention, with additional long-term effects like weight gain and sexual dysfunction [54]. They also may affect cardiac conduction through sodium and calcium channel inhibition, which necessitates an EKG prior to initiating therapy with a TCA for at-risk patients. These effects limit their appropriate use in geriatric populations, patients at risk of developing suicidal ideation, or those with cardiac pathology.

Drug developers designed SSRIs and SNRIs to more precisely target the serotonin and serotonin/norepinephrine receptors, respectively. This reduces their side effect profile but also theoretically some of their efficacy as well [55]; however, there are no rigorous head-to-head trials to demonstrate this. Moreover, for many, SNRIs like duloxetine, venlafaxine, and their derivatives offer the best risk:benefit ratios as a primary or adjunctive medication for neuropathic pain. TCAs, SSRIs, and SNRIs have the obvious benefit of treating depression that is commonly comorbid with chronic pain.

Gabapentin/Pregabalin

Initially developed for the treatment of epilepsy, gabapentin and the later-developed related compound pregabalin are now commonly prescribed agents for neuropathic pain. Gabapentin and pregabalin have notable side effects of weight gain, somnolence, and dizziness and may even potentiate the respiratory drive suppressing effects of medications such as opioids. In addition, pregabalin is a controlled substance in the United States (listed as Schedule V), with both gabapentinoids carrying some risk of abuse [56], particularly pregabalin.

Despite these risks, gabapentinoids treat neuropathic pain through a unique mechanism that makes them potential effective adjunctive medications to others like SNRIs, bupropion, and topical agents [57]. In select populations, they may be combined with TCAs as well, but given the overlapping side effect of somnolence and dizziness, this should be done judiciously particularly for individuals with low fall risk. In fact, the data for gabapentin [58] and pregabalin [59] as monotherapy for neuropathy are mixed and suggest modest benefit overall, making their first-line use less promising given the potential for side effects. As combination therapy, however, lower doses may affect relatively better outcomes with fewer side effects.

Gabapentin and pregabalin offer one additional benefit for the neuropsychiatric pillar of prehabilitation—sleep improvements. Both gabapentin and pregabalin are associated with increased total slow-wave ("deep") sleep and slow-wave sleep as a percentage of sleep in healthy individuals, individuals with chronic pain conditions such as fibromyalgia, and other neurologic conditions such as epilepsy [60, 61]. Research demonstrates a negative impact on REM sleep percentage, however.

Capsaicin

As the primary noxious component of chili peppers, capsaicin acutely induces a burning sensation and, at high doses, potentially sharper pain on mucosal and dermal surfaces. The medicinal benefit lies in the physiology that effectuates these sensations. Regular repeated administration of topical capsaicin depletes neuronal substance P, effectively impairing transmission of other neuropathic pain signals. This is one typical limiting.

Available formulations are designated "low" and "high" concentrations. Low concentration is typically administered as a topical cream that must be applied multiple times per day, whereas high concentration (approximately 100 times the potency) is contained within a patch. For some, the initial administration of the high concentration is particularly painful. Unfortunately, not all patients with various types of neuropathic pain such as peripheral neuropathy, postherpetic neuralgia, and HIV neuropathy respond to treatment. Those that do, however, may report substantial benefit from high-concentration capsaicin [62]. In some cases, these high concentration studies used low-concentration capsaicin as active controls, which is of uncertain benefit [63].

Carbamazepine and Oxcarbazepine

Originally designed for epilepsy and trigeminal neuralgia, carbamazepine and its active metabolite oxcarbazepine have a long history of use with well-documented side effect profiles. These medications are teratogenic, carry risk of inducing Stevens-Johnson syndrome (more commonly in individuals of Asian descent, given HLA-B*1502 inheritance), aplastic anemia or combination of leukopenia/anemia/thrombocytopenia, and hyponatremia. Both medications also induce CYP3A4, which increases the metabolism of other substances metabolized by CYP3A4.

Despite these considerations, carbamazepine and oxcarbazepine warrant consideration in refractory neuropathic pain because they are likely more effective [64] than SNRIs and TCAs [51] although not typically first line except for trigeminal neuralgia due to side effect profile. Also, oxcarbazepine, although structurally similar, has less robust data; however, pooled analysis shows the potential for appreciable benefit in appropriate candidates [65, 66]. Although no longer first-line agents for neuropathic pain, carbamazepine and oxcarbazepine may have benefit in a multimodal pain management program for neuropathy pain refractory to more commonly used anticonvulsants like gabapentin and pregabalin.

Corticosteroids

Corticosteroids like prednisone, methylprednisolone, dexamethasone, triamcinolone, and betamethasone are commonly prescribed orally for systemic anti-inflammatory benefit or injected locally to a site of pain and inflammation. Practitioners may inject these intra-articularly, adjacent to tendons/ligaments, and adjacent to compressed and inflamed nerves such as in acute radiculopathy.

For acute conditions, oral or local steroids may quell a debilitating inflammatory process to permit greater movement and, in appropriate cases, facilitate participation in physical or occupational therapy to correct contributing biomechanical issues. For certain conditions, like acute low back pain without neurologic leg weakness, however, literature suggests steroids are no more effective than placebo in improving pain within 5–7 days [67]. However, if the injury includes focal neurologic findings, which would suggest compression and inflammation of a spinal nerve, epidural steroid injections [68] may be effective in mitigating leg pain and short-term disability.

For spinal stenosis, epidural steroid injections have uncertain benefit [69, 70]. Presumably, this variable effect follows similar principles for predicting successful response to epidural steroid injections for radiculopathy, in that evidence of acutely inflamed nerves (as suggested by symptoms of persistent pain ± weakness) typically suggest better responsiveness to steroids. As lumbar spinal stenosis is uncommonly caused by acute processes, the intervention is therefore less likely to be successful for most patients. They may be considered in select patients, and to better predict a successful outcome, practitioners may consider obtaining objective evidence via electromyography (EMG) though this is not common practice [71].

As one safety consideration, for transforaminal epidural steroid injections, FDA guidelines suggest only using non-particulate injectates like dexamethasone as particulate corticosteroids may increase the risk of cord infarction. However, for severe radicular pain, triamcinolone acetate may be superior to dexamethasone, and there is at least one published case report of a patient suffering infarction after dexamethasone epidural steroid injection [72].

With regard to corticosteroids for peripheral joint disease, one study evaluated the safety of administering intra-articular triamcinolone injections every 3 months for 2 years [73]. The results of the study suggest that at least for the knee, this frequency and duration is safe and unlikely to have any negative impact on the rate of progression for knee osteoarthritis. This is only one trial, in one joint, and for a relatively limited duration. In a systematic review of 40 studies [74], researchers assessed the available evidence regarding the potential impact of intra-articular steroids on articular cartilage. Unsurprisingly, results were mixed, but an intuitive trend was clear; for low doses and low durations, the injections were beneficial to cartilage, likely due to the anti-inflammatory effect permitting recovery from damage. This effect was more notable with triamcinolone, methylprednisolone, and hydrocortisone. At higher doses and durations, the corticosteroids demonstrated chondrotoxicity. The authors suggest a cutoff of approximately <2–3 mg/dose or 8–12 mg/cumulative total doses as a likely safe and potentially beneficial limit. These interpretations should not be presumed to be final and complete. All the studied injectates—prednisolone, hydrocortisone, betamethasone, dexamethasone, and methylprednisolone—except triamcinolone only had in vitro and *animal* in vivo data.

Treating inflamed tendons and ligaments is one final common application for corticosteroids in musculoskeletal medicine. Likely through similar processes as those with their chondrotoxicity effects, repeat administration to pathologic tendon and fascia or direct injection into these tissues increases the risk of rupture [75]. Similarly, oral steroids also increase the risk of fractures, particularly tibial stress fractures. When used sparingly and injected adjacent to inflamed tendons (often into the tendon sheath), corticosteroid injections can support faster resolution of pain and facilitate recovery of function.

Platelet Rich Plasma and Hyaluronic Acid Injections

Currently, the consensus is that having obesity increases the risk of musculoskeletal degenerative processes, particularly in weight-bearing areas of the body, as demonstrated in the increased incidence of osteoarthritis, tendinopathies, and plantar fasciitis. The mechanism is not exclusively limited to the mechanical stress of excess body weight on the supportive structures. Obesity is often regarded as a low-grade inflammatory state, and elevated circulating pro-inflammatory cytokines IL-6, IL-1 beta, and TNF alpha likely contribute to the development of musculoskeletal disease [76]. Amplified by the ancillary sleep disorders that are more common in obesity, this is an ideal setup for developing acute and chronic joint, tendon, or fascial pain.

Therefore, it is important to consider known treatments for musculoskeletal disease in the unique context of metabolic disease and obesity. A study published in the *Journal of Foot and Ankle Surgery* assessed corticosteroid injection versus platelet rich plasma (PRP) for the treatment of plantar fasciitis [77]. PRP, in summary, is an emerging treatment for many musculoskeletal disorders across diverse populations. For this treatment, a centrifuge spins the patient's blood to separate the different components into layers. Using the platelet and certain white blood cell layers to produce a thick, concentrated liquid, the practitioner injects the concentrate into small areas of a poorly healing injury or chronic inflammation, such as tendons, fascia, joints, and ligaments. The premise is that the PRP directly and indirectly provides growth and healing factors, which in the longer term can relieve pain and promote healing.

This mechanism is in contrast with corticosteroid injections which are anti-inflammatory, thus relieving pain but providing limited direct healing benefit. As noted previously, research suggests that repeat and/or high-dose steroid injections into a joint accelerate degenerative processes [74], and repeat injections near/into tendons and muscles may weaken them and risk further injury such as tears and rupture.

When utilized for plantar fasciitis, the practitioner injects either steroid or PRP into the plantar fascia origination site at the calcaneus. In one comparison study of PRP and corticosteroids, both PRP and steroids resulted in significant pain relief at 4 weeks and 24 weeks, but the steroid provided greater relief [77]. However, since corticosteroids may impair healing in the long term and weaken local structures, some practitioners have an absolute limit of one injection for plantar fasciitis in the patient's lifetime due to the risk of rupture of the fascia. In larger joints, medical providers typically limit injections to a frequency of one every 3 months or longer [78], often with a lifetime limit as well.

PRP, instead, provides significant pain relief for plantar fasciitis and is safe for repeat administrations; in fact, as it helps precipitate healing of chronic injuries, following PRP with physical therapy may ultimately lead to the resolution of the conditions for which it is being injected. Of note, the study comparing PRP to steroids for plantar fasciitis also prescribed celecoxib immediately following PRP treatment for three days, as PRP typically increases pain transiently after the injection. This may theoretically have impacted the outcome of the study, as nonsteroidal anti-inflammatory drugs (NSAIDs) overall inhibit platelet function, and platelet function is crucial to the growth factor release after PRP injection. This effect is likely less, however, with celecoxib than other NSAIDs like ibuprofen (Motrin) or naproxen (Aleve) as it selectively inhibits certain enzymes (cyclooxygenase-2 or COX-2) while leaving others that are more present on platelets relatively unaffected (COX-1).

One of the most prevalent areas for joint pathology overall is the knee, and like other joints, the incidence of knee osteoarthritis is higher in patients with obesity. There are three main nonsurgical treatments for knee osteoarthritis—steroid injections as highlighted previously, hyaluronic acid, and PRP. Hyaluronic acid is one of the main ingredients in normal joint fluid and when injected into the knee is considered "viscosupplementation." The premise behind replacing the hyaluronic acid is that it is injected as a thick fluid, providing lubrication inside the damaged joint, relieving stiffness and pain [79]. Like most pain-relieving interventions, one goal is to facilitate increased exercise participation and physical therapy to further reduce pain in the long term. Unfortunately, like steroids, viscosupplementation does not treat arthritis directly. It only relieves the symptoms, and the relief does not last forever. Hyaluronic acid treatment benefits may last a few months longer than steroid injections (6 months vs 2–3 months); however, each patient's response is unique [80].

A recent review and meta-analysis compared the use of hyaluronic acid against platelet-rich plasma in patients with obesity [81]. Aggregating the studies within the review into a meta-analysis, researchers were able to determine the benefit of PRP relative to hyaluronic acid at 3 months, 6 months, and 1 year after the injection for overall pain, stiffness, and physical functioning. Initially, within the first 2–3 months, the results are ambiguous; however, there is a trend toward greater benefit from the PRP—particularly in the domain of physical functioning. As time passes and the benefit of hyaluronic acid decreases, PRP's true advantage becomes evident. At 6 months, patients with obesity who received knee intra-articular PRP injections noted improvement in pain, stiffness, and physical functioning. These results were durable and remained at 1 year relative to hyaluronic acid treatments.

Overall, PRP shows promise in treating many of the conditions for which providers currently use corticosteroid injections. Currently, the data are far from conclusive, which some attribute to the fact that PRP preparations have yet to be standardized. As further research is conducted, a standard protocol for PRP, other blood components, and related therapies like stem cell concentrates will clarify the primary areas of benefit. Currently, cost is the most apparent practical hindrance to PRP adoption. Insurance does not cover the intervention, as presently it is viewed as experimental; therefore, this requires an out-of-pocket expense typically around $600–$700 [82].

Nonsteroidal Anti-inflammatory Drugs (NSAIDs)

NSAIDs yield their analgesic, fever-reducing, and anti-inflammatory benefits by inhibiting the cyclooxygenase (COX) enzymes. Unlike acetaminophen, excessive or high dose use does not directly harm the liver; however, they are contraindicated in individuals with liver disease due to bleeding risks and secondary renal injury [83]. Instead, NSAIDs like ibuprofen, naproxen, and dozens of others can be acutely harmful through their effects on the gastrointestinal tract (which may be symptomatic) and their impact on kidney health, which typically goes unnoticed. The use of NSAIDs reduces prostaglandin synthesis; these proteins are responsible for many important homeostatic functions in the body including protecting the stomach/proximal small bowel from digestive acids and enzymes, regulating blood flow to the kidneys, and mediating pain and inflammation.

The design of COX-2 isoform selective NSAIDs provided drug candidates with better tolerability for patients with an elevated risk of gastrointestinal and renal adverse events; however, with greater COX-2 selectivity, these agents also demonstrated an increased risk of cardiovascular thrombotic events [84]. Trials including early COX-2 selective NSAIDs like rofecoxib and valdecoxib demonstrated significantly increased thromboembolic events, eventually leading to their discontinuation. Celecoxib remains one of the most COX-2 selective NSAIDs available and should be prescribed with caution in individuals with known atherosclerotic cardiovascular disease (ASCVD); alternatively, naproxen provides the least selectivity and is, therefore, safest in these individuals.

Another persistent concern with using NSAIDs is managing postoperative pain, particularly following orthopedic procedures. When acute inflammation primes and directs the immune system to sites of tissue injury, the immune system responds by clearing damaged tissue and debris, fighting any pathogens that may have infiltrated the area, and releasing other chemical mediators to increase blood flow from existing blood vessels and to angiogenesis.

Studies of bony tissue have shown that NSAIDs may slow postoperative healing [85]. Reviewing available literature on research in humans summarized in one review and meta-analysis [86], the findings were conflicting but revealed a potential theme. Generally, short courses (i.e., approximately 1-week duration) of the various studied NSAIDs administered at the lowest doses for pain control did not affect bone healing. Associations between the use of NSAIDs and impaired bone healing were typically apparent in longer courses, with durations on the order of several months. Also, other factors such as smoking and poor nutrition increase the likelihood of poor bone healing, as they will affect blood flow and nutrient availability to the nutritionally demanding bone remodeling process.

Opioids

Early liberal use of opioids to treat both acute and chronic sources of pain contributed to high rates of addiction and overdoses. In response, state regulatory boards and insurance companies implemented strict controls on prescribing these medications. Between these forces and a cultural shift in the medical community, patients whose chronic pain had been managed with opioid medications have been having increasing difficulty finding prescribers to continue the prescription they may require for the rest of their lives. Patients with acute sources of severe pain are also finding their pain inadequately treated, particularly those individuals with prior opioid use [87].

The increasing scrutiny over opioid prescribing practices has likely saved countless lives by preventing exposure to addictive substances by susceptible individuals and by mitigating the diversion of prescription opioids for illegal resale. This scrutiny has left many healthcare providers uncertain about which indications they can justify new opioid medication prescriptions. Most commonly, cancer-associated pain is often managed with opioids given the severity and character of the pain. Otherwise, most indications for use are limited to acute pain. As such, conditions like bone fractures that are expected to steadily improve are managed with a short course of pain medication. Some fractures in particular, such as rib fractures, are more often managed more "aggressively," as behaviors to minimize worsening pain such as shallow breathing increase the risk of acute pulmonary complications like atelectasis and pneumonia [88].

Low-Dose Naltrexone

Naltrexone is a medication with several indications, including for maintaining remission of opioid and alcohol use disorders, in combination with bupropion to help facilitate and maintain weight loss, and, more recently, in lower doses for pain and inflammatory conditions. Naltrexone is typically considered "low dose naltrexone" (LDN) when prescribed in amounts under 5 mg. At these low doses, naltrexone has antagonistic effects of one pathway (toll-like receptor 4 or TLR 4) versus inhibition of the traditional analgesic effects at higher doses via mu-opioid receptor (MOR) antagonism [89]. By antagonizing TLR4 on glial cells, LDN may provoke a subsequent decrease in interferon-beta and TNF-alpha synthesis, lowering neuroinflammation. Independent of this, agonism of central MOR at low doses leads to upregulation of the endogenous endorphin system promoting additional neuropsychological benefits.

Currently, LDN is being trialed in treating numerous neurologic conditions, particularly those with a clear or suspected inflammatory component [90] like multiple sclerosis (MS), complex regional pain syndrome (CRPS), fibromyalgia, inflammatory bowel disease (IBD), and even irritable bowel syndrome (IBS). Evidence for MS is mixed but suggests the potential for improving spasticity and fatigue in some [91]. Similarly, the literature currently suggests potential significant benefits for the sleep disturbances, pain, and dystonia seen in CRPS without major adverse events; however, the bulk of current literature is retrospective [92]. In inflammatory bowel disease, published data are currently very sparse and not well-designed, but the data offer substantial promise [93]. Evidence for efficacy in treating fibromyalgia is also still preliminary. However, given the high prevalence and significant debility fibromyalgia causes for millions, continued research is essential [94, 95]. As LDN is well-tolerated with only minor side effects, practitioners may consider this as an adjunctive medication for symptomatic individuals who have explored conventional avenues. Note that at the time of this writing, LDN is not commercially available and must be compounded for patients.

Cannabis (Marijuana)

The term "cannabis" is often preferred over "marijuana" as the latter was originally used to stigmatize the *Cannabis sativa* plant by making it sound foreign and intimidating in an attempt to sway public opinion. The cannabis plant contains nearly 100 different cannabinoids, but the two in greatest concentrations are THC (tetrahydrocannabinol) and CBD (cannabidiol). THC is psychoactive (i.e., results in alterations in consciousness, cognition, perception, mood, or behavior), whereas CBD is not regarded as psychoactive. Other cannabinoids have some milder psychoactive activity, as well. THC is currently illegal at the federal level in the United States as a Schedule I drug, but currently, the federal government defers to each state to decide on prosecuting individuals for possession and use. CBD, on the other hand, is generally regarded as legal since it may be derived from the legal plant *hemp*, which is essentially cannabis that only contains very small amounts of THC.

Overall, research has shown that cannabis/cannabinoids have small but significant benefits for chronic pain (both cancer-associated and non-cancer pain) and perceived sleep quality [96]. For chronic neuropathic pain, CBD/THC blends may be more effective than either cannabinoid alone; however, for those looking to manage daily neuropathic pain without spending every day mildly intoxicated, CBD may be effective alone or in combination with terpene, non-cannabinoid compounds [97].

For acute pain, such as pain after a surgical or dental procedure, cannabinoids have an inconsistent and modest benefit as standalone medication [98]. However, as a complement to opioid-based pain management regimens, they may augment the benefit of opioids like oxycodone or morphine without increasing the side effect profile. In fact, they may reduce the nausea often associated with opioid use. Presuming that the individual is recovering from a surgical procedure at home and not operating heavy machinery, a mix of multiple cannabinoids (i.e., a THC/CBD blend or medical cannabis) may offer the most effective pain control [99–101].

For sleep and sleep quality, the data are currently limited in offering conclusions. Given the intoxicating nature of THC, many find that it significantly reduces the time for them to fall asleep, which is supported by evidence [102]. Unfortunately, like alcohol, most sedative hypnotics, and other aids, it decreases overall sleep quality likely by impairing the rapid eye movement (REM) sleep stage. CBD, however, may avoid the negative impact on sleep quality while maintaining some benefit for falling/staying asleep [103].

The interaction between cannabis use and weight/weight management is a complex and evolving discussion. Superficially, one's knee-jerk reaction may be to assume cannabis, and the subsequent appetite stimulation ("munchies") is a quick route to long-term weight gain. This makes it difficult to treat pain in individuals with obesity who are often burdened by it. The research, however, does not support this direct link. In fact, the third National Health and Examination Survey (NHANES) showed that in chronic heavy users of cannabis, BMI was actually lower, even when controlling for other variables such as age, gender, education, caloric intake, and cigarette smoking [104]. This suggests that long-term appetite or metabolic changes may occur that offset short-term appetite stimulation.

Cannabis is being increasingly used as one component of a multimodal pain control regimen since it does not have the same risk of overdose and abuse potential seen in opioids and has a novel mechanism that complements other commonly used pain medications without dangerous interactions. Moreover, individuals consume cannabinoids to assist in falling asleep without some of the risks of certain prescription sleep medications such as zolpidem and other "z-drugs." [105] Unfortunately for many, cannabis use is a disqualifying factor when seeking approval for weight loss and other major surgeries.

A recently published systematic review compiled studies evaluating the use of cannabis in the perioperative period in patients undergoing bariatric surgery [106]. The studies demonstrated that approximately 10% of patients admitted to cannabis use in the perioperative period. For comparison, approximately 37% of non-cannabis users and 26% of reported cannabis users in the studies also consume tobacco products despite tobacco utilization having known negative effects on healing after surgery due to its pro-inflammatory and vasoconstrictive effects [107]. One study included in the review found that 6- and 12-month weight loss was significantly higher in the patients who used cannabis; however, the study compared only eight patients who use cannabis with 231 nonusers for statistical analysis. Additionally, the two studies included in the review tracked postoperative complications and found no significant difference in minor or major complications within 90 days suggesting, at least, short-term postoperative safety.

However, a review of the literature and understanding of the breadth of physiologic effects suggests that cannabis use is not entirely harmless in the perioperative period. Chronic users may still have different anesthetic requirements during surgery due to long-term physiologic adaptations to the main cannabinoids. General guidelines based on currently available research suggest delaying any procedure requiring general anesthesia at least 72 h from last use of cannabis/cannabinoid medications for multiple reasons, including both antithrombotic and platelet aggregation effects, temperature dysregulation, cerebral vasodilation or vasospasm, cardiac arrhythmias, and changes in drug metabolism [108]. THC is a potent CYP3A4 and weak CYP2C9 inhibitor. Through these and other mechanisms related to endocannabinoid system changes, cannabis use may increase the dosage requirements of propofol for induction anesthesia while prolonging the action of intravenous anesthetics like barbiturates, ketamine, propanidid, and alfaxolone.

Psychedelic Medicine

Psychedelic substances are regaining recognition as potential treatments for myriad illnesses. Medications such as psilocybin, LSD, and nontraditional psychedelics like ketamine have well-politicized histories that are also layered in rumor and mystery. Psilocybin, a prodrug for psilocin, the main active ingredient in "magic mushrooms" and LSD, was initially heralded as a potential breakthrough in the field of psychiatry. Studies into the benefits for depression and addiction were extremely promising, but the culture surrounding these drugs quickly created a panic among parents and politicians. This ultimately led to their classification as Schedule I substances, a designation implying no recognized medical benefit and a high liability for harm. Despite use in some recreational settings, ketamine never developed the same irredeemable reputation and remains on the WHO list of essential medications for its use as an anesthetic. Unsurprisingly, with ketamine's similar potential benefit for treatment-resistant depression and neuropathic pain [109], research into its efficacy resumed and progressed more quickly.

Currently, the s-enantiomer esketamine is approved for treatment-resistant depression, showing benefits in patients with depression that persisted despite the use of traditional agents such as selective serotonin reuptake inhibitors (SSRIs), serotonin-norepinephrine reuptake inhibitors (SNRIs), and bupropion. Ketamine's unique benefit in treating depression is that its effects are nearly immediate, whereas traditional agents typically take weeks to months for full benefit. Ketamine also may improve refractory chronic pain, as well. Some chronic pain conditions like complex regional pain syndrome (CRPS) are notoriously difficult to treat with all known pain reduction modalities. When treating depression, if an individual will ultimately derive benefit from ketamine therapy in chronic pain, the benefits are often rapid and may be quite significant.

In one meta-analysis [110], researchers assessed the available pool of randomized controlled trials of ketamine at sub-anesthetic doses for its effectiveness in treating multiple types of chronic pain. The studies found a significant reduction in pain with maximum benefit typically occurring between 2 days and 2 weeks from treatment, and they report similar benefits even when comparing low-dose ketamine to high-dose ketamine. Given the probable dose–response relationship between ketamine and unpleasant side effects, this suggests that similar benefits may be achieved at more tolerable lower doses although individual studies and anecdotal reports suggest there may, in fact, be better and longer-lasting pain control with higher doses. More research is needed to clarify this.

When considering specific subtypes of pain, ketamine significantly reduced neuropathic (nerve type such as in nerve injuries, spinal cord injuries, and CRPS) and non-neuropathic (fibromyalgia, ischemic limb pain, and CRPS type I) pain. While the average pain reduction in the former group was −1.75 on a 0–10 scale and the latter group was −1.97 (but with greater variance), a specific analysis comparing the efficacy of treating one type of pain over the other was not statistically different. For CRPS specifically, the pain reduction was greater on average at −2.38 points, but this was not statistically different from non-CRPS pain even though this group had a reduction average of −1.71. At 2 weeks after the initial IV ketamine treatment, pain reduction remained substantial at −2.23 points, but by 4 weeks, the benefit was not significantly different from placebo.

Shifting cultural views on psilocybin as a therapeutic tool has allowed for increasing legitimate research to demonstrate the effects. One small meta-analysis [111] aggregated the few available studies assessing the efficacy of psilocybin for depression and anxiety. In this review, no persistent or serious adverse effects were reported, yet large and significant reductions in anxiety and depression were both independently noted. These benefits remained even at 6-month follow-up. Of note, psilocybin alone has similar efficacy to cognitive behavioral therapy. Therefore, the additive effects of both together could potentially be even greater.

In one final study in which psilocybin therapy was compared with escitalopram, two doses of psilocybin administered 3 weeks apart were as effective in reducing the severity of depression in 6 weeks as escitalopram. Importantly, the psilocybin group had a much quicker response and appeared to have nearly double the rate of full depression remission (over 50% of individuals). Therefore, psilocybin offered a faster-acting and greater benefit with fewer side effects than traditional medications. This research group will publish more follow-up information to determine the length of response in both groups.

There are important caveats when considering the magnitude of these claims as determined by the research. Primarily, researchers are unable to fully “blind” patients in the psilocybin and control groups, as psychedelic therapies have quite distinctive effects, and patients can easily differentiate if they have been given the active drug or placebo. Also, some studies have identified a short-term increased risk of suicidality when used for treating refractory depression [112].

Agmatine

Agmatine, a decarboxylated metabolite of arginine, is regarded as a "neuromodulator" and with concentrations in the CNS similar to other neurotransmitters, it is regulated through vesicular uptake/storage/release like other neurotransmitters. Agmatine also co-localizes in neurons with other neurotransmitters, but as a "neuromodulator", however, agmatine has effects across many neurotransmitter receptor families [113]. Agmatine agonizes nicotinic acetylcholine, serotonin 5-HT_{2A} and $5HT_3$, alpha-2-adrenergic, and I_1 and I_2 imidazoline receptors while also inhibiting NMDA and nitric oxide synthase. Higher levels of endogenous agmatine are associated with physiologic stress, with some hypothesizing that the increased synthesis is a neuronal protective mechanism. While it's possible that the causality could be reversed—meaning agmatine might contribute to or worsen physiological stress—this is unlikely. Dozens of studies have shown agmatine's efficacy in providing neuroprotective benefits in models of brain hypoxia/ischemia; MPTP-, glutamate-, and NMDA-induced neurotoxicity; spinal cord injury; and other pathologies. Interestingly, it also has demonstrated antidepressant, anticonvulsive, and antinociceptive benefits. These benefits are conferred through both related and disparate physiologic pathways by inhibiting apoptosis, inflammation, gliosis, and edema as well as having antioxidant, scavenging, neurogenic, angiogenic, and oligodendrogenic effects.

Current clinical use of agmatine is predominantly dedicated to treating neuropathic pain and depression, particularly with high doses. These specific activities make it a potentially crucial tool in the prehabilitation toolbox. Given its long use in relatively high doses (>1 g) over-the-counter workout supplements without any published accounts of significant adverse events besides gastrointestinal distress, risk/benefit considerations may warrant trials of agmatine for individuals as an adjunctive medication in the treatment of pain or depression/anxiety 113]. Specifically, early clinical studies suggest that agmatine alone has significant benefits for different types of neuropathic pain such as radiculopathy [114] and peripheral neuropathy [115] and, when administered with opioids, has a synergistic effect on increasing analgesia through either antagonizing the NMDA receptor [116] or as an alpha-2-adrenergic receptor agonist [117].

There are no published reports of worsening respiratory depression when used in combination with opioids. The alpha-2-adrenergic activity suggests a theoretical risk of additive effects on hypotension if agmatine behaves like better-studied alpha-2-adrenergic agents such as clonidine. Alternatively, agmatine's demonstrated ability to *reduce* tolerance and dependence to opioids suggests at least some of the effect is mediated through NMDA receptor antagonism. Further research needs to establish the relationship of agmatine with physical dependence on opioids, but known effects suggest the promise of reducing opioid requirements while maintaining or increasing analgesic benefits.

5 In the Research Pipeline for Exercise Performance and Recovery

Myostatin Pathway Inhibitors (Myostatin, Activin, and GDF11)

Myostatin is a protein produced by skeletal muscles (myokine) that inhibits myoblast proliferation and muscle protein synthesis while stimulating protein degradation. This is an evolutionarily conserved function to prevent organisms from expending limited resources to maintain metabolically costly skeletal muscle. This catabolic action opposes anabolic stimuli such as resistance training and high protein consumption. The influence of myostatin increases individuals age through mechanisms including low-grade muscle inflammation and intramuscular fat. As a result, the catabolic/anabolic balance shifts toward a phenotype of anabolic resistance and sarcopenia.

Given the integral role of the myostatin pathway in the pathophysiology of sarcopenia and frailty, researchers are trialing inhibitors of the different proteins in the pathway as treatments for Duchenne muscular dystrophy (DMD), inclusion body myositis, cancer cachexia, and obesity [[118]. Most trials demonstrate significant increases in lean mass, with functional benefits only really seen in elderly/frail populations [119]. One agent, bimagrumab, targets the activin II receptor, which is a regulator within the myostatin pathway. One trial of bimagrumab demonstrated a 20% fat mass decrease with concordant gains in lean mass despite being on a calorie-restricted diet [89], a compositional shift that other weight loss agents are unable to achieve due to indiscriminate loss of fat mass and lean mass. Patients given bimagrumab also demonstrated improvements in insulin sensitivity, leptin sensitivity, and higher adiponectin levels suggesting indirect systemic health benefits as well. At the time of this writing, bimagrumab is in trials for the treatment of obesity.

PPAR Agonists

The peroxisome proliferator-activated receptors (PPARs), a family of enzymes (alpha, beta, gamma, and delta), are expressed in most tissues in the body, and stimulating the various subtypes promotes different metabolic benefits. Currently, PPAR alpha agonists (the fibrate medication class) and gamma agonists (the thiazolidinedione class of medications) are indicated for lowering lipids and insulin sensitization, respectively. The other subtypes remain areas of research, as PPAR delta (in combination with alpha) increases beta-oxidation of fat via changes in mitochondrial profile/density and uncouples oxidative phosphorylation [90]. Researchers are designing new single-/multi-subtype agonists to treat metabolic syndrome (especially MAFLD) and neurodegenerative diseases [91]. These pathways are activated endogenously through exercise and fasting, and given their broad metabolic benefits, PPAR alpha/delta agonists are sometimes regarded as "exercise mimetics."

PPAR family enzymes are integral in downstream mitochondrial biogenesis and differentiation [123], which is how they exert influence in promoting an oxidative phenotype at the mitochondrial level. Tissues express higher proportions of different PPAR isotypes—for example, PPAR alpha in the liver, PPAR gamma in adipocytes, and PPAR delta in muscle fibers [124]. At the whole-person level, activation of PPAR delta may substantially increase tolerance to endurance exercise within weeks [125]. Early PPAR delta–selective agents, however, stimulated tumorigenesis in rodents, and therefore, researchers have yet to identify a safe, selective ligand to unlock the potential benefit. Of note, the angiotensin-receptor-blocker telmisartan also activates PPAR gamma and PPAR delta [126], which likely mediate the known anti-obesity and metabolic benefits of the medication [[127]. This effect is unique to telmisartan relative to other ARBs and may belie its unique protective effects relative to other drugs in the same class [128] and other antihypertensive classes [129].

Selective Androgen Receptor Modulators (SARMs)

Compounds in this class stimulate the androgen receptor with a particular affinity for muscle/bone tissue while avoiding prostatic tissue [130]. This makes the medications anabolic to muscle and catabolic to adipose tissue [131]. Given their androgenic activity, many studies include primarily/exclusively male participants, as the risk of masculinizing effects may preclude use in women. Further, given their androgenic activity, these drugs typically result in negative feedback in the hypothalamic–pituitary–gonadal access, causing suppression of LH/FSH release and subsequent decreases in gonadal testosterone production, which can affect male fertility. These agents may have the greatest utility in males with frailty and negligible or manageable metabolic disease who are not planning on further family planning. In these patients, the benefits for bone density and skeletal muscle mass may outweigh the side effects, but further studies need to demonstrate this risk/benefit profile. Ideally, future drug development would focus on greatly anabolic SARMs with negligible androgenic activity for broader utility and less impact on the HPG axis [132].

Tesofensine

Tesofensine is a medication originally developed for neurodegenerative disorders such as Alzheimer's and Parkinson's diseases. It functions directly as a triple monoamine reuptake inhibitor (dopamine, norepinephrine, and serotonin) while also increasing levels of brain-derived neurotrophic factor (BDNF), a protein that stimulates synaptogenesis and neuronal survival. While it failed to meet endpoints in the initial studies for neurocognitive benefits, one frequently reported side effect in subjects was weight loss. Subsequent research demonstrated an estimated total body weight loss of ~10% [133]. Researchers are currently studying tesofensine in populations with hyperphagia secondary to Prader–Willi syndrome and hypothalamic obesity. With further research, tesofensine could be shown to be an effective adjunct for weight loss, mood, and potential other CNS-mediated pathology such as neuropathic pain, given the efficacy of other monoamine reuptake inhibitors for these conditions.

6 "Do No Harm"

In some situations, the impact a practitioner makes can be greater by the medications avoided than the ones he or she actually prescribes. Specifically, in cases of individuals with obesity who are attempting to better control weight and metabolic disease, common medications to treat psychiatric illness, manage epilepsy, prevent pregnancy, treat cancer and autoimmune disorders, and ironically even mitigate the effects of metabolic disease itself may promote progression of disease.

Antipsychotics

Mechanistically, the same receptors targeted by antipsychotics also mediate their effect on body weight and insulin resistance. Due to the imprecise nature of antipsychotics as antagonists/partial agonists across multiple isoforms of dopamine, 5HT, adrenergic, and muscarinic acetylcholine receptors, the exact mechanism by which they affect metabolic parameters remains unclear [134]. Phenotypically, however, individuals who suffer these negative side effects often report significantly increased appetite and lower energy levels, which contribute to the phenomenon. Transitioning from some of the older atypical agents like olanzapine, clozapine, risperidone, and quetiapine, which more notoriously promote metabolic dysfunction to newer agents such as aripiprazole, paliperidone, lurasidone, cariprazine, and related compounds that have lower rates of these effects [135]. Unfortunately, in many moderate-severe cases of psychiatric disorders, the patient has already trialed these medications and discontinued them due to side effects or inadequate efficacy.

Antidepressants

Some antidepressants may contribute to weight gain, either directly due to appetite-stimulating properties or indirectly from the resolution of previously diminished appetite secondary to the mood disorder. Typically, this effect is less pronounced than from most antipsychotics/mood-stabilizing medications; however, individual cases may vary. Tricyclic antidepressants, atypical antidepressants like mirtazapine, the SSRI paroxetine, the SNRI venlafaxine, some MAOIs, and brexpiprazole are associated with weight gain more than other agents.

Antihyperglycemic Medications

As introduced previously, most new medications developed for type 2 diabetes mellitus (T2DM) are either considered neutral weight (with metabolic benefits beyond glucose control) or support weight loss. For severe or persistent type 2 DM, these measures may be inadequate for glucose control, and the patient requires more aggressive measures such as insulin secretagogues like sulfonylureas and meglitinides or exogenous insulin. While these measures may achieve tighter glycemic control, they also may promote weight gain and, without other interventions, facilitate escalating subsequent insulin requirements.

Corticosteroids, Contraceptive Medications, and Antiestrogen Therapies

Medications like glucocorticoids, medroxyprogesterone acetate (as Depo-Provera), and some oral contraceptive pills are analogous to endogenous hormones such as cortisol, progesterone, and estrogen and have varying impacts on weight and metabolic health. Systemic glucocorticoids may quickly induce an iatrogenic Cushing's syndrome and contraceptives have a risk of weight gain for some. These may negatively impact lipid profiles; though, in a prehabilitation context, this impact is unlikely to have direct acute impacts on procedural outcomes. Similarly, medications used for hormone-responsive cancers like tamoxifen [136] and aromatase inhibitors [137] affect estrogen receptors or the conversion of sex hormones in the body and may be associated with negative metabolic effects and weight gain.

Antihypertensives

As some medications like phentermine, bupropion, and mirabegron promote weight loss and/or improved insulin sensitivity through sympathetic pathway activation, nonselective beta-adrenergic antagonists such as propranolol [138] may directly worsen metabolic health and contribute indirectly by impairing exercise tolerance. Peripheral calcium channel blockers such as amlodipine are not associated with the same degree of weight gain but may cause edema in the extremities that increases body weight.

Antiepileptic Drugs and Mood Stabilizers (AEDs)

Some AEDs/mood-stabilizing medications for bipolar disorder are associated with increased appetite and weight gain. Most notably, valproic acid and divalproex have the greatest weight-promoting effects, followed by gabapentinoids and, questionably carbamazepine as well [139]. Like valproic acid and related medications and carbamazepine, which are prescribed off-label as adjunctive treatments in bipolar disorder, lithium [140] and antipsychotic medications (as described previously) are also associated with weight gain. For some, the use of these medications is unavoidable, but for others, transitioning to medications like zonisamide and topiramate may promote weight loss. Alternatively, lamotrigine, levetiracetam, and phenytoin are neutral weight and may offer similar efficacy in treating neurologic disease as the weight-promoting medications.

References

1. Mavros Y, O'Neill E, Connerty M, Bean JF, Broe K, Kiel DP, et al. Oxandrolone augmentation of resistance training in older women: a randomized trial. Med Sci Sports Exerc. 2015;47(11):2257–67.
2. Orr R, Singh MF. The anabolic androgenic steroid oxandrolone in the treatment of wasting and catabolic disorders. Drugs. 2004;64(7):725–50.
3. Liao Z, Vosberg DE, Pausova Z, Paus T. A shifting relationship between sex hormone-binding globulin and total testosterone across puberty in boys. J Clin Endocrinol Metab. 2022;107(10):e4187–e96.
4. Anawalt BD. Diagnosis and management of anabolic androgenic steroid use. J Clin Endocrinol Metab. 2019;104(7):2490–500.
5. Rossouw JE, Anderson GL, Prentice RL, LaCroix AZ, Kooperberg C, Stefanick ML, et al. Risks and benefits of estrogen plus progestin in healthy postmenopausal women: principal results from the Women's Health Initiative randomized controlled trial. JAMA. 2002;288(3):321–33.
6. Cagnacci A, Venier M. The controversial history of hormone replacement therapy. Medicina (Kaunas). 2019;55(9):602.
7. Weiss NS, Ure CL, Ballard JH, Williams AR, Daling JR. Decreased risk of fractures of the hip and lower forearm with postmenopausal use of estrogen. N Engl J Med. 1980;303(21):1195–8.
8. Islam RM, Bell RJ, Green S, Page MJ, Davis SR. Safety and efficacy of testosterone for women: a systematic review and meta-analysis of randomised controlled trial data. Lancet Diabetes Endocrinol. 2019;7(10):754–66.
9. Smith GI, Yoshino J, Reeds DN, Bradley D, Burrows RE, Heisey HD, et al. Testosterone and progesterone, but not estradiol, stimulate muscle protein synthesis in postmenopausal women. J Clin Endocrinol Metab. 2014;99(1):256–65.
10. Davison SL, Bell RJ, Gavrilescu M, Searle K, Maruff P, Gogos A, et al. Testosterone improves verbal learning and memory in postmenopausal women: results from a pilot study. Maturitas. 2011;70(3):307–11.
11. Pellegrino A, Tiidus PM, Vandenboom R. Mechanisms of estrogen influence on skeletal muscle: mass, regeneration, and mitochondrial function. Sports Med. 2022;52(12):2853–69.
12. Corona G, Rastrelli G, Di Pasquale G, Sforza A, Mannucci E, Maggi M. Testosterone and cardiovascular risk: meta-analysis of interventional studies. J Sex Med. 2018;15(6):820–38.
13. Lunenfeld B, Mskhalaya G, Zitzmann M, Arver S, Kalinchenko S, Tishova Y, et al. Recommendations on the diagnosis, treatment and monitoring of hypogonadism in men. Aging Male. 2015;18(1):5–15.
14. Vilsbøll T, Christensen M, Junker AE, Knop FK, Gluud LL. Effects of glucagon-like peptide-1 receptor agonists on weight loss: systematic review and meta-analyses of randomised controlled trials. BMJ. 2012;344
15. Rubino D, Abrahamsson N, Davies M, Hesse D, Greenway FL, Jensen C, et al. Effect of continued weekly subcutaneous semaglutide vs placebo on weight loss maintenance in adults with overweight or obesity: the STEP 4 randomized clinical trial. JAMA. 2021;325(14):1414–25.
16. Tuchscherer RM, Thompson AM, Trujillo JM. Semaglutide: the newest once-weekly GLP-1 RA for type 2 diabetes. Ann Pharmacother. 2018;52(12):1224–32.

17. Tall Bull S, Nuffer W, Trujillo JM. Tirzepatide: a novel, first-in-class, dual GIP/GLP-1 receptor agonist. J Diabetes Complications. 2022;36(12):108332.
18. Sheahan KH, Wahlberg EA, Gilbert MP. An overview of GLP-1 agonists and recent cardiovascular outcomes trials. Postgrad Med J. 2020;96(1133):156–61.
19. Kristensen SL, Rørth R, Jhund PS, Docherty KF, Sattar N, Preiss D, et al. Cardiovascular, mortality, and kidney outcomes with GLP-1 receptor agonists in patients with type 2 diabetes: a systematic review and meta-analysis of cardiovascular outcome trials. Lancet Diab Endocrinol. 2019;7(10):776–85.
20. Ornellas T, Chavez B. Naltrexone SR/Bupropion SR (Contrave): a new approach to weight loss in obese adults. Pharmacy Therapeut. 2011;36(5):255.
21. Lei X-G, Ruan J-Q, Lai C, Sun Z, Yang X. Efficacy and safety of phentermine/topiramate in adults with overweight or obesity: a systematic review and meta-analysis. Obesity. 2021;29(6):985–94.
22. Acosta A, Camilleri M, Abu Dayyeh B, Calderon G, Gonzalez D, McRae A, et al. Selection of antiobesity medications based on phenotypes enhances weight loss: a pragmatic trial in an obesity clinic. Obesity. 2021;29(4):662–71.
23. Magill RA, Waters WF, Bray GA, Volaufova J, Smith SR, Lieberman HR, et al. Effects of tyrosine, phentermine, caffeine D-amphetamine, and placebo on cognitive and motor performance deficits during sleep deprivation. Nutr Neurosci. 2003;6(4):237–46.
24. Hendricks E, Srisurapanont M, Schmidt S, Haggard M, Souter S, Mitchell C, et al. Addiction potential of phentermine prescribed during long-term treatment of obesity. Int J Obes (Lond). 2014;38(2):292–8.
25. Sahebkar A, Simental-Mendía LE, Reiner Ž, Kovanen PT, Simental-Mendía M, Bianconi V, et al. Effect of orlistat on plasma lipids and body weight: a systematic review and meta-analysis of 33 randomized controlled trials. Pharmacol Res. 2017;122:53–65.
26. Pinto LC, Rados DV, Remonti LR, Kramer CK, Leitao CB, Gross JL. Efficacy of SGLT2 inhibitors in glycemic control, weight loss and blood pressure reduction: a systematic review and meta-analysis. Diabetol Metab Syndr. 2015;7(1):1–2.
27. Briand F, Mayoux E, Brousseau E, Burr N, Urbain I, Costard C, et al. Empagliflozin, via switching metabolism toward lipid utilization, moderately increases LDL cholesterol levels through reduced LDL catabolism. Diabetes. 2016;65(7):2032–8.
28. Blüher M. GLP1 receptor agonist overcomes SGLT2 inhibitor-related overeating. Nat Rev Endocrinol. 2022;18(9):523–4.
29. O'Mara AE, Johnson JW, Linderman JD, Brychta RJ, McGehee S, Fletcher LA, et al. Chronic mirabegron treatment increases human brown fat, HDL cholesterol, and insulin sensitivity. J Clin Invest. 2020;130(5):2209–19.
30. Loh RK, Formosa MF, La Gerche A, Reutens AT, Kingwell BA, Carey AL. Acute metabolic and cardiovascular effects of mirabegron in healthy individuals. Diabetes Obes Metab. 2019;21(2):276–84.
31. Kulkarni AS, Gubbi S, Barzilai N. Benefits of metformin in attenuating the hallmarks of aging. Cell Metab. 2020;32(1):15–30.
32. Zhang J-H, Zhang X-Y, Sun Y-Q, Lv R-H, Chen M, Li M. Metformin use is associated with a reduced risk of cognitive impairment in adults with diabetes mellitus: a systematic review and meta-analysis. Front Neurosci. 2022;16:984559.
33. Koenig AM, Mechanic-Hamilton D, Xie SX, Combs MF, Cappola AR, Xie L, et al. Effects of the insulin sensitizer metformin in Alzheimer's disease: pilot data from a randomized placebo-controlled crossover study. Alzheimer Dis Assoc Disord. 2017;31(2):107.
34. Karise I, Bargut TC, del Sol M, Aguila MB, Mandarim-de-Lacerda CA. Metformin enhances mitochondrial biogenesis and thermogenesis in brown adipocytes of mice. Biomed Pharmacother. 2019;111:1156–65.
35. Konopka AR, Laurin JL, Schoenberg HM, Reid JJ, Castor WM, Wolff CA, et al. Metformin inhibits mitochondrial adaptations to aerobic exercise training in older adults. Aging Cell. 2019;18(1):e12880.

36. Chang R, Tu T-Y, Hung Y-M, Huang J-Y, Chou M-C, Wei JC-C. Metformin use is associated with a lower risk of rotator cuff disease in patients with Type 2 diabetes mellitus. Diabetes Metab. 2022;48(5):101368.
37. Kurtz JA, VanDusseldorp TA, Doyle JA, Otis JS. Taurine in sports and exercise. J Int Soc Sports Nutr. 2021;18(1):39.
38. Waldron M, Patterson SD, Tallent J, Jeffries O. The effects of an oral taurine dose and supplementation period on endurance exercise performance in humans: a meta-analysis. Sports Med. 2018;48(5):1247–53.
39. Kumari N, Prentice H, Wu J-Y. Taurine and its neuroprotective role. Taurine 8: Volume 1: The nervous system, immune system, diabetes and the cardiovascular system; 2013, pp. 19–27.
40. Silva SP, Zago AM, Carvalho FB, Germann L, Colombo GM, Rahmeier FL, et al. Neuroprotective effect of taurine against cell death, glial changes, and neuronal loss in the cerebellum of rats exposed to chronic-recurrent neuroinflammation induced by LPS. J Immunol Res. 2021;2021:7497185.
41. Kim S-J, Gupta RC, Lee HW. Taurine-diabetes interaction: from involvement to protection. Curr Diabetes Rev. 2007;3(3):165–75.
42. Guan L, Miao P. The effects of taurine supplementation on obesity, blood pressure and lipid profile: a meta-analysis of randomized controlled trials. Eur J Pharmacol. 2020;885:173533.
43. Faghfouri AH, Seyyed Shoura SM, Fathollahi P, Shadbad MA, Papi S, Ostadrahimi A, et al. Profiling inflammatory and oxidative stress biomarkers following taurine supplementation: a systematic review and dose-response meta-analysis of controlled trials. Eur J Clin Nutr. 2022;76(5):647–58.
44. de Mendonça FM, de Mendonça GP, Souza LC, Galvao LP, Paiva HS, de Azevedo Marques Périco C, Torales J, Ventriglio A, Maurício Castaldelli-Maia J, Sousa Martins Silva A. Benzodiazepines and sleep architecture: a systematic review. CNS Neurol Disord Drug Targets. 2023;22(2):172–9.
45. Curado DF, et al. Dependence on hypnotics: a comparative study betweenchronic users of benzodiazepines and Z-drugs. Braz J Psychiatry. 2021;44(3):248–56.
46. Geller AS. Benzodiazepine oncogenesis as mediated via diminished restorative sleep effect-edsympathoadrenal activation. Mayo Clin Proc. 2012;87(10):1034–5. Elsevier
47. Zheng Y, Lv T, Wu J, Lyu Y. Trazodone changed the polysomnographic sleep architecture in insomnia disorder: a systematic review and meta-analysis. Sci Rep. 2022;12(1):14453.
48. Wiegand MH. Antidepressants for the treatment of insomnia: a suitable approach? Drugs. 2008;68:2411–7.
49. Sharp T, Collins H. Mechanisms of SSRI therapy and discontinuation. In: Emerging neurobiology of antidepressant treatments; 2023. p. 21–47.
50. Fornasari D. Pharmacotherapy for neuropathic pain: a review. Pain Ther. 2017;6(1):25–33.
51. Wong MC, Chung JW, Wong TK. Effects of treatments for symptoms of painful diabetic neuropathy: systematic review. BMJ (Clin Res Ed). 2007;335(7610):87.
52. Obata H. Analgesicmechanisms of antidepressants for neuropathic pain. Int J Mol Sci. 2017;18(11):2483.
53. Stepanenko YD, Sibarov DA, Shestakova NN, Antonov SM. Tricyclic antidepressant structure-related alterations in calcium-dependent inhibition and open-channel block of NMDA receptors. Front Pharmacol. 2022;14(12):815368.
54. Ulrich S, et al. Efficacy and adverse effects of tranylcypromine and tricyclic antidepressants in the treatment of depression: a systematic review and comprehensive meta-analysis. J Clin Psychopharmacol. 2020;40(1):63–74.
55. Anderson IM. Selective serotonin reuptake inhibitors versus tricyclic antidepressants: a meta-analysis of efficacy and tolerability. J Affect Disord. 2000;58(1):19–36.
56. Spence D. Bad medicine: gabapentin and pregabalin. Br Med J. 2013;347:f6747.
57. Holbech JV, Jung A, Jonsson T, Wanning M, Bredahl C, Bach FW. Combination treatment of neuropathic pain: Danish expert recommendations based on a Delphi process. J Pain Res. 2017;10:1467–75.

58. Moore RA, Wiffen PJ, Derry S, Rice ASC. Gabapentin for chronic neuropathic pain and fibromyalgia in adults. Cochrane Database Syst Rev. 2014;4
59. Moore RA, Straube S, Wiffen PJ, Derry S, McQuay HJ. Pregabalin for acute and chronic pain in adults. Cochrane Database Syst Rev. 2009;8(3):CD007076.
60. Hindmarch I, Dawson J, Stanley N. A double-blind study in healthy volunteers to assess the effects on sleep of pregabalin compared with Alprazolam and placebo. Sleep. 2005;28(2):187–94.
61. Yeh W-C, Lu S-R, Wu M-N, Lee K-W, Chien C-F, Fong Y-O, et al. The impact of antiseizure medications on polysomnographic parameters: a systematic review and meta-analysis. Sleep Med. 2021;81:319–26.
62. Derry S, Rice ASC, Cole P, Tan T, Moore RA. Topical capsaicin (high concentration) for chronic neuropathic pain in adults. Cochrane Database Syst Rev. 2017;1(1):CD007393.
63. Derry S, Moore RA. Topical capsaicin (low concentration) for chronic neuropathic pain in adults. Cochrane Database Syst Rev. 2012;2012(9):CD010111.
64. Wiffen PJ, Derry S, Moore RA, Kalso EA. Carbamazepine for chronic neuropathic pain and fibromyalgia in adults. Cochrane Database Syst Rev. 2014;2014(4):CD005451.
65. Zhou M, Chen N, He L, Yang M, Zhu C, Wu F. Oxcarbazepine for neuropathic pain. Cochrane Database Syst Rev. 2017;12(12):CD007963.
66. Magenta P, Arghetti S, Di Palma F, Jann S, Sterlicchio M, Bianconi C, et al. Oxcarbazepine is effective and safe in the treatment of neuropathic pain: pooled analysis of seven clinical studies. Neurol Sci. 2005;26:218–26.
67. Eskin B, Shih RD, Fiesseler FW, Walsh BW, Allegra JR, Silverman ME, et al. Prednisone for emergency department low back pain: a randomized controlled trial. J Emerg Med. 2014;47(1):65–70.
68. Oliveira CB, Maher CG, Ferreira ML, Hancock MJ, Oliveira VC, McLachlan AJ, et al. Epidural corticosteroid injections for sciatica: an abridged cochrane systematic review and meta-analysis. Spine. 2020;45(21):E1405–E15.
69. Chou R, Hashimoto R, Friedly J, Fu R, Bougatsos C, Dana T, et al. Epidural corticosteroid injections for radiculopathy and spinal stenosis: a systematic review and meta-analysis. Ann Intern Med. 2015;163(5):373–81.
70. Carassiti M, Pascarella G, Strumia A, Russo F, Papalia GF, Cataldo R, et al. Epidural steroid injections for low back pain: a narrative review. Int J Environ Res Public Health. 2022;19(1):231.
71. Lin CK, Borresen A, Kroll M, Annaswamy TM. Predicting response to epidural steroid injections for lumbar spinal stenosis with biomarkers and electromyography. PM&R. 2020;12(7):663–70.
72. Tagowski M, Lewandowski Z, Hodler J, Spiegel T, Goerres GW. Pain reduction after lumbar epidural injections using particulate versus non-particulate steroids: intensity of the baseline pain matters. Eur Radiol. 2019;29(7):3379–89.
73. Raynauld J-P, Buckland-Wright C, Ward R, Choquette D, Haraoui B, Martel-Pelletier J, et al. Safety and efficacy of long-term intraarticular steroid injections in osteoarthritis of the knee: A randomized, double-blind, placebo-controlled trial. Arthritis Rheum. 2003;48(2):370–7.
74. Wernecke C, Braun HJ, Dragoo JL. The effect of intra-articular corticosteroids on articular cartilage: a systematic review. Orthop J Sports Med. 2015;3(5):2325967115581163.
75. Nichols AW. Complications associated with the use of corticosteroids in the treatment of athletic injuries. Clin J Sport Med. 2005;15(5):E370.
76. Wang T, He C. Pro-inflammatory cytokines: the link between obesity and osteoarthritis. Cytokine Growth Factor Rev. 2018;44:38–50.
77. Tabrizi A, Dindarian S, Mohammadi S. The effect of corticosteroid local injection versus platelet-rich plasma for the treatment of plantar fasciitis in obese patients: a single-blind, randomized clinical trial. J Foot Ankle Surg. 2020;59(1):64–8.
78. Blankstein M, Lentine B, Nelms NJ. Common practices in intra-articular corticosteroid injection for the treatment of knee osteoarthritis: a survey of the American association of hip and knee surgeons membership. J Arthroplasty. 2021;36(3):845–50.

79. Phillips M, Bhandari M, Grant J, Bedi A, Trojian T, Johnson A, Schemitsch E. A systematic review of current clinical practice guidelines on intra-articular hyaluronic acid, corticosteroid, and platelet-rich plasma injection for knee osteoarthritis: an international perspective. Orthop J Sports Med. 2021;9(8):23259671211030272.
80. Bannuru RR, Natov NS, Dasi UR, Schmid CH, McAlindon TE. Therapeutic trajectory following intra-articular hyaluronic acid injection in knee osteoarthritis–meta-analysis. Osteoarthritis Cartilage. 2011;19(6):611–9.
81. Luo P, Xiong Z, Sun W, Shi L, Gao F, Li Z. How to choose platelet-rich plasma or hyaluronic acid for the treatment of knee osteoarthritis in overweight or obese patients: a meta-analysis. Pain Res Manag. 2020;2020(1):7587936.
82. Tiao J, Wang K, Herrera M, Ren R, Rosenberg AM, Cassie R, Poeran J. There is wide variation in platelet-rich plasma injection pricing: a United States nationwide study of top orthopaedic hospitals. Clin Orthop Relat Res. 2024;482(4):675–84.
83. Risser A, Donovan D, Heintzman J, Page T. NSAID prescribing precautions. Am Fam Physician. 2009;80(12):1371–8.
84. Mosler C. Cardiovascular risk associated with NSAIDs and COX-2 inhibitors. US Pharm. 2014;39(3):35–8.
85. Wheatley BM, Nappo KE, Christensen DL, Holman AM, Brooks DI, Potter BK. Effect of NSAIDs on bone healing rates: a meta-analysis. J Am Acad Orthop Surg. 2019;27(7):e330–6.
86. Borgeat A, Ofner C, Saporito A, Farshad M, Aguirre J. The effect of nonsteroidal anti-inflammatory drugs on bone healing in humans: a qualitative, systematic review. J Clin Anesth. 2018;1(49):92–100.
87. Roberto A, Greco MT, Uggeri S, Cavuto S, Deandrea S, Corli O, et al. Living systematic review to assess the analgesic undertreatment in cancer patients. Pain Pract. 2022;22(4):487–96.
88. Dowell D,.Haegerich TM, Chou R. CDC guideline for prescribing opioids for chronic pain—United States, 2016. JAMA. 2016;315(15):1624–45.
89. Toljan K, Vrooman B. Low-dose naltrexone (LDN)—review of therapeutic utilization. Med Sci. 2018;6(4):82.
90. Kim PS, Fishman MA. Low-dose naltrexone for chronic pain: update and systemic review. Curr Pain Headache Rep. 2020;24(10):64.
91. Gironi M, Martinelli-Boneschi F, Sacerdote P, Solaro C, Zaffaroni M, Cavarretta R, Moiola L, Bucello S, Radaelli M, Pilato V, Rodegher ME. A pilot trial of low-dose naltrexone in primary progressive multiple sclerosis. Mul Scler. 2008;14(8):1076–83.
92. Soin A, Soin Y, Dann T, Buenaventura R, Ferguson K, Atluri S, et al. Low-dose naltrexone use for patients with chronic regional pain syndrome: a systematic literature review. Pain Physician. 2021;24(4):E393.
93. Parker CE, Nguyen TM, Segal D, MacDonald JK, Chande N. Low dose naltrexone for induction of remission in Crohn's disease. Cochrane Database Syst Rev. 2018;4(4):CD010410.
94. Parkitny L, Younger J. Reduced pro-inflammatory cytokines after eight weeks of low-dose naltrexone for fibromyalgia. Biomedicine. 2017;5(2):16.
95. Colomer-Carbonell A, Sanabria-Mazo JP, Hernández-Negrín H, Borràs X, Suso-Ribera C, García-Palacios A, et al. Study protocol for a randomised, double-blinded, placebo-controlled phase III trial examining the add-on efficacy, cost–utility and neurobiological effects of low-dose naltrexone (LDN) in patients with fibromyalgia (INNOVA study). BMJ Open. 2022;12(1):e055351.
96. Wang L, Hong PJ, May C, Rehman Y, Oparin Y, Hong CJ, et al. Medical cannabis or cannabinoids for chronic non-cancer and cancer related pain: a systematic review and meta-analysis of randomised clinical trials. BMJ (Clin Res Ed). 2021;374:n1034.
97. Maayah ZH, Takahara S, Ferdaoussi M, Dyck JR. The molecular mechanisms that underpin the biological benefits of full-spectrum cannabis extract in the treatment of neuropathic pain and inflammation. Biochim Biophys Acta Mol Basis Dis. 2020;1866(7):165771.
98. Beaulieu P. Cannabinoids and acute/postoperative pain management. Pain. 2021;162(8):2309.

99. Maayah ZH, Takahara S, Ferdaoussi M, Dyck JRB. The molecular mechanisms that underpin the biological benefits of full-spectrum cannabis extract in the treatment of neuropathic pain and inflammation. Biochim Biophys Acta (BBA) Mol Basis Dis. 2020;1866(7):165771.
100. Maayah ZH, Takahara S, Ferdaoussi M, Dyck JRB. The anti-inflammatory and analgesic effects of formulated full-spectrum cannabis extract in the treatment of neuropathic pain associated with multiple sclerosis. Inflamm Res. 2020;69(6):549–58.
101. Anand U, Pacchetti B, Anand P, Sodergren MH. Cannabis-based medicines and pain: a review of potential synergistic and entourage effects. Pain Manage. 2021;11(4):395–403.
102. Babson KA, Sottile J, Morabito D. Cannabis, cannabinoids, and sleep: a review of the literature. Curr Psychiatry Rep. 2017;19(4):23.
103. Kisiolek JN, Flores VA, Ramani A, Butler B, Haughian JM, Stewart LK. Eight weeks of daily cannabidiol supplementation improves sleep quality and immune cell cytotoxicity. Nutrients. 2023;15(19):4173.
104. Alshaarawy O, Anthony JC. Are cannabis users less likely to gain weight? Results from a national 3-year prospective study. Int J Epidemiol. 2019;48(5):1695–700.
105. Wong CK, Marshall NS, Grunstein RR, Ho SS, Fois RA, Hibbs DE, Hanrahan JR, Saini B. Spontaneous adverse event reports associated with zolpidem in the United States 2003–2012. J Clin Sleep Med. 2017;13(2):223–34.
106. Jung F, Lee Y, Manzoor S, Hong D, Doumouras AG. Effects of perioperative cannabis use on bariatric surgical outcomes: a systematic review. Obes Surg. 2021;31:299–306.
107. Hawn MT, Houston TK, Campagna EJ, Graham LA, Singh J, Bishop M, Henderson WG. The attributable risk of smoking on surgical complications. Ann Surg. 2011;254(6):914–20.
108. Echeverria-Villalobos M, Todeschini AB, Stoicea N, Fiorda-Diaz J, Weaver T, Bergese SD. Perioperative care of cannabis users: a comprehensive review of pharmacological and anesthetic considerations. J Clin Anesth. 2019;57:41–9.
109. Maher DP, Chen L, Mao J. Intravenous ketamine infusions for neuropathic pain management: a promising therapy in need of optimization. Anesth Analg. 2017;124(2):661–74.
110. Orhurhu V, Orhurhu MS, Bhatia A, Cohen SP. Ketamine infusions for chronic pain: a systematic review and meta-analysis of randomized controlled trials. Anesth Analg. 2019;129(1):241–54.
111. Goldberg SB, Pace BT, Nicholas CR, Raison CL, Hutson PR. The experimental effects of psilocybin on symptoms of anxiety and depression: a meta-analysis. Psychiatry Res. 2020;284:112749.
112. Goodwin GM, Aaronson ST, Alvarez O, Arden PC, Baker A, Bennett JC, Bird C, Blom RE, Brennan C, Brusch D, Burke L. Single-dose psilocybin for a treatment-resistant episode of major depression. N Engl J Med. 2022;387(18):1637–48.
113. Freitas AE, Neis VB, Rodrigues ALS. Agmatine, a potential novel therapeutic strategy for depression. Eur Neuropsychopharmacol. 2016;26(12):1885–99.
114. Keynan O, Mirovsky Y, Dekel S, Gilad VH, Gilad GM. Safety and efficacy of dietary agmatine sulfate in lumbar disc-associated radiculopathy. an open-label, dose-escalating study followed by a randomized, double-blind, placebo-controlled trial. Pain Med. 2010;11(3):356–68.
115. Piletz JE, Aricioglu F, Cheng JT, Fairbanks CA, Gilad VH, Haenisch B, Halaris A, Hong S, Lee JE, Li J, Liu P. Agmatine: clinical applications after 100 years in translation. Drug Discov Today. 2013;18(17-18):880–93.
116. Peterson CD, Kitto KF, Verma H, Pflepsen K, Delpire E, Wilcox GL, Fairbanks CA. Agmatine requires GluN2B-containing NMDA receptors to inhibit the development of neuropathic pain. Mol Pain. 2021;17:17448069211029171.
117. Halaris A, Plietz J. Agmatine: metabolic pathway and spectrum of activity in brain. CNS Drugs. 2007;21:885–900.
118. Lee S-J. Targeting the myostatin signaling pathway to treat muscle loss and metabolic dysfunction. J Clin Investig. 2021;131(9)
119. Consitt LA, Clark B. The vicious cycle of myostatin signaling in sarcopenic obesity: myostatin role in skeletal muscle growth, insulin signaling and implications for clinical trials. J Frailty Aging. 2018;7(1):21–7.

120. Heymsfield SB, Coleman LA, Miller R, Rooks DS, Laurent D, Petricoul O, et al. Effect of bimagrumab vs placebo on body fat mass among adults with type 2 diabetes and obesity: a phase 2 randomized clinical trial. JAMA Netw Open. 2021;4(1):e2033457.
121. Lee CH, Olson P, Hevener A, Mehl I, Chong LW, Olefsky JM, et al. PPARdelta regulates glucose metabolism and insulin sensitivity. Proc Natl Acad Sci U S A. 2006;103(9):3444–9.
122. Tailleux A, Wouters K, Staels B. Roles of PPARs in NAFLD: potential therapeutic targets. Biochim Biophys Acta (BBA) Mol Cell Biol Lipids. 2012;1821(5):809–18.
123. Remels AHV, Langen RCJ, Schrauwen P, Schaart G, Schols AMWJ, Gosker HR. Regulation of mitochondrial biogenesis during myogenesis. Mol Cell Endocrinol. 2010;315(1):113–20.
124. Barish GD, Narkar VA, Evans RM. PPARδ: a dagger in the heart of the metabolic syndrome. J Clin Invest. 2006;116(3):590–7.
125. Narkar VA, Downes M, Ruth TY, Embler E, Wang Y-X, Banayo E, et al. AMPK and PPARδ agonists are exercise mimetics. Cell. 2008;134(3):405–15.
126. Rawish E, Nickel L, Schuster F, Stölting I, Frydrychowicz A, Saar K, et al. Telmisartan prevents development of obesity and normalizes hypothalamic lipid droplets. J Endocrinol. 2020;244(1):95–110.
127. Takagi H, Niwa M, Mizuno Y, Goto S-N, Umemoto T, Group A. Telmisartan as a metabolic sartan: the first meta-analysis of randomized controlled trials in metabolic syndrome. J Am Soc Hypertens. 2013;7(3):229–35.
128. Liu C-H, Sung P-S, Li Y-R, Huang W-K, Lee T-W, Huang C-C, et al. Telmisartan use and risk of dementia in type 2 diabetes patients with hypertension: a population-based cohort study. PLoS Med. 2021;18(7):e1003707.
129. Lee CJ, Sung J-H, Kang T-S, Park S, Lee S-H, Kim J-Y, et al. Effects of high-intensity statin combined with telmisartan versus amlodipine on glucose metabolism in hypertensive atherosclerotic cardiovascular disease patients with impaired fasting glucose: a randomized multicenter trial. Medicine. 2022;101(36):e30496.
130. Venkatesh VS, Grossmann M, Zajac JD, Davey RA. The role of the androgen receptor in the pathogenesis of obesity and its utility as a target for obesity treatments. Obes Rev. 2022:e13429.
131. Navarro G, Allard C, Xu W, Mauvais-Jarvis F. The role of androgens in metabolism, obesity, and diabetes in males and females. Obesity. 2015;23(4):713–9.
132. Solomon ZJ, Mirabal JR, Mazur DJ, Kohn TP, Lipshultz LI, Pastuszak AW. Selective androgen receptor modulators: current knowledge and clinical applications. Sex Med Rev. 2019;7(1):84–94.
133. Axel AMD, Mikkelsen JD, Hansen HH. Tesofensine, a novel triple monoamine reuptake inhibitor, induces appetite suppression by indirect stimulation of α1 adrenoceptor and dopamine D1 receptor pathways in the diet-induced obese rat. Neuropsychopharmacology. 2010;35(7):1464–76.
134. Carli M, Kolachalam S, Longoni B, Pintaudi A, Baldini M, Aringhieri S, Fasciani I, Annibale P, Maggio R, Scarselli M. Atypical antipsychotics and metabolic syndrome: from molecular mechanisms to clinical differences. Pharmaceuticals. 2021;14(3):238.
135. Akinola PS, Tardif I, Leclerc J. Antipsychotic-induced metabolic syndrome: a review. Metab Syndr Relat Disord. 2023;21(6):294–305.
136. Pemmaraju N, Munsell M, Hortobagyi G, Giordano S. Retrospective review of male breast cancer patients: analysis of tamoxifen-related side-effects. Ann Oncol. 2012;23(6):1471–4.
137. Buch K, Gunmalm V, Andersson M, Schwarz P, Brøns C. Effect of chemotherapy and aromatase inhibitors in the adjuvant treatment of breast cancer on glucose and insulin metabolism—a systematic review. Cancer Med. 2019;8(1):238–45.
138. Pischon T, Sharma A. Use of beta-blockers in obesity hypertension: potential role of weight gain. Obes Rev. 2001;2(4):275–80.
139. Ben-Menachem E. Weight issues for people with epilepsy—a review. Epilepsia. 2007;48:42–5.
140. Baptista T, Teneud L, Contreras Q, Alastre T, Burguera J, De Burguera M, et al. Lithium and body weight gain. Pharmacopsychiatry. 1995;28(02):35–44.

Enhanced Recovery and Prehabilitation in the Perioperative Setting

Stephen A. Esper, Jennifer Holder-Murray,
and Aman Mahajan

1 Why Perioperative Care?

Remarkable innovations within surgery over the last two centuries have roots firmly planted in the specialty of anesthesiology. The journey began on October 16, 1846 when William T.G. Morton (1819–1868) conquered one of humankind's greatest fears—the pain of surgery—using inhaled ether gas as the first successful and safe anesthetic [1]. Anesthesiologists have made enormous advancements in reducing intraoperative risk over the years, and their continued engagement with patients and collaboration with various partners across the realm of surgical care will lead to long-term enhancements in healthcare. Thanks to the innovations in medications and safety and equipment protocols over the past 50 years, fatal events from the administration of anesthesia in American Society of Anesthesiology (ASA) Class 1 and 2 patients are as rare as 1 in 1,000,000, making anesthesiology as safe as commercial jet aviation and the nuclear industry, and far safer than traveling in a road vehicle [2].

Simultaneously, there are other unmet needs in perioperative care. For instance, cardiac surgery in ASA Class III–V patients is only slightly safer than mountaineering in the Himalayas above 8000 m, but less safe than traveling by planes, trains, and cars, and over 1000 fold less safe than the nuclear industry [2]. Postoperative mortality is not a category in the Center for Disease Control and Prevention (CDC) mortality tables; in the United States (US), prior to COVID-19, 30-day postoperative mortality was approximated as the third leading contributor

S. A. Esper (✉) · A. Mahajan
Department of Anesthesiology and Perioperative Medicine, University of Pittsburgh School of Medicine, Pittsburgh, PA, USA
e-mail: espersa@upmc.edu; mahajana@upmc.edu

J. Holder-Murray
Department of Surgery, University of Pittsburgh School of Medicine, Pittsburgh, PA, USA
e-mail: holdermurrayjm@upmc.edu

A. Watson, K. Barr (eds.), *A Prehabilitation Guide for All Providers*,
https://doi.org/10.1007/978-3-031-72862-4_4

of all causes of death [3]. An estimated 48.4 million surgical procedures are performed annually in the US [4]. Thirty-day postoperative complications may develop in up to 15% of patients. These complications are estimated to cost hospitals more than $11,000 per case, totaling well over $31.35 billion nationally per year [5, 6]. How healthcare professionals administer treatments or employ less-invasive approaches to surgery is not necessarily the advent of new technologies. Perhaps it is a return to human health basics, the benefits of exercise and diet that best optimize patients to be as near as possible to their peak performance before any procedure. Mortality after peptic ulcer disease surgery in 1936 was 3.5% for well-nourished patients versus 33% for malnourished patients. Mortality in 2011 for the same procedure was 4% versus 23%, and this has not changed significantly in over 70 years. Looking at this from another angle, the two greatest advancements that increased life expectancy had nothing to do with surgical/anesthesia technology, pain relievers, or sedatives. It was simpler: the arrival of antibiotics/vaccines and clean water. Life expectancy increased from an average of 39 years across males and females to an average of 73 years from 1918 to 1980—a 34-year change in about 60 years [7]. The current life expectancy is 77 years (from 1981 until 2021), demonstrating marginal progress despite technological advances. Innovation should not be for every patient to undergo surgery using the latest equipment, but how to use the best approaches to ensure patients are in the best condition for surgery and how to get them in the best condition. To decrease surgical complications and increase good postoperative outcomes, providers' focus on preoperative and perioperative management has moved to care for patients with modifiable risk factors and higher risks for postoperative mortality and complications. Hence, there are critical opportunities to improve perioperative health, including (1) categorizing patients (complexity-based care delivery); (2) using digital technology and data to improve quality; (3) standardizing in-hospital perioperative care and value-based pathways; (4) modifying lifestyle before surgery; and (5) reaching full recovery post-surgery.

Among the ~100,000 surgical procedures performed in the US every day, approximately 20% involved patients with modifiable risk factors that heighten perioperative complications [8]. Presurgery risk predictors of postoperative adverse outcomes are categorized into three groups: healthcare characteristics, patient characteristics, and socioeconomic characteristics [9]. Healthcare characteristics encompass surgery type and intensity, anesthetic type, blood pressure, heart rate, goal-directed fluid therapy, and other factors. Socioeconomic characteristics include patient support systems like employment, education, family, income, and community. Patient characteristics are further divided into sub-categories of fixed and modifiable characteristics. Fixed characteristics are non-modifiable traits like genetics, chromosomal makeup, and age. Clinicians concentrate on acquired and modifiable risk factors like diabetes, anemia, chronic pain, nutritional status, chronic obstructive pulmonary disease, heart disease, obstructive sleep apnea, coagulation, nutrition, alcohol/tobacco/drug use, mental health, and physical activity [9].

2 Examples of Modifiable Risk Factors to Address in the Perioperative Period

Anemia

Nearly 40% of preoperative patients have anemia from chronic disease, nutrient deficiency, or inherent blood-borne disorders [10]. Patients with preoperative anemia have lower 5-year survival rates; one study showed that non-anemic patients had a 67% survival rate versus 48% for anemic patients ($p < 0.001$) [11]. Preoperative anemia is associated with a 2.29 odds ratio of 30-day postoperative mortality in patients undergoing noncardiac surgery [12]. Actually, according to research published in *JAMA*, for every hematocrit point under 39, 30-day postoperative mortality risk increases by 1.6% in patients undergoing noncardiac surgery [13]. Although anemia may be considered an objective sign of another illness, it is still an independent risk factor for mortality in patients who have it [14]. In the general surgical population, even receiving one to two units of packed red blood cells is associated with surgical site infections and higher 30-day mortality [15]. Programs for the management of preoperative anemia are shown to reduce the need for blood transfusion, total cost of care, length of intensive care unit (ICU) and hospital stay, 30-day readmission, and discharge disposition.

Nutrition

About 40% of the in-hospital patient population suffers from malnutrition; patient nutrition erodes further overtime during their hospital stay [16]. The NSQIP database shows that albumin lower than 3.5 is the fourth leading risk factor associated with 30-day postoperative mortality [17]. Furthermore, trauma, burns, and major illnesses in the setting of protein energy malnourishment have a significantly higher association with mortality from 30 days to at least 9 months after insult [18, 19]. In a 2015 study, athlete post-marathon glycogen scores were compared to post-surgery/critical illness scores; the authors found that, in many cases, critical illness/surgery depleted the same energy as that from an athlete running three consecutive marathons [20]. Numerous studies have shown that better nutrition is associated with fewer infections and complications and less sepsis, as well as shorter length of hospital stay [21, 22]. Certainly, in some settings, basal metabolic rate doubles and protein catabolism quadruples during critical illness and surgery as a muscular substrate is used to heal the surgical injury. Surgery involves tissue injury, essentially. Despite the positive benefits, surgery triggers an entire hormonal and neurotransmitter cascade. The hypothalamus releases adrenocorticotropic hormone (ACTH), which acts on the adrenals to release cortisol, epinephrine, and norepinephrine. The pancreas releases glucagon, and the innate and adaptive immune systems release tumor necrosis factor and interleukins. These secretions result in hypermetabolism, adipocyte lipolysis, skeletal muscle protein degradation, hepatic acute phase protein synthesis, hepatic gluconeogenesis, and pyrexia, as well as blood loss. These facts lend credence to the theory that, while many patients think of surgical anesthesia as a short nap to get some "good rest," the stress and hormonal release from these surgeries are actually equivalent to those from running a race.

Opioid Use

Pain is defined by the International Association for the Study of Pain (IASP) as "an unpleasant sensory and emotional experience associated with actual or potential tissue damage, or described in terms of such damage" [23]. This raises important implications: pain is completely subjective and pain is whatever the patient says it is. These implications affect how anesthesiologists treat sympathetic stimulation in the operating room (OR). In the past, anesthesiologists treated elevations in blood pressure and heart rate with opioids because these sympathetic markers had been considered signs of patients experiencing pain under general anesthesia. However, other approaches, such as beta-blockers and deepening anesthesia without administering opioids, while the patient is unable to experience pain, can be used to treat the sympathetic response to surgery. Consider how many of us are treated for hypertension with oxycodone rather than atenolol or hydrochlorothiazide for treatment.

In alleviating pain, the standard historical approach has relied nearly exclusively on opioids, especially with the use of patient-controlled analgesia devices (PCAs). However, limiting perioperative opioids confers a substantial benefit. While opioids immediately decrease pain after dosage, pain scores diminish after opioids wear off. Postoperative opioid requirements increase, and opioids subsequently escalate nausea and vomiting, reduce gastrointestinal motility, depress respiratory drive, induce endocrine dysfunction, worsen urinary retention, and suppress the immune system [24]. Several randomized controlled trials have shown a positive correlation between postoperative nausea and vomiting/pain scores and opioid administration [25–32]. Exposure to any opioid or fentanyl in the OR worsens postoperative pain scores. PCAs containing opioids have been the standard method used for opioid administration due to their efficacy and safety [33] in controlling opioid administration in patients. However, since PCAs offer only opioid medication, it is possible that the desired analgesic effect will be associated with the aforementioned opioid-related complications.

Decreasing opioids in the perioperative setting, using multimodal analgesia (see the following), and preoperative counseling to lessen catastrophizing are all very important not just for perioperative health, but also for general patient health.

Mood Disorders

In lung transplant patients, perioperative anxiety and depression are associated with 40% higher 1-year postoperative morbidity and mortality [34]. In cardiac surgery patients, depression occurs at a rate three times higher than that of the general population and is associated with a significantly higher risk of morbidity and mortality

[35]. In cancer patients, depression rates in cancer patients are, again, three times higher than those in the population at large, and mortality is 25% higher for those experiencing depressive symptoms and 39% higher in those with minor or major depression [36]. Perioperatively treating anxiety and depression is extremely critical to decrease postoperative morbidity and mortality.

Frailty

Frailty is the clinical syndrome of reduced physiological reserve, where small deficits accumulate in multiple adaptive systems, any one of which might be clinically insignificant alone, but when combined with other deficits, produce significant vulnerability to stress that can lead to catastrophic decompensation. The prevalence of reduced physiological reserve is 4–16% in community-dwelling women and men older than 65. When frailty was defined, the prevalence was 9.9%, but when including psychosocial aspects, the prevalence grew to 13.6%. Frailty and pre-frailty rates are 25–56% and 28–44%, respectively, in elderly surgical patients greater than 65 years of age [37–41]. Factors like lower educational level, being unmarried, use of postmenopausal hormone therapy, being a current smoker, depression, older age, intellectual disability, and race are all causes and contributors. In almost all cases, frailty is marked by decreased endurance, nutrition, strength, and cognitive capacity. This concept is more complex than a patient's age or sum of comorbidities [42, 43].

Over 60,000 elective surgeries were performed in 2015 at a single university-based tertiary referral hospital; 8000 (13%) were deemed high risk based on patients' coexisting medical conditions and underlying physical status. Despite the utmost efforts with current medical and surgical approaches, morbidity and mortality with the prevalence of low-value care are considerable. High-risk patients account for 90% of the care provided during hospitalization more than 30% of ICU admissions, and 70% of postoperative deaths. In value-based healthcare, identifying and mitigating morbid and mortal patient risks are critical for patients, families, providers, and healthcare systems. Further, data from the Veteran's Affairs Surgical Quality Initiative Program show that regardless of the magnitude of the surgery, frail patients are high risk and suffer mortality rates much higher than the 1% 30-day mortality that is typically deemed the threshold for high-risk surgery. Frail (RAI 30–39) and very frail (RAI ≥40) patients experience distressingly high rates of mortality, even for low and moderate-stress surgeries, as rated using the validated Operative Stress Score [44, 45].

This concept is reflected in the literature. Among patients who underwent breast surgeries such as lumpectomy (which the American Heart Association typically considers a low-risk procedure), patients with frailty/from skilled nursing facilities have a 30-day post-surgery mortality rate of 8.5% and a 1-year mortality rate of 31% [46], with a distinct functional decline in 58% of surviving patients. A study from 2016 describes a consistent positive correlation between mortality and measured frailty across all service lines [47].

Many frailty scales are used, including the Clinical Frailty Scale, the Fried Phenotype Scale, the Surgical Risk Analysis Index (RAI), and the Edmonton Frail Scale [48]. The University of Pittsburgh Medical Center (UPMC) uses the RAI, which has good accuracy and is based upon a survey of 14 factors including sex, age, loss of appetite, weight loss, heart failure, shortness of breath, malignancy, renal disease, ability to perform activities of daily living, and living arrangements [42]. A prospective study of more than 36,000 patients at UPMC showed that surgical RAI was significantly associated with higher mortality, 30- and 90-day readmission, and a more than 7-day length of hospital stay. In the most frail patients, an odds ratio of 5.12 was shown for mortality, as well as a 10.13 odds ratio for length of hospital stay greater than 7 days [49].

3 Prehabilitation in the Perioperative Period

Prehabilitation is defined as "the process of enhancing the functional capacity of the individual to enable him or her to withstand a stressful event" [50, 51]. Exercise and prehabilitation, which had historically focused on cardiopulmonary rehab before surgery, are both very important for outcomes. A *Canadian Journal of Anaesthesiology* article discussed perioperative cardiopulmonary exercise testing and prehabilitation related to perioperative programs globally [52]. In the discussion in the article, reduction of fitness before surgery is associated with higher postoperative morbidity and mortality. Patients who exercise even with documented hypertension, heart failure, coronary artery disease, chronic obstructive pulmonary disease, diabetes, dementia, cancer, stroke, and depression have better outcomes [53–66]. Moreover, other publications support the considerable benefits of exercise and cardiopulmonary exercise therapy before and after major surgery. These exercise therapies can decrease the length of hospital stay, hospital-associated complications, infections, and postoperative mortality [67].

A significant body of evidence indicates that exercise training is suitable and safe in patients with various severe pulmonary and cardiac diseases, many of whom need surgery to manage other diseases. A randomized controlled trial of 246 low-risk cardiac surgery patients showed a one-day reduction in ICU stay and a shorter length of hospital stay in the intervention group [68]. The authors found cardiopulmonary fitness to be a strong independent predictor of survival after lung surgery, especially for those with non-small cell lung cancer [69]. Non-randomized, preliminary data from elective rectal cancer surgery patients within enhanced recovery programs show the feasibility of delivering a structured, responsive cardiopulmonary exercise interval training program three times a week for 6 weeks in a hospital setting after neoadjuvant chemoradiotherapy and prior to surgery [70]. Most importantly, the time after neoadjuvant therapy allows patients to participate in an exercise program. Neoadjuvant therapy provides a unique window of time to enhance patients' nutrition and fitness; these patients are often some of the most debilitated. While some elective surgeries can be postponed to improve the patient's tolerance to preoperative exercise, many surgeries for oncologic or infectious diseases cannot be delayed. Adding physical activity and fitness to the preoperative course for elderly major abdominal surgery patients significantly improved the length of hospital stay, discharge destination (home versus inpatient rehabilitation versus skilled nursing facility), and mortality prediction [71]. While this study demonstrated that patients benefited from 60-min sessions 2–4 weeks before surgery, even shorter regimens ranging from 1 to 7 days before major abdominal surgery are associated with a significant drop in postoperative complications [72, 73].

Prehabilitation interventions have tiered approaches [74]. Considering only exercise and nutrition, the primary approach is universal interventions for everyone leading up to surgery. This approach includes balancing diet macronutrients, encouraging protein consumption to help support exercise and decrease muscular atrophy, and screening for malnutrition and physical inactivity with advice on how to increase activity with exercise at home and in therapy programs. The next level involves a targeted, specific approach to risk factors, where a dietitian must evaluate the patient for malnutrition when suspected/confirmed, with prescribed supplements and menus for macro/micronutrient deficiency. In addition, patients must undergo supervised exercise programs with some level of monitoring. Last, prescribed supplementation when an oral route is unavailable may be necessary for some specialized complex patients, as well as HIIT/monitored exercise in high-risk patients.

Medical experts have known about the relationship between optimal nutrition/exercise and good surgical outcomes for some time. However, what about other conditions that are more difficult to diagnose like frailty or delirium? Is prehabilitation possible for these patients? One study showed that 47% of frail cardiac patients developed delirium in comparison to 2.6% of robust patients, and the relative risk of delirium was 18 times higher for frail patients, suggesting frailty identifies patients at high risk for delirium [75]. Cognitive impairment also heightens the chances of postoperative delirium. The MiniCog screening test showed that cognitive impairment in surgical patients increases with age, from 5% prevalence in 70–79-year-olds to 33% in those aged above 85. In addition, 67% of patients with cognitive impairment are discharged to a facility, 21% experience postoperative delirium, and their length of hospital stay is 1.12 days longer [75–77]. Pathways to prevent delirium have been developed to treat these patients throughout the perioperative period. The ASA supports these guidelines and pathways through the perioperative brain health initiative [78, 79]. However, these time-intensive tests could be replaced by different technologically advanced programs that could more easily predict delirium, cognitive impairment, and postoperative cognitive dysfunction.

For example, BrainCheck® (Houston, Texas) developed a validated application that tests attention, memory, reaction times, executive functions, and motor functions. The BrainCheck® application has been demonstrated to detect forms of cognitive impairment in various populations like COVID-19 survivors and cancer and traumatic brain injury patients [80–83]. By focusing attention on this measurement of cognitive impairment, providers can perform cognitive prehabilitation to decrease delirium in these patients, as proposed in a 2021 article showing that patients who engaged in tablet-based preoperative cognitive exercises (games) targeting speed, memory, flexibility, attention, and problem-solving functions for 10 h before surgery were less likely to have delirium than those who did not participate in the cognitive exercises.

4 Institutional Approaches to Perioperative Care and Prehabilitation

Nevertheless, hospitals are complex adaptive systems, not factories. Standard system processes and risk stratification should be implemented to help address complications efficiently. For instance, anesthesiologists cannot agree on how much crystalloid solution to administer to patients intraoperatively. In a two-center, retrospective analysis of 6000 patients examining total crystalloid administration during abdominal surgery, crystalloid administration ranged anywhere from 2.3 to 14 cc/kg/h [84]. Another study showed significant interinstitutional differences in failure to rescue patients from complications after surgery. Amongst some US hospitals, types and rates of postsurgical complications were similar (24–26%), but mortality rates ranged from 12.5% to 21.4% [85]. How can healthcare providers improve this?

Segmenting patients based on complexity and risk is critical. While many routine patient care processes can be standardized or run on a focused factory model with established protocols, some patients and processes are significantly complex and require a complex adaptive system approach [86]. "Solution-shops" are defined as hospitals that are shops "structured to diagnose and recommend solutions to unstructured problems" [87]. When this term is applied to medicine, it usually means that decision-making relies on training, experience, and intuition to define the course of care [88]. One study showed two different hospital surgical populations with two distinct opportunities [86]. In the study, one population was lower-risk patients at institutions participating in high-volume surgeries with low variance; this population would achieve the best gains through efficient and standardized processes for consistency. The second population demonstrated the complex adaptive system, institutions with a relatively lower volume of surgeries with a high variance and a high incidence of postoperative complications, where best gains would be achieved through improving clinical outcomes through a network of experts and pathways created to address causes of complications.

Hospitals are organized generally as networks optimized for interaction between experts within multiple specialties/individuals/groups [86]. Programs should capitalize on teams of experts who develop protocols and decision logic, based upon current evidence, that can be executed on large groups of patients without intensive resource utilization, a prime example of which is the American College of Cardiology/American Heart Association approach to perioperative cardiac assessment for coronary artery disease [89]. Patient risk and required assessment are categorized by severity of illness and procedure. Linear processes can drive standardized care for non-complex patients. However, more complex patients need multiple nuanced interactions using a tailored approach as in an adaptive system [86]. The standard or factor approach involves surgeries that with low complexity and lower risk occur in higher volumes, and have lower variance in the procedure, where potential benefits are related to care coordination, high efficiency, and discharge planning. Higher complexity procedures are those in which the population may have a higher incidence and variance of postoperative complications and in which improved clinical outcomes are facilitated by a network of experts. For instance, orthopedic surgeries like total joint replacements occur in high volumes and are lower-risk procedures, even though many older elective orthopedic surgical patients most likely have some level of preoperative cognitive impairment. Such impairment is associated with the development of postoperative delirium, longer hospital stays, reduced likelihood of discharge to home [77], and a delayed return to cognitive health. This "at risk" patient subset needs a more adaptive approach. This approach can also be used to determine the best care location. These patients can be stratified preoperatively, but innovation in intraoperative care is extremely important for their postoperative recovery.

Three terrific examples have been reported. Mayo Clinic implemented a focused factory model for cardiac surgery with five stages: population identification and segmentation; clinical pathway and protocol creation for all areas of care; design, building, and adoption of health information technology systems for communication and decision support, empowerment of bedside providers to advance (de-escalate) care by such protocols, when appropriate, and keeping patients with similar complexities near one and other [90]. They found a significant reduction in mortality across their population and considerable improvement in complication rates for renal failure, pneumonia, and sepsis.

Another report describes the segmentation of transaortic valve replacement (TAVR) patients based on underlying risks into distinct pathways for intraoperative conscious sedation, general anesthesia care, and postoperative clinical care, in an effort to reduce cost and improve outcomes [91]. The authors reported that conscious sedation for TAVR was safe and could considerably decrease cost and improve outcomes (reduced length of hospital and ICU stay) with favorable patient parameters, which included a transfemoral approach, no perfusion or OR nurses on standby, and a surgeon in house but not scrubbed, with a fast-track recovery plan. This tactic frees up personnel for other cases as necessary.

Finally, the journal *Anesthesiology* published a study on the value of patient segmentation in improving intra/perioperative care delivery and OR throughput in orthopedic surgery [92]. The investigators demonstrated that with appropriately selected patients, spinal anesthesia for arthroplasties and parallel processing using induction rooms can result in a patient out-of-room time of only 14 min and an increase in the number of cases per OR per day. This style of OR management can be highly efficient because of patient selection/segmentation. Selection criteria for more facile patients included those undergoing primary joint replacement, patients with an anticipated easy spinal anesthetic without contra-indication, and patient willingness. Patients who did not meet these criteria had to receive treatment in regular ORs with more personalized care.

These examples comprise only a small subset of all surgeries, and risk assessment is required in all specialties. Establishing such a risk assessment algorithm that can accurately predict postoperative mortality and complications with anesthesia and surgery requires significant information technology, design, building, and testing. Recent reports suggest the successful development of such risk models using various machine-learning approaches. Several anesthesiology and perioperative care groups have developed adaptive models using "deep learning" to predict 30-day mortality [93, 94]. However, at the current time, few studies have reported a change in care delivery or clinical practice results after the implementation of these models. The ability to diagnose complications in the OR well before they happen would revolutionize intraoperative care, prevent significant events, and further enhance postoperative recovery.

Risk stratifying patients, educating them, giving them realistic expectations, and empowering them to understand that they are the most important person in their care and recovery are only the start of the clinical pathway. Challenges remain in both the intra and postoperative arena. Requirements include integrating care outside of the hospital before and after surgery, standardizing intraoperative care, and effective use of in-hospital resources in the postoperative period. This brings about the concept of vertical and horizontal integration of pathways [95]. Each surgical service line has a pathway by which they care for their patients. However, certain disease states and treatment methodologies will cross all surgical service lines, guided by the same tenets. Patients with diabetes or hyperglycemia still require glucose control. Congestive heart failure patients still need specific care whether they are having a total joint replacement or a Whipple procedure. Patients will still experience discomfort and need pain management regardless of their procedure.

Enhanced recovery protocols (ERPs) are an excellent example of innovation within intraoperative and postoperative care [96–106], based on the five major principles of limiting preoperative fasting, minimally invasive surgical procedures, multimodal analgesia, early feeding, and early ambulation, ERPs cross multiple surgeries. At Kaiser, an ERP clinical pathway with certain minor differences based upon surgery type, was prospectively implemented in a controlled manner for orthopedic and colorectal surgery patients. They found significant decreases in length of hospital stay, mortality, and postoperative complications [107]. At UPMC, utilization of an ERP across eight service lines in approximately 6000 patients was significantly associated with improved discharge disposition and a reduction in mortality at 30 days, 1 year, and 2 years. Compliance with only five or more elements of the ERP was associated with better outcomes [108].

Clinical pathways are not only important for hospital systems and patients; there is also a significant value added for society in general. Over 100 million Americans suffer from chronic pain, and pain treatments cost upward of US $635 billion, twice the amount spent on cancer and heart disease combined ($552 billion) [109]. In 2014, 21.5 million American patients were diagnosed with substance use disorder, and 10% of those cases involved prescription pain medications [110]. Physicians write 259 million opioid prescriptions every year, more than enough to give every American adult their own bottle of pills [110]. Drug overdose has been the leading cause of accidental death in the US; the opioid epidemic is partially caused by these prescription opioids, many of which are given after surgery [111]. Anesthesiologists can have a direct impact on this epidemic by coordinating perioperative pain medicine within the preoperative arena, partnering with surgical teams to coordinate team-based treatments, offering opioid-sparing/opioid-free analgesia through regional anesthesia teams, and developing a postsurgical and postdischarge pain plan for patients. Two excellent examples from the literature show that anesthesiology-led acute and chronic pain services as part of a perioperative surgical home/comprehensive program play a significant role in improving outcomes and improving the opioid epidemic [112, 113]. Acute postoperative pain is usually well controlled in institutions with an anesthesia pain management service (APS). The inclusion of complimentary regional anesthesia and multimodal analgesia has transformed perioperative care and can decrease opioid use for postoperative pain [114]. Importantly, pain is often less well controlled on general medical wards, even at institutions with an APS, since the service usually focuses on managing peripheral nerve catheters and epidural analgesia. Improving pain assessment and treatment for all hospitalized patients is a significant opportunity for anesthesiologists to improve patient outcomes and decrease overall healthcare costs, thus improving value. Lastly, providers can extend this value by establishing pathways for patients discharged with opioids and dictate the quantity of opioids they should have when they go home. Anesthesiologists can train in palliative care and become able to offer a more diverse repertoire of treatments to patients undergoing palliative procedures. Collectively, these approaches create significant value for healthcare systems and for all of society.

5 Technological Contributions to Perioperative Care

The ability to collect reliable and meaningful data is crucial to the successful implementation of these integrative pathways. This data will help inform us whether to continue or discontinue a current path. Transitioning to an electronic medical record (EMR) promised a free flow of data for rapid healthcare transformation. The current dystopic state of somewhat poorly recorded and difficult-to-access medical record data is a major barrier to defining success metrics. Healthcare data analytics and information technology are required for any sustainable performance improvement initiative and the data gathered should be used as a strength and advantage to help departments and organizations compete more effectively. Anesthesiologists with direct knowledge about perioperative mortality, complications, and other metrics that impact performance can affect an insurance payer's and hospital's ability to compete in a value-based system.

In that regard, anesthesiology departments can use their expertise and knowledge in the perioperative domain to help build or partner with hospitals' information technology groups to create validated and scalable clinical and financial data dashboards and marts to implement value-based care initiatives [115]. These tools can also help identify clinical comorbidities that departments and hospitals can use to help risk-adjust their value-based payments.

With the continued growth of software applications and digital technology for health improvements, many programs have integrated clinical decision support systems into their clinical practices, either as tools built within their institution's EMR or as stand-alone applications that interface with EMRs. Digital health solutions can enable the implementation of clinical pathways and compliance monitoring, all of which can help to positively affect the course of patient success. For instance, clinical decision support was used to calculate patient risk for postoperative nausea and vomiting (PONV) based on EMR data [116]. After the implementation of this support, there was a clear reduction in PONV with high pathway compliance. Machine learning can improve intraoperative clinical decision support and predict adverse hemodynamic events and other crises, a reality in critical care units [117], in patients intraoperatively, leading to the practice of "proactive" instead of "reactive" OR medicine [118]. These types of models have been developed at the University of California, Los Angeles [94, 119, 120] and Duke University [5].

6 The Role of Perioperative Care Centers and Enhanced Recovery Protocols

In most systems, the perioperative journey is impersonal and complex. Patients do not have access to a customized preparation plan, despite a large body of evidence that supports the idea that surgery optimization drives lower costs and outcomes, including preventing 50% of surgical complications and $25–45B in wasteful spending from avoidable, unnecessary readmissions and complications [121–123]. Preoperative clinics (PCs) have undergone a functional evolution, starting with their initial core functions, which were to gather and summarize all available and relevant information to optimize OR throughput. The next step is risk assessment to coordinate the perioperative process and reduce silo-driven care with the early involvement of perioperative and operative teams. Next, those risks can be modified with allergy de-labeling, obesity management, smoking cessation, and identifying and managing medical conditions, while also understanding the patient's needs, goals, lifestyle, and values to make their health care work within their framework. PCs have multiple organizational tiers. Some hospitals have no PC, pain service, or other hospital-based structure. In some places, the anesthesiology service has a formal relationship with a hospital-based PC, and in others, anesthesiology manages preoperative assessment. In upper-level, integrated tiers, the anesthesiology service can have a comprehensive optimization, pain, and postoperative service that can be closely coordinated with institutional population health programs and is completely integrated within a health care system [124]. Duke has one such integrated center, the perioperative enhancement team at their Preoperative Anesthesia and Surgical Screening Clinic. Duke's center uses prescriptive preoperative screening, manages modifiable comorbid conditions, facilitates communication and education, coordinates surgical care, and enacts population health of at-risk patients [125].

A risk model developed at the UPMC was tested and validated on over 1 million patients and demonstrated an ability to predict 30-day mortality and major adverse cardiac and cerebrovascular events with a high degree of accuracy (>95% area under the curve) [126]. This helps identify high-risk patients scheduled for surgery and, when feasible, facilitates preoperative optimization by medical and perioperative teams, including the UPMC Center for Perioperative Care (CPC), which comprises a host of outpatient and inpatient perioperative services aimed to not only optimize a patient for a procedure but also help them establish better habits for their life [127]. Providers stratify patients into low-, intermediate-, and high-risk categories and use multiple methods to ensure patients receive the personalized care they require. This allows features like a fast-track path for low-risk healthier patients, and these patients are appropriate for electronic consultation. When a surgical clinic orders an electronic consultation, the perioperative team follows testing guidelines and recommends/orders pathways, and these patients do not require further workup. Intermediate-risk patients receive medical optimization and other, more in-depth clinical pathways. Finally, high-risk patients, in addition to the steps described for low and intermediate-risk patients, receive shared decision-making discussions as well as goals of care and values to ensure that the pursued treatment is the most appropriate. This system is applicable to practice population health, performing screenings for multiple diseases including anemia and diabetes. Patients seen in the CPC have significantly less mortality than patients who do not pass through the CPC (0.4% versus 1.2% at 30 days, 1.1% versus 3.2% at 90 days).

Importantly, health system providers and patients have different points of view. Patients feel a lack of clear direction; often receive little tailored guidance on surgery prep; are stressed to keep instructions and appointments organized before surgery; value emotionally shared accountability, motivation, and support; and want tools to support surgical efforts and understand risks. Health system providers feel there is not enough bandwidth to counsel patients and bemoan a lack of visibility into patient progress and efforts. Even the most well-meaning patient can forget preoperative instructions and heavily rely on nursing teams to communicate with patients, but again, acknowledges thin bandwidth. Health system providers are skeptical that patients will make meaningful behavioral modifications to lower risks; it is critical for patients to understand and follow 48-h protocols, which affect scheduling and clinical and economic outcomes.

To help with this process, there are digital perioperative care platforms that engage in personalized coaching. For example, the perioperative improvement program by PIP Care is a company that partners closely with healthcare systems to ensure that surgery patients are engaged, prepared, and optimized for surgery and recovery through the use of one-on-one health coaching, protocols, and process trackers with educational content, personalized clinical interventions, and integration of predictive analytics, risk management, and outcomes reporting. These platforms use an app and text messaging to provide encouragement and accountability to improve protocol adherence. In a recent study, the implementation of this digital health application was not only highly rated by patients but also showed significant reductions in length of stay [128]. Digitized protocols are provided for practical advice and adherence to value-based clinical pathways, including ERPs, personalized to each patient [128]. These ERPs and value-based care pathways are very important for patient optimization and outcomes, which represent a good example of innovation within the intraoperative and postoperative arena [96–106]. Based on the five major tenets of limiting preoperative fasting, minimally invasive surgical procedures, multimodal analgesia, early feeding, and early ambulation, these ERPs cross multiple surgeries. At Kaiser, two populations, colorectal and orthopedic surgery patients, saw the controlled and prospective implementation of an ERP, with certain minor differences based on the type of surgery. Kaiser found significantly reduced length of stay, reduced mortality, and reduced postoperative complications [107]. At UPMC, utilization of an ERP across eight service lines in approximately 6000 patients was significantly associated with improved discharge disposition and a reduction in mortality at 30 days, 1 year, and 2 years, and compliance with only five or more elements of the ERP was associated with better outcomes [108]. But again, ERPs are not defined by only early ambulation or by multimodal analgesia, but by compliance with most of the measures in the pathway itself [129]. The longitudinal care cycle, which can be weeks to months long, encompasses the patient's responsibility toward their health through the distant postoperative future and their continued engagement to stay healthy. This is far more important than the operative episode of only a few hours or days. Focusing only on the system's "inputs and outputs" of these short episodic levels obscures the true relationship from a patient perspective, making the shorter cycle of care far less important than the longer cycle of care [130, 131]. This includes the decision to perform the procedure or surgery itself. In more direct terms, once the decision is made to perform a surgery, the use of isoflurane versus sevoflurane during operative care may not matter nearly as much as the patient's decrease in body mass index which may reduce the risk of malnutrition, diabetes, cardiovascular disease, stroke, and polypharmacy, all of which can stop the patient from requiring the next, more invasive procedure. Reactive medicine (helping to manage the patient from one episode to another) then becomes preventative medicine and the surgical encounter, in many cases, becomes the first touchpoint for a patient to participate in their own medical care.

Funding Support Dr. Mahajan is supported by National Institutes of Health awards RO1 HL136836 and R44 DA049630.

Conflicts of Interest None.

References

1. Robinson DH, Toledo AH. Historical development of modern anesthesia. J Investig Surg. 2012;25(3):141–9.
2. Amalberti R, Auroy Y, Berwick D, Barach P. Five system barriers to achieving ultrasafe health care. Ann Intern Med. 2005;142(9):756–64.
3. Bartels K, Karhausen J, Clambey ET, Grenz A, Eltzschig HK. Perioperative organ injury. Anesthesiology. 2013;119(6):1474–89.
4. Hall MJ, Schwartzman A, Zhang J, Liu X. Ambulatory surgery data from hospitals and ambulatory surgery centers: United States, 2010. Natl Health Stat Report. 2017;102:1–15.

5. Corey KM, Kashyap S, Lorenzi E, Lagoo-Deenadayalan SA, Heller K, Whalen K, et al. Development and validation of machine learning models to identify high-risk surgical patients using automatically curated electronic health record data (Pythia): a retrospective, single-site study. PLoS Med. 2018;15(11):e1002701.
6. Healey MA, Shackford SR, Osler TM, Rogers FB, Burns E. Complications in surgical patients. Arch Surg. 2002;137(5):611–7; discussion 7–8.
7. Department of Health and Human Services NCfHS. National vital statistics reports. Centers for Disease Control and Prevention; 2012.
8. Fleisher LA, Lee TH. Anesthesiology and anesthesiologists in the era of value-driven health care. Healthc (Amst). 2015;3(2):63–6.
9. Aronson S, Murray S, Martin G, Blitz J, Crittenden T, Lipkin ME, et al. Roadmap for transforming preoperative assessment to preoperative optimization. Anesth Analg. 2020;130(4):811–9.
10. Munoz Gomez M, Leal Noval SR. [Perioperative anemia correction in patient blood management programs: lights and shadows]. Rev Esp Anestesiol Reanim. 2015;62(8):421–4.
11. Kikuchi M, Inagaki T, Shinagawa N. Five-year survival of older people with anemia: variation with hemoglobin concentration. J Am Geriatr Soc. 2001;49(9):1226–8.
12. Beattie WS, Karkouti K, Wijeysundera DN, Tait G. Risk associated with preoperative anemia in noncardiac surgery: a single-center cohort study. Anesthesiology. 2009;110(3):574–81.
13. Wu WC, Schifftner TL, Henderson WG, Eaton CB, Poses RM, Uttley G, et al. Preoperative hematocrit levels and postoperative outcomes in older patients undergoing noncardiac surgery. JAMA. 2007;297(22):2481–8.
14. Musallam KM, Tamim HM, Richards T, Spahn DR, Rosendaal FR, Habbal A, et al. Preoperative anaemia and postoperative outcomes in non-cardiac surgery: a retrospective cohort study. Lancet. 2011;378(9800):1396–407.
15. Bernard AC, Davenport DL, Chang PK, Vaughan TB, Zwischenberger JB. Intraoperative transfusion of 1 U to 2 U packed red blood cells is associated with increased 30-day mortality, surgical-site infection, pneumonia, and sepsis in general surgery patients. J Am Coll Surg. 2009;208(5):931–7, 937.e1–2; discussion 938–9.
16. Barker LA, Gout BS, Crowe TC. Hospital malnutrition: prevalence, identification and impact on patients and the healthcare system. Int J Environ Res Public Health. 2011;8(2):514–27.
17. Hu WH, Cajas-Monson LC, Eisenstein S, Parry L, Cosman B, Ramamoorthy S. Preoperative malnutrition assessments as predictors of postoperative mortality and morbidity in colorectal cancer: an analysis of ACS-NSQIP. Nutr J. 2015;14:91.
18. Cederholm T, Jagren C, Hellstrom K. Outcome of protein-energy malnutrition in elderly medical patients. Am J Med. 1995;98(1):67–74.
19. Cederholm TE, Hellstrom KH. Reversibility of protein-energy malnutrition in a group of chronically-ill elderly outpatients. Clin Nutr. 1995;14(2):81–7.
20. Wischmeyer PE, San-Millan I. Winning the war against ICU-acquired weakness: new innovations in nutrition and exercise physiology. Crit Care. 2015;19(Suppl 3):S6.
21. Mazaki T, Ishii Y, Murai I. Immunoenhancing enteral and parenteral nutrition for gastrointestinal surgery: a multiple-treatments meta-analysis. Ann Surg. 2015;261(4):662–9.
22. Drover JW, Dhaliwal R, Weitzel L, Wischmeyer PE, Ochoa JB, Heyland DK. Perioperative use of arginine-supplemented diets: a systematic review of the evidence. J Am Coll Surg. 2011;212(3):385–99, 399.e1
23. International Association for the Study of Pain Task Force on Taxonomy. Part III: pain terms, a current list with definitions and notes on usage. In: Merskey H, Bogduk N, editors. Classification of chronic pain. 2nd ed. Seattle: IASP Press; 1994. p. 209–14.
24. Barash PG, Cullen BF, Stoelting RK. Clinical anesthesia. Philadelphia: Lippincott Williams & Wilkins; 2006, 1 p.
25. Chia YY, Liu K, Wang JJ, Kuo MC, Ho ST. Intraoperative high dose fentanyl induces postoperative fentanyl tolerance. Can J Anaesth. 1999;46(9):872–7.
26. Collard V, Mistraletti G, Taqi A, Asenjo JF, Feldman LS, Fried GM, et al. Intraoperative esmolol infusion in the absence of opioids spares postoperative fentanyl in patients undergoing

ambulatory laparoscopic cholecystectomy. Anesth Analg. 2007;105(5):1255–62, table of contents.
27. Coloma M, Chiu JW, White PF, Armbruster SC. The use of esmolol as an alternative to remifentanil during desflurane anesthesia for fast-track outpatient gynecologic laparoscopic surgery. Anesth Analg. 2001;92(2):352–7.
28. Crawford MW, Galton S, Naser B. Postoperative morphine consumption in children with sickle-cell disease. Paediatr Anaesth. 2006;16(2):152–7.
29. Gottschalk A, Durieux ME, Nemergut EC. Intraoperative methadone improves postoperative pain control in patients undergoing complex spine surgery. Anesth Analg. 2011;112(1):218–23.
30. Guignard B, Bossard AE, Coste C, Sessler DI, Lebrault C, Alfonsi P, et al. Acute opioid tolerance: intraoperative remifentanil increases postoperative pain and morphine requirement. Anesthesiology. 2000;93(2):409–17.
31. Mendel HG, Guarnieri KM, Sundt LM, Torjman MC. The effects of ketorolac and fentanyl on postoperative vomiting and analgesic requirements in children undergoing strabismus surgery. Anesth Analg. 1995;80(6):1129–33.
32. Sukhani R, Vazquez J, Pappas AL, Frey K, Aasen M, Slogoff S. Recovery after propofol with and without intraoperative fentanyl in patients undergoing ambulatory gynecologic laparoscopy. Anesth Analg. 1996;83(5):975–81.
33. Nicholson A, Lowe MC, Parker J, Lewis SR, Alderson P, Smith AF. Systematic review and meta-analysis of enhanced recovery programmes in surgical patients. Br J Surg. 2014;101(3):172–88.
34. Dew MA, Rosenberger EM, Myaskovsky L, DiMartini AF, DeVito Dabbs AJ, Posluszny DM, et al. Depression and anxiety as risk factors for morbidity and mortality after organ transplantation: a systematic review and meta-analysis. Transplantation. 2015;100(5):988–1003.
35. Thombs BD, de Jonge P, Coyne JC, Whooley MA, Frasure-Smith N, Mitchell AJ, et al. Depression screening and patient outcomes in cardiovascular care: a systematic review. JAMA. 2008;300(18):2161–71.
36. Satin JR, Linden W, Phillips MJ. Depression as a predictor of disease progression and mortality in cancer patients: a meta-analysis. Cancer. 2009;115(22):5349–61.
37. Bandeen-Roche K, Xue QL, Ferrucci L, Walston J, Guralnik JM, Chaves P, et al. Phenotype of frailty: characterization in the women's health and aging studies. J Gerontol A Biol Sci Med Sci. 2006;61(3):262–6.
38. Cawthon PM, Marshall LM, Michael Y, Dam TT, Ensrud KE, Barrett-Connor E, et al. Frailty in older men: prevalence, progression, and relationship with mortality. J Am Geriatr Soc. 2007;55(8):1216–23.
39. Fried LP, Tangen CM, Walston J, Newman AB, Hirsch C, Gottdiener J, et al. Frailty in older adults: evidence for a phenotype. J Gerontol A Biol Sci Med Sci. 2001;56(3):M146–56.
40. Kiely DK, Cupples LA, Lipsitz LA. Validation and comparison of two frailty indexes: the MOBILIZE Boston Study. J Am Geriatr Soc. 2009;57(9):1532–9.
41. Woods NF, LaCroix AZ, Gray SL, Aragaki A, Cochrane BB, Brunner RL, et al. Frailty: emergence and consequences in women aged 65 and older in the Women's Health Initiative Observational Study. J Am Geriatr Soc. 2005;53(8):1321–30.
42. Hall DE, Arya S, Schmid KK, Blaser C, Carlson MA, Bailey TL, et al. Development and initial validation of the risk analysis index for measuring frailty in surgical populations. JAMA Surg. 2017;152(2):175–82.
43. Hall DE, Arya S, Schmid KK, Carlson MA, Lavedan P, Bailey TL, et al. Association of a frailty screening initiative with postoperative survival at 30, 180, and 365 days. JAMA Surg. 2017;152(3):233–40.
44. Shinall MC Jr, Shireman PK, Hall DE. Implications of preoperative patient frailty on stratified postoperative mortality-reply. JAMA Surg. 2020;155(7):670–1.
45. Shinall MC Jr, Arya S, Youk A, Varley P, Shah R, Massarweh NN, et al. Association of preoperative patient frailty and operative stress with postoperative mortality. JAMA Surg. 2020;155(1):e194620.

46. Tang V, Zhao S, Boscardin J, Sudore R, Covinsky K, Walter LC, et al. Functional status and survival after breast cancer surgery in nursing home residents. JAMA Surg. 2018;153:1090.
47. Mosquera C, Spaniolas K, Fitzgerald TL. Impact of frailty on surgical outcomes: the right patient for the right procedure. Surgery. 2016;160(2):272–80.
48. Imamura K, Yamamoto S, Suzuki Y, Yoshikoshi S, Harada M, Osada S, et al. Comparison of the association between six different frailty scales and clinical events in patients on hemodialysis. Nephrol Dial Transplant. 2022;38:455.
49. Varley PR, Borrebach JD, Arya S, Massarweh NN, Bilderback AL, Wisniewski MK, et al. Clinical utility of the risk analysis index as a prospective frailty screening tool within a multi-practice, multi-hospital integrated healthcare system. Ann Surg. 2020;274:e1230.
50. Ditmyer MM, Topp R, Pifer M. Prehabilitation in preparation for orthopaedic surgery. Orthop Nurs. 2002;21(5):43–51; quiz 2–4.
51. Topp R, Ditmyer M, King K, Doherty K, Hornyak J 3rd. The effect of bed rest and potential of prehabilitation on patients in the intensive care unit. AACN Clin Issues. 2002;13(2):263–76.
52. Levett DZ, Grocott MP. Cardiopulmonary exercise testing, prehabilitation, and Enhanced Recovery After Surgery (ERAS). Can J Anaesth. 2015;62(2):131–42.
53. Thompson PD, Franklin BA, Balady GJ, Blair SN, Corrado D, Estes NA 3rd, et al. Exercise and acute cardiovascular events placing the risks into perspective: a scientific statement from the American Heart Association Council on Nutrition, Physical Activity, and Metabolism and the Council on Clinical Cardiology. Circulation. 2007;115(17):2358–68.
54. Thompson PD, Buchner D, Pina IL, Balady GJ, Williams MA, Marcus BH, et al. Exercise and physical activity in the prevention and treatment of atherosclerotic cardiovascular disease: a statement from the Council on Clinical Cardiology (Subcommittee on Exercise, Rehabilitation, and Prevention) and the Council on Nutrition, Physical Activity, and Metabolism (Subcommittee on Physical Activity). Circulation. 2003;107(24):3109–16.
55. Belardinelli R, Georgiou D, Cianci G, Purcaro A. Randomized, controlled trial of long-term moderate exercise training in chronic heart failure: effects on functional capacity, quality of life, and clinical outcome. Circulation. 1999;99(9):1173–82.
56. Mandic S, Myers J, Selig SE, Levinger I. Resistance versus aerobic exercise training in chronic heart failure. Curr Heart Fail Rep. 2012;9(1):57–64.
57. O'Connor CM, Whellan DJ, Lee KL, Keteyian SJ, Cooper LS, Ellis SJ, et al. Efficacy and safety of exercise training in patients with chronic heart failure: HF-ACTION randomized controlled trial. JAMA. 2009;301(14):1439–50.
58. Cornelissen VA, Buys R, Smart NA. Endurance exercise beneficially affects ambulatory blood pressure: a systematic review and meta-analysis. J Hypertens. 2013;31(4):639–48.
59. Cornelissen VA, Smart NA. Exercise training for blood pressure: a systematic review and meta-analysis. J Am Heart Assoc. 2013;2(1):e004473.
60. Hayashino Y, Jackson JL, Fukumori N, Nakamura F, Fukuhara S. Effects of supervised exercise on lipid profiles and blood pressure control in people with type 2 diabetes mellitus: a meta-analysis of randomized controlled trials. Diabetes Res Clin Pract. 2012;98(3):349–60.
61. Thomas DE, Elliott EJ, Naughton GA. Exercise for type 2 diabetes mellitus. Cochrane Database Syst Rev. 2006;(3):CD002968.
62. Waschki B, Kirsten A, Holz O, Muller KC, Meyer T, Watz H, et al. Physical activity is the strongest predictor of all-cause mortality in patients with COPD: a prospective cohort study. Chest. 2011;140(2):331–42.
63. Cooney GM, Dwan K, Greig CA, Lawlor DA, Rimer J, Waugh FR, et al. Exercise for depression. Cochrane Database Syst Rev. 2013;(9):CD004366.
64. Forbes D, Thiessen EJ, Blake CM, Forbes SC, Forbes S. Exercise programs for people with dementia. Cochrane Database Syst Rev. 2013;(12):CD006489.
65. Saunders DH, Sanderson M, Brazzelli M, Greig CA, Mead GE. Physical fitness training for stroke patients. Cochrane Database Syst Rev. 2013;(10):CD003316.
66. Des Guetz G, Uzzan B, Bouillet T, Nicolas P, Chouahnia K, Zelek L, et al. Impact of physical activity on cancer-specific and overall survival of patients with colorectal cancer. Gastroenterol Res Pract. 2013;2013:340851.

67. Hoogeboom TJ, Dronkers JJ, Hulzebos EH, van Meeteren NL. Merits of exercise therapy before and after major surgery. Curr Opin Anaesthesiol. 2014;27(2):161–6.
68. Arthur HM, Daniels C, McKelvie R, Hirsh J, Rush B. Effect of a preoperative intervention on preoperative and postoperative outcomes in low-risk patients awaiting elective coronary artery bypass graft surgery. A randomized, controlled trial. Ann Intern Med. 2000;133(4):253–62.
69. Jones LW, Watson D, Herndon JE, Eves ND, Haithcock BE, Loewen G, et al. Peak oxygen consumption and long-term all-cause mortality in nonsmall cell lung cancer. Cancer. 2010;116(20):4825–32.
70. West MA, Lythgoe D, Barben CP, Noble L, Kemp GJ, Jack S, et al. Cardiopulmonary exercise variables are associated with postoperative morbidity after major colonic surgery: a prospective blinded observational study. Br J Anaesth. 2014;112(4):665–71.
71. Dronkers JJ, Chorus AMJ, van Meeteren NLU, Hopman-Rock M. The association of preoperative physical fitness and physical activity with outcome after scheduled major abdominal surgery. Anaesthesia. 2013;68(1):67–73.
72. Fagevik Olsen M, Hahn I, Nordgren S, Lonroth H, Lundholm K. Randomized controlled trial of prophylactic chest physiotherapy in major abdominal surgery. Br J Surg. 1997;84(11):1535–8.
73. Kundra P, Vitheeswaran M, Nagappa M, Sistla S. Effect of preoperative and postoperative incentive spirometry on lung functions after laparoscopic cholecystectomy. Surg Laparosc Endosc Percutan Tech. 2010;20(3):170–2.
74. Durrand J, Singh SJ, Danjoux G. Prehabilitation. Clin Med (Lond). 2019;19(6):458–64.
75. Brown CH 4th, Max L, LaFlam A, Kirk L, Gross A, Arora R, et al. The association between preoperative frailty and postoperative delirium after cardiac surgery. Anesth Analg. 2016;123(2):430–5.
76. Culley DJ, Flaherty D, Fahey MC, Rudolph JL, Javedan H, Huang CC, et al. Poor performance on a preoperative cognitive screening test predicts postoperative complications in older orthopedic surgical patients. Anesthesiology. 2017;127(5):765–74.
77. Culley DJ, Flaherty D, Reddy S, Fahey MC, Rudolph J, Huang CC, et al. Preoperative cognitive stratification of older elective surgical patients: a cross-sectional study. Anesth Analg. 2016;123(1):186–92.
78. Practice guidelines for preoperative fasting and the use of pharmacologic agents to reduce the risk of pulmonary aspiration: application to healthy patients undergoing elective procedures: an updated report by the American Society of Anesthesiologists Task Force on Preoperative Fasting and the Use of Pharmacologic Agents to Reduce the Risk of Pulmonary Aspiration. Anesthesiology. 2017;126(3):376–93.
79. American Society of Anesthesiologists. Perioperative delirium. American Society of Anesthesiologists; 2022. https://www.asahq.org/brainhealthinitiative/tools/infographics.
80. Henneghan AM, Lewis KA, Gill E, Kesler SR. Cognitive impairment in non-critical, mild-to-moderate COVID-19 survivors. Front Psychol. 2022;13:770459.
81. Ye S, Sun K, Huynh D, Phi HQ, Ko B, Huang B, et al. A computerized cognitive test battery for detection of dementia and mild cognitive impairment: instrument validation study. JMIR Aging. 2022;5(2):e36825.
82. Yang S, Flores B, Magal R, Harris K, Gross J, Ewbank A, et al. Diagnostic accuracy of tablet-based software for the detection of concussion. PLoS One. 2017;12(7):e0179352.
83. Franco-Rocha OY, Mahaffey ML, Matsui W, Kesler SR. Remote assessment of cognitive dysfunction in hematologic malignancies using web-based neuropsychological testing. Cancer Med. 2022;12:6068.
84. Lilot M, Ehrenfeld JM, Lee C, Harrington B, Cannesson M, Rinehart J. Variability in practice and factors predictive of total crystalloid administration during abdominal surgery: retrospective two-centre analysis. Br J Anaesth. 2015;114(5):767–76.
85. Ghaferi AA, Birkmeyer JD, Dimick JB. Variation in hospital mortality associated with inpatient surgery. N Engl J Med. 2009;361(14):1368–75.
86. Mahajan A, Islam SD, Schwartz MJ, Cannesson M. A hospital is not just a factory, but a complex adaptive system-implications for perioperative care. Anesth Analg. 2017;125(1):333–41.

87. Skinner W. The focused factory. Harv Bus Rev. 1974;52(3):113.
88. Christensen CM, Grossman JH, Hwang J. The innovator's prescription: a disruptive solution for health care. McGraw-Hill; 2009.
89. Fleisher LA, Fleischmann KE, Auerbach AD, Barnason SA, Beckman JA, Bozkurt B, et al. 2014 ACC/AHA guideline on perioperative cardiovascular evaluation and management of patients undergoing noncardiac surgery: a report of the American College of Cardiology/American Heart Association Task Force on Practice Guidelines. Circulation. 2014;130(24):e278–333.
90. Cook D, Thompson JE, Habermann EB, Visscher SL, Dearani JA, Roger VL, et al. From 'solution shop' model to 'focused factory' in hospital surgery: increasing care value and predictability. Health Aff (Millwood). 2014;33(5):746–55.
91. Toppen W, Johansen D, Sareh S, Fernandez J, Satou N, Patel KD, et al. Improved costs and outcomes with conscious sedation vs general anesthesia in TAVR patients: time to wake up? PLoS One. 2017;12(4):e0173777.
92. Smith MP, Sandberg WS, Foss J, Massoli K, Kanda M, Barsoum W, et al. High-throughput operating room system for joint arthroplasties durably outperforms routine processes. Anesthesiology. 2008;109(1):25–35.
93. Fritz BA, Cui Z, Zhang M, He Y, Chen Y, Kronzer A, et al. Deep-learning model for predicting 30-day postoperative mortality. Br J Anaesth. 2019;123(5):688–95.
94. Hill BL, Brown R, Gabel E, Rakocz N, Lee C, Cannesson M, et al. An automated machine learning-based model predicts postoperative mortality using readily-extractable preoperative electronic health record data. Br J Anaesth. 2019;123(6):877–86.
95. Cannesson M, Mahajan A. Vertical and horizontal pathways: intersection and integration of enhanced recovery after surgery and the perioperative surgical home. Anesth Analg. 2018;127(5):1275–7.
96. Boisen ML, McQuaid AJ, Esper SA, Holder-Murray J, Zureikat AH, Hogg ME, et al. Intrathecal morphine versus nerve blocks in an enhanced recovery pathway for pancreatic surgery. J Surg Res. 2019;244:15–22.
97. Holder-Murray J, Esper SA, Boisen ML, Gealey J, Meister K, Medich DS, et al. Postoperative nausea and vomiting in patients undergoing colorectal surgery within an institutional enhanced recovery after surgery protocol: comparison of two prophylactic antiemetic regimens. Korean J Anesthesiol. 2019;72(4):344–50.
98. Khalil A, Ganesh S, Hughes C, Tevar AD, Hasche JJ, Esper S, et al. Evaluation of the enhanced recovery after surgery protocol in living liver donors. Clin Transpl. 2018;32(8):e13342.
99. Kowalsky SJ, Zenati MS, Steve J, Esper SA, Lee KK, Hogg ME, et al. A combination of robotic approach and ERAS pathway optimizes outcomes and cost for pancreatoduodenectomy. Ann Surg. 2018;269:1138.
100. Arumainayagam N, McGrath J, Jefferson KP, Gillatt DA. Introduction of an enhanced recovery protocol for radical cystectomy. BJU Int. 2008;101(6):698–701.
101. Balzano G, Zerbi A, Braga M, Rocchetti S, Beneduce AA, Di Carlo V. Fast-track recovery programme after pancreaticoduodenectomy reduces delayed gastric emptying. Br J Surg. 2008;95(11):1387–93.
102. Bardram L, Funch-Jensen P, Jensen P, Crawford ME, Kehlet H. Recovery after laparoscopic colonic surgery with epidural analgesia, and early oral nutrition and mobilisation. Lancet. 1995;345(8952):763–4.
103. Beamish AJ, Chan DS, Blake PA, Karran A, Lewis WG. Systematic review and meta-analysis of enhanced recovery programmes in gastric cancer surgery. Int J Surg. 2015;19:46–54.
104. Braga M, Pecorelli N, Ariotti R, Capretti G, Greco M, Balzano G, et al. Enhanced recovery after surgery pathway in patients undergoing pancreaticoduodenectomy. World J Surg. 2014;38(11):2960–6.
105. Scheib SA, Thomassee M, Kenner JL. Enhanced recovery after surgery in gynecology: a review of the literature. J Minim Invasive Gynecol. 2019;26(2):327–43.

106. Singh PM, Panwar R, Borle A, Goudra B, Trikha A, van Wagensveld BA, et al. Efficiency and safety effects of applying ERAS protocols to bariatric surgery: a systematic review with meta-analysis and trial sequential analysis of evidence. Obes Surg. 2017;27(2):489–501.
107. Liu VX, Rosas E, Hwang J, Cain E, Foss-Durant A, Clopp M, et al. Enhanced recovery after surgery program implementation in 2 surgical populations in an integrated health care delivery system. JAMA Surg. 2017;152(7):e171032.
108. Esper SA, Holder-Murray J, Subramaniam K, Boisen M, Kenkre TS, Meister K, et al. Enhanced recovery protocols reduce mortality across eight surgical specialties at academic and university-affiliated community hospitals. Ann Surg. 2020. Epub ahead of print; https://doi.org/10.1097/SLA.0000000000004642.
109. Relieving pain in America: a blueprint for transforming prevention, care, education, and research. Washington DC: The National Academies Collection: Reports Funded by National Institutes of Health; 2011.
110. Centers for Disease Control and Prevention. Opioid painkiller prescribing, where you live makes a difference. 2014.
111. Center for Behavioral Health Statistics and Quality. Behavioral health trends in the United States: results from the 2014 National Survey on Drug Use and Health. Substance Abuse and Mental Health Services Administration; 2015.
112. Pozek JJ, De Ruyter M, Khan TW. Comprehensive acute pain management in the perioperative surgical home. Anesthesiol Clin. 2018;36(2):295–307.
113. Khan TW, Manion S. Perioperative surgical home for the patient with chronic pain. Anesthesiol Clin. 2018;36(2):281–94.
114. Brandal D, Keller MS, Lee C, Grogan T, Fujimoto Y, Gricourt Y, et al. Impact of enhanced recovery after surgery and opioid-free anesthesia on opioid prescriptions at discharge from the hospital: a historical-prospective study. Anesth Analg. 2017;125(5):1784–92.
115. Hofer IS, Gabel E, Pfeffer M, Mahbouba M, Mahajan A. A systematic approach to creation of a perioperative data warehouse. Anesth Analg. 2016;122(6):1880–4.
116. Gabel E, Shin J, Hofer I, Grogan T, Ziv K, Hong J, et al. Digital quality improvement approach reduces the need for rescue antiemetics in high-risk patients: a comparative effectiveness study using interrupted time series and propensity score matching analysis. Anesth Analg. 2019;128(5):867–76.
117. Yoon JH, Pinsky MR. Predicting adverse hemodynamic events in critically ill patients. Curr Opin Crit Care. 2018;24(3):196–203.
118. Wiley K, Davies J, Canadian Patient Safety Institute. Getting ahead of harm before it happens: a guide about proactive analysis for improving surgical care safety. US Department of Health and Human Services, Agency for Healthcare Research and Quality; 2017.
119. Misic VV, Gabel E, Hofer I, Rajaram K, Mahajan A. Machine learning prediction of postoperative emergency department hospital readmission. Anesthesiology. 2020;132(5):968–80.
120. Hofer IS, Cheng D, Grogan T, Fujimoto Y, Yamada T, Beck L, et al. Automated assessment of existing patient's revised cardiac risk index using algorithmic software. Anesth Analg. 2019;128(5):909–16.
121. McDonald SR, Heflin MT, Whitson HE, Dalton TO, Lidsky ME, Liu P, et al. Association of integrated care coordination with postsurgical outcomes in high-risk older adults: the perioperative optimization of senior health (POSH) initiative. JAMA Surg. 2018;153(5):454–62.
122. Slakey DP, Silver DS, Chazin SM, Katoozian PY, Sikora KS, Ruther MM. Making enhanced recovery the norm not the exception. Am J Surg. 2020;219(3):472–6.
123. Mouch CA, Kenney BC, Lorch S, Montgomery JR, Gonzalez-Walker M, Bishop K, et al. Statewide prehabilitation program and episode payment in medicare beneficiaries. J Am Coll Surg. 2020;230(3):306–13.e6.
124. Aronson S, Grocott MPW, Mythen MMG. Preoperative patient preparation, programs, and education in the United States: state of the art, state of the science, and state of affairs. Adv Anesth. 2019;37:127–43.

125. Aronson S, Westover J, Guinn N, Setji T, Wischmeyer P, Gulur P, et al. A perioperative medicine model for population health: an integrated approach for an evolving clinical science. Anesth Analg. 2018;126(2):682–90.
126. Mahajan A, Esper S, Oo TH, McKibben J, Garver M, Artman J, et al. Development and validation of a machine learning model to identify patients before surgery at high risk for postoperative adverse events. JAMA Netw Open. 2023;6(7):e2322285.
127. Mahajan A, Esper SA, Cole DJ, Fleisher LA. Anesthesiologists' role in value-based perioperative care and healthcare transformation. Anesthesiology. 2021;134(4):526–40.
128. Esper SA, Holder-Murray J, Meister KA, Lin HS, Hamilton DK, Groff YJ, et al. A novel digital health platform with health coaches to optimize surgical patients: feasibility study at a large academic health system. JMIR Perioper Med. 2024;7:e52125.
129. Holder-Murray JE, Esper S, Wang Z, Cui Z, Wang X. Optimizing perioperative care: enhanced recovery and Chinese medicine. In: Brunicardi FC, editor. Schwartz's principles of surgery. 11th ed. New York: McGraw-Hill; 2018.
130. Grocott MP, Mythen MG. Perioperative medicine: the value proposition for anesthesia? A UK perspective on delivering value from anesthesiology. Anesthesiol Clin. 2015;33(4):617–28.
131. Porter ME. What is value in health care? N Engl J Med. 2010;363(26):2477–81.

Prehabilitation in Spine Surgery and Joint Arthroplasty

James E. Eubanks Jr, Esther R. C. Janssen, Krish Bharat, and Chandler Bolles

1 Why Prehabilitation?

Prehabilitation as a concept was first mentioned in 1945 in the *British Medical Journal* in the context of training military personnel to prevent injury [1]. Prehabilitation in spinal care was initially used in rehabilitation medicine to prevent injury by developing strength, flexibility, and aerobic fitness. The history of prehabilitation in spinal medicine dates back to 1985 when a study by Teitz et al. recognized the importance of anticipating possible areas of injury through preventative "prehabilitation" exercises to avert common sports injuries [2]. In the following decades, prehabilitation in the context of spine and orthopedics was only mentioned in relation to the prevention of (sports) injury, not for the purpose of surgical preparation. More recently, prehabilitation has expanded from the prevention of injury to improving surgical outcomes, particularly in the case of spine surgeries. The first mentions of preoperative exercise for the prevention of postoperative complications can be found as early as 1977 [3].

A study conducted by Ditmyer et al. in 2002 titled "Prehabilitation in Preparation for Orthopaedic Surgery" showed that by improving an individual's functional

J. E. Eubanks Jr (✉)
Medical University of South Carolina (MUSC), Charleston, SC, USA
e-mail: eubankja@musc.edu

E. R. C. Janssen
Post-doc Allied Healthcare Sciences, Radboud University Medical Center IQ Health, Nijmegen, Netherlands
e-mail: esther.rc.janssen@radboudumc.nl

K. Bharat
University of Pittsburgh Medical Center, Pittsburgh, PA, USA
e-mail: bharatk@upmc.edu

C. Bolles
Edward Via College of Osteopathic Medicine, Spartanburg, SC, USA
e-mail: cbolles@vcom.edu

A. Watson, K. Barr (eds.), *A Prehabilitation Guide for All Providers*,
https://doi.org/10.1007/978-3-031-72862-4_5

capacity through increased physical activity before an anticipated orthopedic procedure, patients could maintain a higher level of functional ability and recover more rapidly in the postoperative rehabilitation process [4]. The first study on prehabilitation prior to spinal surgery was conducted by Nielsen et al. in 2008 and demonstrated that prehabilitation was more cost-effective compared to standard care [5]. The number of publications investigating prehabilitation applications before surgery has continued increasing since these early publications, and prehabilitation research has gained popularity, especially in the last decade.

This surge in prehabilitation literature is not coincidental. In recent years, there has been a paradigm shift in clinical surgical practice from a predominantly reactive approach in perioperative care toward a more proactive and preventative model. The introduction of enhanced recovery after surgery (ERAS) in the 1990s was a key concept driving this transition [6]. This change in approach recognizes the importance of optimizing patient health and fitness before surgery to improve clinical outcomes and the patient experience. As evidence accumulates showing the benefits of prehabilitation, providers are increasingly incorporating this into clinical practice. Within spine and orthopedics, prehabilitation is gaining a notable role within bundled payments as part of value-based care [7].

2 Significance of Prehabilitation in the Context of the Burden of Disease in Musculoskeletal Disorders

The burden of musculoskeletal disorders globally and in the United States (US) is high. They are the leading contributor to disability according to the WHO, with low back pain being the leading cause of years lived in disability [8]. Low back pain is highly prevalent in the global population, affecting an estimated 80% of adults at some point during their lives [9]. Spine-related disorders are the most costly health conditions in the United States across out-of-pocket costs as well as both public and private insurance costs [10]. The prevalence of musculoskeletal complaints rises with population aging, along with the costs associated with the care of these conditions. Over the past two decades, there has been a substantial rise in the rate of spine and joint replacement surgeries [11]. A systematic review on the cost-effectiveness of prehabilitation before major surgery shows the potential for cost-reduction through shortening the length of hospital stay, improving preoperative quality of life, delaying surgery, or even eliminating the need for surgery, altogether [12, 13]. In spine surgery, the length of stay can be reduced by 1–2 days in certain populations [12, 14, 15].

Driven by the same paradigm shift seen in perioperative care for other conditions, the standard of practice is increasingly implementing an evidence-based, proactive, multimodal, biopsychosocial-oriented approach [16]. Prehabilitation utilizes this approach to deliver timely, high-value care to optimize patient outcomes with emphasis placed on mitigating postoperative complications and improving the patient experience. Complications of orthopedic procedures place a significant burden on the health of patients and healthcare systems [17]. As a result, hospital administrators and policymakers have a vested interest in reducing hospital length of stay.

3 Continuum of Care

This chapter details the preoperative and perioperative phases of care for patients undergoing spine surgery. Similar principles are observed for these two populations—spine and joint surgery patients, and underlying prehabilitation themes will be discussed.

Presurgical Phase

Before considering spine surgery (defined here as decompression and fusion) as a treatment option, patients typically have undergone various conservative treatment measures. The stepped care approach is a treatment strategy commonly used in the management of spine and musculoskeletal disorders. Stepped care attempts to align the intensity of healthcare resources with the level of care necessary to achieve an optimal outcome [18]. Stepped care involves starting with the least invasive and least resource-intensive interventions and progressing to more intensive treatments as needed. Common treatment options for conservative treatment of spine and joint pain include lifestyle modifications, physical therapy, oral medications, injections, and other treatments directed toward decreasing pain to achieve a satisfactory surgical outcome. Recognizing the intricate interaction between behavioral, psychological, and social factors that influence pain perception and disability, a biopsychosocial approach to care informs the ideal personalized treatment plan for these patients.

Although care does not always proceed in this fashion, in this model surgery is reserved for patients who have exhausted all other treatment options. The decision to undergo elective surgery should involve shared decision-making between the patient and their healthcare provider, considering the patient's preferences and risk factors if conservative treatment fails to provide adequate pain relief and quality of life improvement. Shared decision-making plays a crucial role in the treatment process. Spine surgery in particular carries significant health risks including permanent neurological sequelae with variable outcomes due to unique patient circumstances, making it particularly important for patients to be well-informed and actively involved in the decision-making process. Additionally, expectation management is vital in shared decision-making as it involves discussing the anticipated outcomes, potential limitations, and any misconceptions. This commitment to shared decision-making is an ongoing process throughout the perioperative phase of spine surgery. This means that it is not just a one-time conversation made before surgery, but rather a continuous dialogue between the patient and his or her entire healthcare team before, during, and after the surgical procedure. Ultimately, the goal of shared decision-making is to ensure patients are active participants in their care, leading to better outcomes, increased satisfaction, and improved quality of life.

If this model were faithfully followed, the intensity of prehabilitation would be minimal, as patients would already be engaging in regular exercise and would have made other lifestyle changes known to improve these conditions, such as optimizing nutrition, achieving a more ideal body weight, and managing tobacco/substance use disorders. However, in reality, patients have not always accomplished these lifestyle modifications before surgery is planned [19].

As with all types of major surgery, spinal surgery carries a risk of adverse events and reoperation. Although mortality rates for spinal surgery are low (~1%) there is a substantial risk for complications, between 10% and 24% depending on the complexity of surgery [20, 21]. With joint arthroplasty, complication rates are similarly variable due to differences in risk between large joint procedures, but overall the incidence of complications ranges between ~7% and 10% in some studies, with elevated risk in non-white populations [22] and patients with other chronic diseases [23]. In addition, major surgery induces a systemic stress response, resulting in an inflammatory reaction that drives metabolic, hormonal, and immunological processes in the body [24]. These processes are necessary to stimulate tissue repair but are also accompanied by increased oxygen demand. To tolerate this increase, patients need an adequate physiological reserve to prevent complications including delayed recovery. Particularly if he or she experiences complications, a patient may experience an accelerated functional decline due to the hospital stay as well as the psychological burden of illness [25]. Notably, patients with baseline frailty, deconditioning, and/or advanced age typically experience the most trouble in coping with the physiological and mental stressors of surgery and hospitalization, as their reserves are inherently limited. Although recent advances in surgery and anesthesiology may help reduce intraoperative stressors, some patients are at greater risk than others for adverse events due to differences in their physiological and psychological capacities and reserves.

Preoperative Phase

Turning "waiting lists" for elective surgery into "preparation lists" is a concept gaining popularity in healthcare systems worldwide. Once a patient has opted for spine or joint surgery, there is an immediate opportunity for the surgical team to initiate optimal surgical preparation of the patient while he or she is most emotionally invested. A passive waiting period before joint replacement surgery can cause a decline in a patient's physical capacity by 25%, a decline in quality of life by 53%, and aggravation of pain in over 80% of patients [26]. As the waiting period for elective procedures varies greatly from one country to the next, this 'waiting' time may dictate the time spent in prehabilitation, as well. Ultimately, the details of this preparatory period are dependent on a patient's specific needs and risk factors.

There are many different concepts and pathways that intend to streamline patient optimization prior to spine surgery. The best-known concept is ERAS (enhanced recovery after surgery), which was first introduced by Bardram et al. in 1995 in which the authors proposed an evidence-based approach to care to reduce the impact of surgery [27]. ERAS has historically focused on pre- and postoperative optimization, while in more recent years focus has shifted toward preoperative optimization, through a more proactive and preventative approach. As outlined in the 2015 study by Hulzebos and van Meeteren, the preoperative period should involve early identification of patients who are at risk of adverse outcomes [28]. This involves implementing tailored interventions aimed at mitigating those risks within a proactive home and clinical culture.

Preoperative Risk Screening

The highly variable outcomes of spine surgery are influenced by factors including the type of surgery, indication, and the patient's characteristics. The percentage of patients reaching a minimal clinically important improvement in pain 1–2 years after spine surgery ranges between 37.5% and 82.4% depending on their diagnosis [29]. In some studies after joint replacement, greater than 75% of patients reported clinically relevant improvements in pain 5 years after surgery [30]. Various patient and surgery characteristics such as age, intraoperative blood loss, smoking, and the American Society of Anesthesiologists (ASA) score are known predictors of postoperative outcomes after surgery. Despite the identification of known predictors for postoperative outcomes in spine surgery, the prediction accuracy of the models has been somewhat limited, likely due to the clinical complexity of spine-related pain and spine surgery. Nonetheless, the benefits of risk reduction focused on modifiable targets such as obesity, smoking, and uncontrolled diabetes are of great interest at this time [31].

The perioperative period provides an opportunity to assess and stratify risks in patients undergoing surgery. Mitigating mortality and morbidity among high-risk individuals is a priority. Various risk-scoring systems are used to evaluate the risks associated with surgery. Cardiovascular risk assessment can be conducted following established guidelines. Utilizing individual preoperative risk assessment tools can help identify high-risk patients and guide risk-based stratification. There is a growing body of evidence to support frailty indices for risk-stratifying patients as well.

Frailty is defined by the WHO Clinical Consortium on Healthy Aging Report as "…a clinically recognizable state in which the ability of older people to cope with every day or acute stressors is compromised by an increased vulnerability brought by age-associated declines in physiological reserve and function across multiple organ systems." This points toward a biopsychosocial model for frailty, whilst in spinal literature a disease-based approach to frailty is often adopted. Many different frailty definitions and assessment tools are used in the literature. Regardless of the specific definition or assessment tool used, the presence and degree of frailty are associated with outcomes of spine surgery [32, 33].

Preoperative Interventions

Education and Expectation Management in Spine Surgery

Patient expectations have been shown to be an independent predictor of outcomes in the surgical population [34]. Greater fulfillment of preoperative expectations is associated with higher postoperative satisfaction [35]. As such, education and expectation management play critical roles in the success of prehabilitation programs and elective surgery in general. Prehabilitation programs often involve educating patients about their conditions, the upcoming surgery, and what they can expect during the recovery process. However, in clinical practice, there is large variability in delivery methods and the content of information provided to patients about their recovery and expected outcomes [36–38]. In a recent scoping review by Eubanks et al., six studies were identified that detailed education interventions prior to major surgery [38]. These studies used different prehabilitation education strategies including indepth information about the surgical procedure, reasons for having the surgery, expectations, risks, limitations, recovery process, and pain experience. In addition, studies delivered prehabilitation education in various ways, such as in-person explanations, phone calls, online educational sessions, recorded videos, illustrative images, and/or specific surveys. When applying such educational interventions in the preoperative period, patients have expressed satisfaction with as little as a single in-person physical therapy visit in conjunction with written and recorded educational materials [39].

Web-based audiovisual systems have also been effective in improving patients' understanding of general preoperative and postoperative care with the added benefit of convenience for surgical teams, as well [38]. In addition to reducing LOS, preoperative spinal education programs produce documented improvements in patients' overall biophysiological, functional, social, ethical, and financial knowledge. One study demonstrated that introducing ERAS principles to patients undergoing spinal surgery and general education enhanced patients' motivation to become mobile, and most patients found this process very useful during their preoperative and postoperative periods [40]. Poor reporting in the literature of differences in preoperative education across orthopedic surgery limits generalizability. At the time of this writing, the quality of reporting content, rationale, and frameworks remains a significant area of improvement to better understand the value of these interventions [41].

Education and Expectation Management in Joint Replacement

Just as "spine surgery" comprises an exceptionally heterogeneous group of back surgeries with variable risks of surgery and "opportunity cost" of inaction, "joint replacement" includes multiple large joint arthroplasties with highly disparate educational considerations. Specifically, a patient undergoing spine surgery or hip replacement may plan for a few days or weeks of decreased mobility, yet these patients are encouraged to ambulate to *some* extent during this period. As such, in most cases the required lifestyle modifications and caregiver support are limited.

Contrast this with typical total shoulder replacements that often mandate immobilization typically for 4–6 weeks [42]. Since shoulder glenohumeral osteoarthritis occurs frequently in patients' dominant arms, their basic understanding of these implications is a critical component of pre-procedural education [43, 44]. While non-complicated single hip replacements allow individuals to return home without heavy dependence on caregivers, standard shoulder replacements, rotator cuff repairs, and other procedures with prolonged postoperative immobilization necessitate planning ahead and potential inpatient rehabilitation. Although not frequently performed, simultaneous multi-joint procedures further increase reliance on others and likely have a higher incidence of postoperative complications like pulmonary embolism and 90-day readmission [45, 46].

One final aspect of pre-procedural education involves the discussion of secondary treatments in the event of infections like hardware infections. While likely not necessary for all individuals undergoing straightforward joint arthroplasty, high-risk individuals such as those with elevated BMIs, multiple comorbidities like diabetes, and/or advanced age may benefit from brief conversations regarding contingencies if faced with potential complications. These may include the need for subsequent interventions like reoperation with washout, IV antibiotics, or potentially even hardware replacement, and this review of surgical risk can serve as motivation for adherence to pre-procedural optimization recommendations [47].

4 Nutrition

The WHO defines malnutrition as deficiencies or excesses in nutrient intake, imbalance of essential nutrients, or impaired nutrient utilization. As such, "malnutrition" encompasses both under and overnutrition, although research has mainly focused on identifying and treating undernutrition before surgery. In orthopedic surgeries, malnutrition is associated with higher risks for complications like surgical site infections (SSIs) and increased hospital length of stay [48]. Clinicians can quantify malnutrition using serologic markers, anthropometric measurements, and screening tools, but currently, there is no accepted gold standard for diagnosing undernutrition. Serum albumin/prealbumin and transferrin are some of the most popular serological markers used for screening undernutrition in clinical settings, though these have limitations in certain situations like inflammation or acute change in nutritional status [49–51]. It is also worth considering overnutrition, which can manifest as metabolic syndrome, comprised of diabetes mellitus, hypercholesterolemia, hyperlipidemia, and similar conditions. Laboratory markers including HbA1c and/or fructosamine, lipid panels, and oral glucose tolerance test (OGTT) assessments should all be considered with aims to target tight glucose control and, of less certain significance, optimize lipid and cholesterol levels to prevent adverse outcomes including postoperative infections. Low serum transferrin preoperatively in orthopedic surgeries is also associated with delayed wound healing [52].

Major spine surgeries have been shown to significantly decrease postoperative nutritional parametric outcomes [53]. Physiologically, our bodies have significant energy expenditure during surgery necessitating higher than normal basal energy requirements leading to increased morbidity, increasing hospital length of stay, and delaying wound healing. Following spinal surgery, many patients become objectively malnourished as demonstrated by hypoalbuminemia with overall decreased lymphocyte count [54]. Aiming for albumin levels above at least 3.5 mg/dL and prealbumin levels of at least >20 mg/dL is ideal prior to undergoing elective spine surgery [55]. Often, recommendations are to achieve this through high-protein drinks or shakes. A daily supplement of 36 g of protein started 48 h before spine fusion surgery and continued for 30 days increased the cross-sectional area of paraspinal muscles and reduced muscle atrophy, with associated decreased pain and disability 30 days postoperatively. In addition, aiming for a TLC (total lymphocyte count) of >1500/mm^3 is another marker of immune competence and is decreased in malnourished patients [56]. Correcting iron-deficiency anemia is another meaningful intervention to include in the preoperative phase. Malnourished patients tend to have longer lengths of stay, often due to additional procedures.

Though the current standard of care is to fast patients (keep NPO) after midnight prior to the surgery, evidence suggests that carbohydrate treatments may replicate advantageous metabolic responses by stimulating endogenous insulin release and decrease peripheral insulin resistance, ultimately ameliorating key aspects of the surgical stress response [57]. A clear liquid beverage containing 12.5 g of carbohydrates/100 mL (containing 50 kcal/100 mL, 290 mOsm/kg, pH of 5.0) with polymers of carbohydrates that reduce osmotic load and do not delay gastric emptying can be considered in liberalized protocols 6 h before the initiation of anesthesia up to 2 h prior to surgery in select patients who are not high risk for postsurgical anesthesia-induced aspiration complications. Some evidence suggests this nutritional strategy can result in reduced length of stay with no significantly increased postoperative complications [58]. Gustafsson showed that type 2 diabetic patients demonstrated no difference in gastric emptying rates compared to healthy controls administered preoperative oral carbohydrate loading (CHO), indicating a low risk of hyperglycemia or preoperative aspiration [59, 60]. However, it is important to note that preoperative oral carbohydrate treatment may not be suitable for patients with confirmed delayed gastric emptying, gastrointestinal motility disorders, or those undergoing emergency surgery [59].

From a spine and musculoskeletal prehabilitation standpoint, newer studies have detailed a presurgical pathway to help optimize patients from a nutritional standpoint. A study by Briguglio et al. introduced the concepts of critical control points (CCP) [61]. They propose 3 CCP with the initial point consisting of evaluation 4–6 weeks to 1–2 months prior to the procedure. During this time, certain risk factors including iron status, excessive body weight, reduced muscle mass, poor protein intake, and poor dietary habits are initially identified. CCP also seeks to identify conditions where risk and severity necessitate monitoring. Closer to the surgery, priorities shift to focus more on balanced food choices such as whole grains, fruits vegetables, and proteins over issues like weight loss. The point in this example is that sufficient preoperative evaluation permits sufficient lead time to identify nutritional deficits and address them in time for surgery.

With regard to supplements, standardized recommendations before spine or joint surgeries are limited. However, given the favorable safety profile of creatine monohydrate [62], it may afford untrained individuals an additive benefit when combined with other hypertrophy-promoting strategies. One review identified the effects of creatine on muscle strength, lean mass, and functional capacity, but proposed daily low-dose supplementation for at least 12 weeks paired with resistance training as the necessary exposure timeline [63]. Other RCTs did not consistently reproduce the effect, however [64], but this may be related to age-dependent effects on response to supplementation with creatine [65].

5 Weight Control Interventions

Spinal Surgery and Weight Loss

Obesity among patients opting for spinal surgery presents a significant challenge in the preoperative phase as higher BMI is a risk factor for worse postoperative outcomes and higher complication rates [66–68]. While bariatric weight loss surgery before spine surgery may be indicated in patients with Class III obesity (formerly regarded as "morbid" obesity), surgeons should consider if it outweighs the potential risks, as weight loss surgery may increase the risk of postoperative complications by 10% in some assessments [69]. Furthermore, the procedure elevates the risk of undernutrition, due to reduced food intake and deliberate reduced nutrient absorption capacity, thereby potentially jeopardizing bone mineral density [70]. A conservative approach to weight control through diet and exercise should be prioritized for weight control in patients opting for spinal surgery, at least in the near term. Non-surgical weight loss interventions can achieve similar outcomes within a relatively short time frame of 3–12 months, especially given the advent of gastrointestinal peptide analog medications like semaglutide, tirzepatide, and others in development at the time of this writing [71]. Now, patients can obtain weight loss amounts previously seen only with bariatric surgery, improving their candidacy for forthcoming surgeries without first necessitating an initial surgery. This weight loss is specifically relevant prior to spine surgery, given the improvement in back pain patients will likely obtain even before surgery. Some patients will experience significant, clinically meaningful improvements in low back and knee pain with "only" 5+% body weight loss [72]. With pain reduction, patients receive subjective feedback on the effects of their initial efforts, fostering ongoing adherence to these and other recommendations. While the structural abnormalities will remain—i.e., prehab does not obviate the need for surgery—individuals' residual time before surgery is more tolerable, allowing for compounding benefits on outcomes from the eventual surgery.

Joint Replacement and Weight Loss

The benefits of weight loss applied in joint replacement candidate contexts are similar, as noted above. This illustrates the growing view of joint osteoarthritis as a metabolic disease as much as the previous perspective of it being "wear and tear." So, not only can metabolic disease control improve surgical outcomes for high-risk individuals [73], but it also may slow further progression in the interim and reduce pain [74, 75]. However, individuals discontinue antiobesity medications typically at least 2 weeks prior to surgery, and, for individuals who underwent bariatric surgery, short-term complication risk may be higher due to increased protein/micronutrient intake requirements [76].

Postoperatively, the earlier weight loss affords reduced weight stress through transplanted joints, likely facilitating earlier weight bearing and faster return to prior gait mechanics [77]. Weight loss preoperatively also reduces the need for post-operative opioid pain medication. With regards to certain weight loss strategies, some medications afford anti-inflammatory benefits outside of the direct effects of weight loss [78] and decreased risk of OA progression [79]. These medications may then improve joint pain through multiple mechanisms preoperatively.

6 Exercise Interventions

The process of prehabilitative exercise interventions carried out through a robust preoperative therapy-based regimen has been shown in several studies to optimize patient recovery following spine surgery [80]. Positive outcomes in postoperative pain and disability indices including the Oswestry Disability Index (ODI), Beck disability index, aerobic capacity, and muscular strength (e.g., quadriceps strength, trunk strength, and lumbar extension and flexion) as well as joint range of motion (ROM) have been observed and demonstrate that exercise-based prehabilitation programs that are individualized or tailored to the patient's needs are especially effective [38]. There is no one-size-fits-all physical exercise regimen, and each regimen's composition is dependent on the patient's function, strength, and pain tolerance. As noted in traditional (non-prehabilitation) lifestyle programs, the best available evidence continues to suggest that the ideal exercises for prehabilitation purposes in orthopedic surgeries are "the ones that patients will do"—i.e., implying consistency is more critical than exercise type.

Within joint arthroplasty prehabilitation, patients with structural risk factors for worsening joint health include pathology in dynamic stabilizers of the joint. For example, in the setting of glenohumeral osteoarthritis, individuals may have concomitant rotator cuff tendinopathy, thereby potentially accelerating the progression of joint disease [81, 82]. Similarly, weak gluteus medius muscles result in a trendelenburg gait that might worsen hip arthritis pain. Essentially, this secondary impact is analogous to weak hip girdle muscles adding to low back strain in patients with lumbar spinal stenosis [83].

In these cases, exercise and physical therapy can benefit chronic joint pain by targeting tendon pathology and dynamic stabilizers of joints. Further, physical therapy as a component of prehabilitation focuses on strengthening limbs that have likely been consciously or unconsciously offloaded for months or years. With deliberate disuse of a limb, even distal muscles experience underutilization, potentially contributing to functional impairment, pain, and fall risk. As such, prehabilitation therapies often include strengthening for immediate pain-relieving benefits as well as improved postoperative pain and function.

Aerobic Capacity Interventions

The ability to undergo physical stress and maintain consistent physiological reserve are both significant concepts for prehabilitation. Functional capacity is normally determined by cardiopulmonary exercise testing (CPET) and has been consistently associated with surgical outcome measures. Patients with poorer cardiorespiratory fitness tend to have worse postsurgical outcomes, which may include surgery-related morbidity and mortality, increased length of stay in the hospital or in sub-acute rehabilitation, and postoperative complications requiring readmissions [28]. From a respiratory health standpoint, the effects of prolonged anesthesia and analgesia as well as the location of the surgical incision are important to consider. Research has identified parametric meaningful changes including changes in lung volumes, decreased respiratory muscle strength, changes in ventilatory patterns, diaphragmatic dysfunction, and alterations in concentrations of carbon dioxide and oxygen exchanges in the lungs. Preoperative high-intensity interval training (HIIT) shows significant improvement in oxygen uptake at peak exercise (VO_{2peak}) in patients undergoing elective abdominal surgery [84]. In spinal fusion surgery, a pilot study showed similar improvements in preoperative aerobic capacity of 21% using a HITT intervention [12]. Improving aerobic capacity improved both LOS as well as inpatient recovery time.

Spine Surgery Resistance Training

Nonetheless, researchers have sought to identify specific programs with the greatest benefit for patients prior to spine surgeries. Marchand et al. noted significant improvements in a regimen involving five exercise phases consisting of concentric or isometric phases specifically tailored to the participants' progress, aiming to improve muscles and structures involved in ambulation [85]. These exercises included trunk stabilization and posterior chain strengthening exercises such as bridges and bird dogs, lower extremity strengthening exercises such as squats and leg lifts, and cycling, and aerobic endurance exercises. Figure 1 demonstrates typical trunk stabilizing and posterior chain strengthening exercises. Another physical therapy program featured in Fors et al. focused on improving walking distance in patients undergoing spine surgery and reported significant improvements in pain indices and muscle strength preoperatively. It has also been shown that regular physical exercise and sports participation improve postoperative outcomes in patients undergoing spine surgery [86]. There is growing evidence that exposure to programs such as f-HIIT programs (functional high-intensity interval training) can help improve the time to functional recovery in postsurgical spine patients [12]. Additionally, newer studies have shown improvements in ODI scores, timed up and go tests (TUGT), trunk flexor and extensor muscle strength, lumbopelvic stability, and lumbar multifidus muscle thickness after structured early aquatic exercise programs for patients who have undergone lumbar fusions [87].

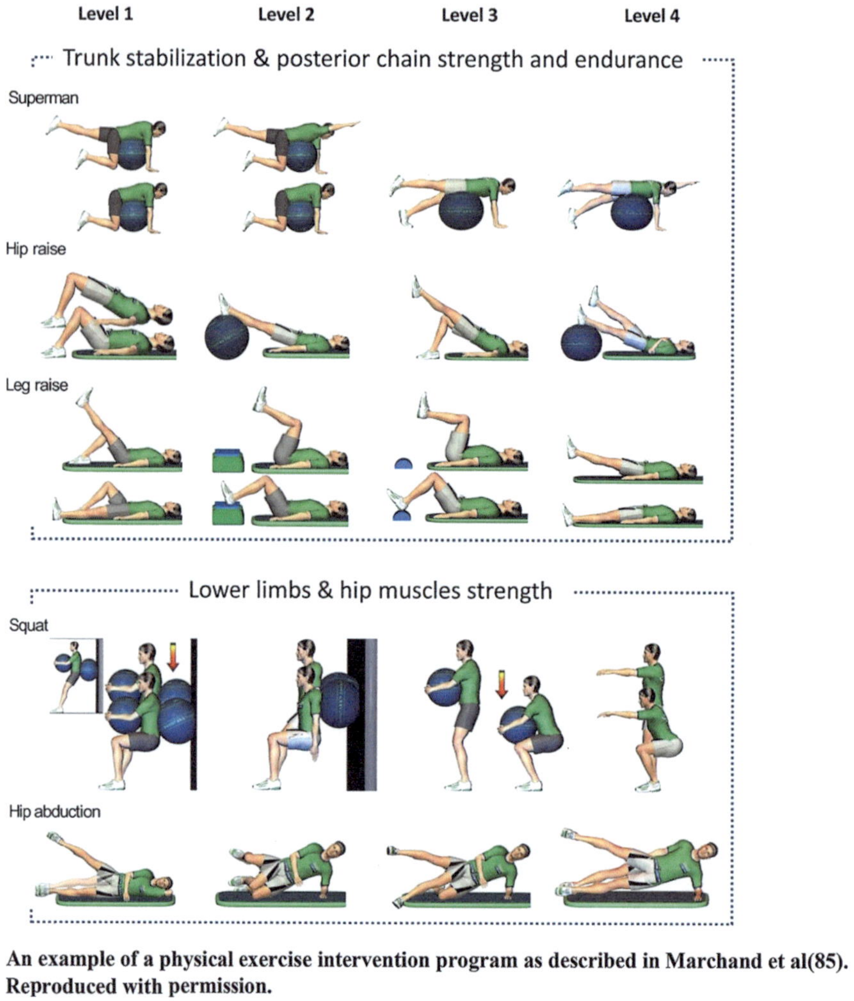

Fig. 1 An example of a physical exercise intervention program as described in Marchand et al. [85]. (Reproduced with permission)

Joint Replacement Resistance Training

As suggested earlier, health optimization strategy differences between spine versus joint replacement surgeries are often less related to one strategy's direct superiority and more about feasibility in the setting of pain. Specifically, heavy loads are difficult to bear on an arthritic joint. Considering this, joint replacement prehabilitation can become achievable with load (weight) reducing strategies such as higher-length partial repetitions and/or blood flow restriction therapy.

By reducing the range of motion and focusing exclusively on the eccentric phase when the muscle is at a longer length—i.e., the "deep stretch" portion of repetition, working muscles can maximize hypertrophic stimulus while limiting a painful range of motion [88]. This maximizes hypertrophy while likely maintaining greater joint stability during the working sets and improved flexibility in as little as 4–5 weeks of training [89, 90]. Although not well studied in this context, eccentric loading may have additional benefits with regard to preferentially strengthening myotendinous tissue and dynamic stabilizers around an arthritic joint, providing a theoretical benefit in this specific context [91].

Blood flow restriction training, as introduced in chapter "Basic Prehabilitation Pillars," uses a semi-occlusive tourniquet to impair venous outflow while leaving arterial inflow to a limb unaffected. In doing this, working muscles remain bathed in metabolic byproducts adding a chemical hypertrophic stimulus to mechanical stimuli [92]. If paired with other strategies like partial, long-length eccentric repetitions, any muscles distal to the tourniquet can achieve a growth stimulus with lower weight, thus minimizing joint-related discomfort.

7 Psychoeducative Interventions and Cognitive Behavioral Therapy (CBT)

Addressing patients' expectations and fears and managing underlying psychiatric issues including depression and anxiety have been shown to have positive outcomes in patients undergoing spine surgery including improved pain satisfaction scores, reduced pain catastrophizing, and facilitated faster return to regular physical activities [38]. Simply providing general education about the upcoming surgery including indepth information about the surgical procedure, reasons for having the surgery, expectations, risks, limitations, recovery process, and pain experience have been associated with improved outcomes [93]. These outcomes include improved patient satisfaction, greater functional improvements, reduced back pain, and decreased emergency department visits [94]. These studies have shown success in delivering prehabilitation education in various ways including in-person explanations, phone calls, online sessions, recorded videos, illustrative images, and/or specific surveys. These educational interventions may improve patients' understanding of postoperative care and management as well as patient satisfaction [95].

Edwards et al. showed that a preoperative spinal education (POSE) program consisting of a single, psychoeducative preparatory intervention involving a 60-min focus group designed to normalize pain expectations, talk patients through the process of physical rehabilitation, and hospital procedures, minimize anxieties, and support postsurgical recovery has shown promising success in post-operative outcomes [96]. This intervention involved a multi-disciplinary approach facilitated by two experienced senior clinicians in a live group with a pre-recorded spinal consultant video presentation, interactive discussion, and accompanying written literature. Pain neuroscience-based educational interventions are premised on a cognitive-behavioral framework and involve the process of making patients aware of the underlying processes governing pain through techniques such as metaphors, pictures, and examples to explain the biological complexity of pain in a comprehensive way to influence the patient's interpretation of their pain. This has been shown to improve surgical experience, reduce overall health costs, and even reduce postoperative health utilization [97].

One recommendation is to provide preoperative CBT that includes a comprehensive overview of information about how to interpret pain, pacing principles, return to work, and coping strategies in addition to surgical details. Typically, the effects of CBT are not seen within the immediate postoperative phase but instead improve disability postoperatively at the 1-year mark [98]. Focused CBT programs may also improve mobility and reduce analgesic use compared to usual care [99]. Additionally, a study by Lotske et al. suggested CBT may even have positive effects on health-related quality of life (HRQoL) measures even a week prior to surgery [100].

In the context of joint replacement, preoperative CBT provides similar benefits and may not require intensive interventions. One study of 4-week and 8-week telehealth-based preoperative cognitive behavioral therapy programs significantly reduced pain catastrophizing preoperatively. Conveniently, 4 weeks was not inferior to an 8-week program [101], potentially reducing resource constraints. However, by 3 months postoperatively, pain outcomes for both intervention groups and the control group were no longer significantly different, suggesting the benefit of CBT may be limited to the preoperative period. Even if this limitation is reproduced in other studies, improved preoperative pain perception is likely a valuable target, as it may improve participation in other prehabilitation therapies. A subsequent systematic review and meta-analysis elucidated this relationship further, identifying the primary benefit of preoperative CBT as short-term (<3 months) pain relief when compared with the "usual care" group, though not universally across all assessments. Longer duration pain relief was similar between groups [102].

8 Pain Management

Opioid Use and Preoperative Pain Control in Spine Surgery

The time immediately following spine surgery represents a challenging phase during the surgical continuum, especially while addressing postoperative pain. Chronic opioid use is associated with poorer postsurgical outcomes. Additionally, greater surgical invasiveness, anxiety, revision surgery, and greater preoperative opioid use are significantly associated with increased postoperative opioid dependence [103]. Opioids are also associated with well-established short- and long-term side effects, including perioperative nausea/vomiting, ileus, pruritus, respiratory depression, urinary retention, and somnolence. Chronic opioid use is associated with increased postoperative pain, opioid dependence, increased burden on healthcare resources, hyperalgesia, sexual dysfunction, bone fracture, and increased risk of myocardial infarction [104].

Controlling patient anxiety, depression, pain catastrophizing and pain sensitivity, as well as preoperative opioid consumption can reduce the incidence of chronic pain and chronic opioid dependence following surgery [105]. Around 4–6 weeks prior to surgery, it is crucial to control some of these factors. A comprehensive psychosocial prehabilitation intervention including CBT (ideally facilitated by a pain psychologist) emphasizing the importance of minimizing opioid use, addressing physical fitness through a robust PT program, and promoting good nutrition have been shown to reduce post-operative pain, improve general well-being and pain satisfaction, reduce opioid utilization, and reduce the utilization of the emergency department postoperatively [106–108]. In addition, the utilization of multimodal analgesia including alternatives to systemic opioids such as NSAIDs, acetaminophen, gabapentin, and pregabalin has demonstrated utility in decreasing postoperative opioid use. In patients undergoing spine surgery, it is recommended to provide NSAIDs along with a lower dose of opioids in patients who are already receiving opioids preoperatively [109]. This practice is associated with reduced VAS scores and opioid dependence postoperatively [110]. In addition, utilization of adjunctive oral or IV acetaminophen has shown efficacy in decreasing pain scores during the acute preoperative phase. Gabapentin and pregabalin may decrease preoperative pain intensity, reduce opioid dependence, and improve functional outcomes postoperatively [104]. Finally, alpha2 agonist medications like clonidine, tizanidine, and dexmedetomidine may reduce perioperative opioid use as well as symptomatic muscle spasms without the risk of dependence seen in benzodiazepines, serotonergic interactions as noted with cyclobenzaprine, and limitations in renal impairment seen with baclofen [111]. Ultimately, a multimodal analgesic approach to pre- and post-operative pain is recommended. A common preoperative regimen of acetaminophen, NSAIDs, and gabapentinoid, with standardized intraoperative and postoperative pain control has demonstrated efficacy in minimizing postoperative opioid use, improving ODI scores, and reducing time to mobilization [112–114].

Lumbar spinal stenosis with neurogenic claudication is responsive to one additional, unique mechanistic target. As neurogenic claudication is presumed to be at least partially the result of vascular compromise in the spine, medications to directly target this pathophysiology have suitability in this subset of patients. Limaprost is a prostaglandin E1 analog that promotes vasodilation of small vessels and can significantly improve neurogenic claudication [115]. Other analogs like misoprostol may have similar efficacy; though, the evidence supporting this isn't as robust.

Preoperative Pain Control in Joint Replacement

As spine surgery prehabilitation affords unique pain control targets, so too does joint replacement. Specifically, in addition to systemically active oral medications, clinicians can target joint pain from advanced osteoarthritis using local injections of different medications and preparations. Intra-articular injections of corticosteroids, NSAIDs, hyaluronic acid, and "orthobiologic" therapies like platelet-rich plasma and others, described in greater detail in chapter "Basic Prehabilitation Pillars," each offers unique risks, benefits, and uncertainties. For example, corticosteroids are potent anti-inflammatories, but are chondrotoxic and impair immune function, typically necessitating a waiting period after injection before elective joint replacement, though the literature is unclear on this requirement [116]. NSAIDs like ketorolac may reduce pain as well with less risk to cartilage health and immune response.

Hyaluronic acid (HA) is a naturally occurring substance in joint spaces, and original intra-articular use focused on the substance's viscosity and, to a lesser extent, potential antioxidant and anti-inflammatory properties [117]. However, HA has utility as a delivery vector by acting as a component of nanoparticles surrounding other anti-inflammatory medications. By potentially mediating uptake, HA nanoparticles may improve the targeting of inflamed tissues in a time-release fashion [118, 119]. HA preparations currently are FDA-approved predominantly for knee osteoarthritis, and despite studies supporting efficacy in other joints with osteoarthritis like the glenohumeral joint, lack of FDA approval permits insurance companies to consider these treatments "experimental" and deny coverage [120].

Platelet-rich plasma (PRP) injections and newer orthobiologic injections like exosome therapy are similarly considered experimental and are not typically reimbursed by insurance providers. Research in the context of prehabilitation is limited, but one review of PRP for knee osteoarthritis did not identify outcomes or benefits with regard to procedure-specific endpoints [121]. However, in patients with knee pain after TKA, it may provide significant pain relief for some [122] and may delay the need for joint replacement [123].

9 Smoking and Alcohol Use

There is high-quality evidence for poor post-surgical outcomes in patients with active alcohol and tobacco use disorders. The postoperative morbidity is said to be increased by nearly two to three-fold with regular alcohol overconsumption, and it is also associated with an increased risk of general infections, poor wound healing, pulmonary complications, increased reoperation rates, prolonged stay at the hospital, and increased rates of ICU admission [6, 124, 125]. It is recommended that at least 1 month of abstinence prior to surgery is adequate for reducing complications [126]. Smoking is also associated with a 25% increased chance of death, increased risk of nonunion and pseudoarthrosis in spinal fusion surgeries, and worse pain indices scores including ODI, EuroQoL, and Short-Form 36 surveys. Smoking has also been associated with increased risk of infection, perioperative respiratory problems, and wound complications [59]. Smoking cessation should be encouraged as early as possible as longer periods without smoking have been associated with a decreasing risk of postoperative complications. Generally, however, at least 4–6 weeks of smoking cessation is recommended preoperatively and is strongly recommended through at least up to 6 months after surgery [127].

10 Summary and Key Points

- Although ideally implemented as part of conservative care for spine and joint conditions before surgery is considered, in practice many patients pursuing elective orthopedic surgeries have deficits in knowledge, fitness, and nutrition that should be addressed preoperatively to improve surgical outcomes.
- Appropriate prehabilitation activities include exercises to support aerobic conditioning (often assessed through VO_{2max}) and muscle hypertrophy.
- Nutritional recommendations should be tailored to the appropriate time frame before surgery: longer time periods allow for more comprehensive interventions that focus on issues such as weight loss, glucose control, and sarcopenia reversal for improvements in body composition. In shorter time frames, recommendations should focus on achievable short-term goals such as sufficient protein intake and carbohydrate restriction when necessary in the days-weeks leading up to surgery.
- Smoking cessation is a key lifestyle factor that improves postoperative outcomes but may worsen respiratory symptoms in the initial weeks.
- Multimodal pain management in the prehabilitation period coupled with appropriate postoperative pain control can decrease postoperative opioid use and reduce time to mobilization, potentially reducing secondary complications.

References

1. Banugo P, Amoako D. Prehabilitation. BJA Educ. 2017;17(12):401–5.
2. Teitz CC, Cook DM. Rehabilitation of neck and low back injuries. Clin Sports Med. 1985;4(3):455–76.
3. Brady L. A multifaceted approach to prevention of thromboembolism: a report of 529 cases. South Med J. 1977;70(5):546–8.
4. Ditmyer MM, Topp R, Pifer M. Prehabilitation in preparation for orthopaedic surgery. Orthop Nurs. 2002;21(5):43–54.
5. Nielsen PR, Andreasen J, Asmussen M, Tønnesen H. Costs and quality of life for prehabilitation and early rehabilitation after surgery of the lumbar spine. BMC Health Serv Res. 2008;8:1–7.
6. Kehlet H. Multimodal approach to control postoperative pathophysiology and rehabilitation. Br J Anaesth. 1997;78(5):606–17.
7. Rana AJ, Bozic KJ. Bundled payments in orthopaedics. Clin Orthop Relat Res. 2015;473(2):422–5.
8. Cieza A, Causey K, Kamenov K, Hanson SW, Chatterji S, Vos T. Global estimates of the need for rehabilitation based on the Global Burden of Disease Study 2019: a systematic analysis for the Global Burden of Disease Study 2019. Lancet. 2020;396(10267):2006–17.
9. Urits I, Burshtein A, Sharma M, Testa L, Gold PA, Orhurhu V, et al. Low back pain, a comprehensive review: pathophysiology, diagnosis, and treatment. Curr Pain Headache Rep. 2019;23:1–10.
10. Dieleman JL, Cao J, Chapin A, Chen C, Li Z, Liu A, et al. US health care spending by payer and health condition, 1996-2016. JAMA. 2020;323(9):863–84.
11. Yelin E, Weinstein S, King T. The burden of musculoskeletal diseases in the United States. Semin Arthritis Rheum. 2016;46(3):259–60.

12. Janssen ER, Punt IM, Biemans CF, van Rhijn L, Willems PC, van Meeteren NL. Preoperative community based functional high intensity interval training (f-HIIT) with high-risk patients opting for lumbar spinal fusion: a pilot study. Disabil Rehabil. 2023;45(5):805–13.
13. Rombey T, Eckhardt H, Kiselev J, Silzle J, Mathes T, Quentin W. Cost-effectiveness of prehabilitation prior to elective surgery: a systematic review of economic evaluations. BMC Med. 2023;21(1):265.
14. Nielsen PR, Jørgensen LD, Dahl B, Pedersen T, Tønnesen H. Prehabilitation and early rehabilitation after spinal surgery: randomized clinical trial. Clin Rehabil. 2010;24(2):137–48.
15. Garrison SR, Schneider KE, Singh M, Pogodzinski J. Preoperative physical therapy results in shorter length of stay and discharge disposition following total knee arthroplasty: a retrospective study. J Rehabil Med Clin Commun. 2019;2:2.
16. Johnson CD, Haldeman S, Chou R, Nordin M, Green BN, Côté P, et al. The Global Spine Care Initiative: model of care and implementation. Eur Spine J. 2018;27:925–45.
17. McIsaac DI, Gill M, Boland L, Hutton B, Branje K, Shaw J, et al. Prehabilitation in adult patients undergoing surgery: an umbrella review of systematic reviews. Br J Anaesth. 2022;128(2):244–57.
18. NICE Guideline NG226. Osteoarthritis in over 16s: diagnosis and management. Methods. 2022.
19. Grotle M, Småstuen MC, Fjeld O, Grøvle L, Helgeland J, Storheim K, et al. Lumbar spine surgery across 15 years: trends, complications and reoperations in a longitudinal observational study from Norway. BMJ Open. 2019;9(8):e028743.
20. Poorman GW, Moon JY, Wang C, Horn SR, Beaubrun BM, Bono OJ, et al. Rates of mortality in lumbar spine surgery and factors associated with its occurrence over a 10-year period: a study of 803,949 patients in the nationwide inpatient sample. Int J Spine Surg. 2018;12(5):617–23.
21. Zaina F, Tomkins-Lane C, Carragee E, Negrini S. Surgical versus non-surgical treatment for lumbar spinal stenosis. Cochrane Database Syst Rev. 2016;2016(1):CD010264.
22. Upfill-Brown A, Paisner N, Sassoon A. Racial disparities in post-operative complications and discharge destination following total joints arthroplasty: a national database study. Arch Orthop Trauma Surg. 2023;143(4):2227–33.
23. Malkani JA, Heimroth JC, Ong KL, Wilson H, Price M, Piuzzi NS, et al. Complications and readmission incidence following Total hip arthroplasty in patients who have end-stage renal failure. J Arthroplast. 2020;35(3):794–800.
24. Margraf A, Ludwig N, Zarbock A, Rossaint J. Systemic inflammatory response syndrome after surgery: mechanisms and protection. Anesth Analg. 2020;131(6):1693–707.
25. Gagliardi AR, Yip CY, Irish J, Wright FC, Rubin B, Ross H, et al. The psychological burden of waiting for procedures and patient-centred strategies that could support the mental health of wait-listed patients and caregivers during the COVID-19 pandemic: a scoping review. Health Expect. 2021;24(3):978–90.
26. Ackerman IN, Bennell KL, Osborne RH. Decline in health-related quality of life reported by more than half of those waiting for joint replacement surgery: a prospective cohort study. BMC Musculoskelet Disord. 2011;12:1–9.
27. Bardram L, Funch-Jensen P, Jensen P, Kehlet H, Crawford M. Recovery after laparoscopic colonic surgery with epidural analgesia, and early oral nutrition and mobilisation. Lancet. 1995;345(8952):763–4.
28. Hulzebos E, Van Meeteren N. Making the elderly fit for surgery. J Br Surg. 2016;103(2):e12–5.
29. Glassman SD, Carreon LY, Djurasovic M, Dimar JR, Johnson JR, Puno RM, et al. Lumbar fusion outcomes stratified by specific diagnostic indication. Spine J. 2009;9(1):13–21.
30. Neuprez A, Neuprez AH, Kaux J-F, Kurth W, Daniel C, Thirion T, et al. Total joint replacement improves pain, functional quality of life, and health utilities in patients with late-stage knee and hip osteoarthritis for up to 5 years. Clin Rheumatol. 2020;39(3):861–71.
31. Kee JR, Mears SC, Edwards PK, Barnes CL. Modifiable risk factors are common in early revision hip and knee arthroplasty. J Arthroplast. 2017;32(12):3689–92.

32. Mohamed B, Ramachandran R, Rabai F, Price CC, Polifka A, Hoh D, et al. Frailty assessment and prehabilitation before complex spine surgery in patients with degenerative spine disease: a narrative review. J Neurosurg Anesthesiol. 2023;35(1):19–30.
33. Bai Y, Zhang X-M, Sun X, Li J, Cao J, Wu X. The association between frailty and mortality among lower limb arthroplasty patients: a systematic review and meta-analysis. BMC Geriatr. 2022;22(1):702.
34. Swarup I, Henn CM, Gulotta LV, Henn RF III. Patient expectations and satisfaction in orthopaedic surgery: a review of the literature. J Clin Orthop Trauma. 2019;10(4):755–60.
35. Soroceanu A, Ching A, Abdu W, McGuire K. Relationship between preoperative expectations, satisfaction, and functional outcomes in patients undergoing lumbar and cervical spine surgery: a multicenter study. Spine. 2012;37(2):E103–8.
36. Janssen ER, Scheijen EE, van Meeteren NL, de Bie RA, Lenssen AF, Willems PC, et al. Determining clinical practice of expert physiotherapy for patients undergoing lumbar spinal fusion: a cross-sectional survey study. Eur Spine J. 2016;25:1533–41.
37. Rushton A, Wright C, Heap A, White L, Eveleigh G, Heneghan N. Survey of current physiotherapy practice for patients undergoing lumbar spinal fusion in the United Kingdom. Spine. 2014;39(23):E1380–7.
38. Eubanks JE, Carlesso C, Sundaram M, Bejarano G, Smeets RJ, Skolasky R, et al. Prehabilitation for spine surgery: a scoping review. PM R. 2023;15(10):1335–50.
39. Eubanks JE, Cupler ZA, Gliedt JA, Bejarano G, Skolasky RL, Smeets RJ, et al. Preoperative spinal education for lumbar spinal stenosis: a feasibility study. PM R. 2024;16:992.
40. Fleege C, Arabmotlagh M, Almajali A, Rauschmann M. Pre-and postoperative fast-track treatment concepts in spinal surgery: patient information and patient cooperation. Orthopade. 2014;43:1062–9.
41. Furtado R, MacDermid JC, Ziebart C, Bryant D, Faber KJ. Preoperative patient education programs for orthopaedic surgery: what do the programs include? How are they delivered? What are the knowledge gaps? A scoping review of 46 studies. J Orthop Sports Phys Ther. 2022;52(9):572–85.
42. Hagen MS, Allahabadi S, Zhang AL, Feeley BT, Grace T, Ma CB. A randomized single-blinded trial of early rehabilitation versus immobilization after reverse total shoulder arthroplasty. J Shoulder Elb Surg. 2020;29(3):442–50.
43. Ibounig T, Simons T, Launonen A, Paavola M. Glenohumeral osteoarthritis: an overview of etiology and diagnostics. Scand J Surg. 2021;110(3):441–51.
44. Schoenfeldt TL, Trenhaile S, Olson R. Glenohumeral osteoarthritis: frequency of underlying diagnoses and the role of arm dominance—a retrospective analysis in a community-based musculoskeletal practice. Rheumatol Int. 2018;38(6):1023–9.
45. Yeager AM, Ruel AV, Westrich GH. Are bilateral total joint arthroplasty patients at a higher risk of developing pulmonary embolism following total hip and knee surgery? J Arthroplast. 2014;29(5):900–2.
46. Sheth DS, Cafri G, Paxton EW, Namba RS. Bilateral simultaneous vs staged total knee arthroplasty: a comparison of complications and mortality. J Arthroplast. 2016;31(9 Suppl):212–6.
47. Layon DR, Johns WL, Morrell AT, Perera R, Patel NK, Golladay GJ, et al. Does adherence to preoperative surgical selection criteria reduce the rate of prosthetic joint infection in primary and revision total knee arthroplasties? Arthroplast Today. 2020;6(3):410–3.
48. Cass AR, Charlton KE. Prevalence of hospital-acquired malnutrition and modifiable determinants of nutritional deterioration during inpatient admissions: a systematic review of the evidence. J Hum Nutr Diet. 2022;35(6):1043–58.
49. Keller U. Nutritional laboratory markers in malnutrition. J Clin Med. 2019;8(6):775.
50. Ranasinghe RN, Biswas M, Vincent RP. Prealbumin: the clinical utility and analytical methodologies. Ann Clin Biochem. 2022;59(1):7–14.
51. Alcorta MD, Alvarez PC, Cabetas RN, Martín MJA, Valero M, Candela CG. The importance of serum albumin determination method to classify patients based on nutritional status. Clin Nutr ESPEN. 2018;25:110–3.

52. Gherini S, Vaughn BK, Lombardi AVJ, Mallory TH. Delayed wound healing and nutritional deficiencies after total hip arthroplasty. Clin Orthop Relat Res (1976–2007). 1993;293:188.
53. Lalueza MP, Colomina MJ, Bagó J, Clemente S, Godet C. Analysis of nutritional parameters in idiopathic scoliosis patients after major spinal surgery. Eur J Clin Nutr. 2005;59(5):720–2.
54. Khalooeifard R, Shariatpanahi ZV, Ahani A, Keykhaee M, Oraee-Yazdani M, Zali A, et al. Effect of protein supplement on paraspinal muscles in spine fusion surgery: a randomized, double-blind, placebo-controlled trial. Int J Spine Surg. 2021;15(1):47–54.
55. Klein JD, Hey LA, Yu CS, Klein BB, Coufal FJ, Young EP, et al. Perioperative nutrition and postoperative complications in patients undergoing spinal surgery. Spine. 1996;21(22):2676–82.
56. Mandelbaum BR, Tolo VT, McAfee PC, Burest P. Nutritional deficiencies after staged anterior and posterior spinal reconstructive surgery. Clin Orthop Relat Res. 1988;234:5–11.
57. Ljungqvist O, Søreide E. Preoperative fasting. J Br Surg. 2003;90(4):400–6.
58. Smith MD, McCall J, Plank L, Herbison GP, Soop M, Nygren J. Preoperative carbohydrate treatment for enhancing recovery after elective surgery. Cochrane Database Syst Rev. 2014;(8):CD009161.
59. Licina A, Silvers A, Laughlin H, Russell J, Wan C. Pathway for enhanced recovery after spinal surgery-a systematic review of evidence for use of individual components. BMC Anesthesiol. 2021;21:1–21.
60. Gustafsson U, Nygren J, Thorell A, Soop M, Hellström P, Ljungqvist O, et al. Pre-operative carbohydrate loading may be used in type 2 diabetes patients. Acta Anaesthesiol Scand. 2008;52(7):946–51.
61. Briguglio M, Wainwright TW. Nutritional and physical prehabilitation in elective orthopedic surgery: rationale and proposal for implementation. Ther Clin Risk Manag. 2022;18:21–30.
62. de Guingand DL, Palmer KR, Snow RJ, Davies-Tuck ML, Ellery SJ. Risk of adverse outcomes in females taking oral creatine monohydrate: a systematic review and meta-analysis. Nutrients. 2020;12(6):1780.
63. Stares A, Bains M. The additive effects of creatine supplementation and exercise training in an aging population: a systematic review of randomized controlled trials. J Geriatr Phys Ther. 2020;43(2):99–112.
64. Candow DG, Chilibeck PD, Gordon J, Vogt E, Landeryou T, Kaviani M, et al. Effect of 12 months of creatine supplementation and whole-body resistance training on measures of bone, muscle and strength in older males. Nutr Health. 2021;27(2):151–9.
65. Burke R, Piñero A, Coleman M, Mohan A, Sapuppo M, Augustin F, et al. The effects of creatine supplementation combined with resistance training on regional measures of muscle hypertrophy: a systematic review with meta-analysis. Nutrients. 2023;15(9):2116.
66. Ross DA, Iyer S, Ross MN. Trends in weight and body mass index after spinal surgery for degenerative disease. Int J Spine Surg. 2021;15(4):834–9.
67. Janssen ER, Punt IM, van Kuijk SM, Hoebink EA, van Meeteren NL, Willems PC. Development and validation of a prediction tool for pain reduction in adult patients undergoing elective lumbar spinal fusion: a multicentre cohort study. Eur Spine J. 2020;29:1909–16.
68. Higgins DM, Mallory GW, Planchard RF, Puffer RC, Ali M, Gates MJ, et al. Understanding the impact of obesity on short-term outcomes and in-hospital costs after instrumented spinal fusion. Neurosurgery. 2016;78(1):127–32.
69. Rudy HL, Cho W, Oster BA, Tarpada SP, Moran-Atkin E. Rapid bodyweight reduction before lumbar fusion surgery increased postoperative complications. Asian Spine J. 2020;14(5):613.
70. Epstein NE. Bariatric bypasses contribute to loss of bone mineral density but reduce axial back pain in morbidly obese patients considering spine surgery. Surg Neurol Int. 2017;8:13.
71. Wing RR, Hill JO. Successful weight loss maintenance. Annu Rev Nutr. 2001;21(1):323–41.
72. Dunlevy C, MacLellan GA, O'Malley E, Blake C, Breen C, Gaynor K, et al. Does changing weight change pain? Retrospective data analysis from a national multidisciplinary weight management service. Eur J Pain. 2019;23(8):1403–15.

73. Lau LCM, Chan PK, Lui TWD, Choi SW, Au E, Leung T, et al. Preoperative weight loss interventions before total hip and knee arthroplasty: a systematic review of randomized controlled trials. Arthroplasty. 2024;6(1):30.
74. Seward MW, Briggs LG, Bain PA, Chen AF. Preoperative nonsurgical weight loss interventions before total hip and knee arthroplasty: a systematic review. J Arthroplast. 2021;36(11):3796–806.e8.
75. Liljensøe A, Laursen J, Bliddal H, Søballe K, Mechlenburg I. Weight loss intervention before total knee replacement: a 12-month randomized controlled trial. Scand J Surg. 2021;110(1):3–12.
76. Liu JX, Paoli AR, Mahure SA, Bosco J III, Campbell KA. Preoperative bariatric surgery utilization is associated with increased 90-day postoperative complication rates after total joint arthroplasty. J Am Acad Orthop Surg. 2020;28(5):e206–12.
77. Stock LA, Brennan JC, Turcotte JJ, King PJ. Effect of weight change on patient-reported outcomes following total joint arthroplasty. J Arthroplast. 2022;37(10):1991–7.e1.
78. Baser O, Isenman L, Baser S, Samayoa G. Impact of semaglutide on osteoarthritis risk in patients with obesity: a retrospective cohort study. Obes Sci Pract. 2024;10(3):e762.
79. Zhu H, Zhou L, Wang Q, Cai Q, Yang F, Jin H, et al. Glucagon-like peptide-1 receptor agonists as a disease-modifying therapy for knee osteoarthritis mediated by weight loss: findings from the Shanghai Osteoarthritis Cohort. Ann Rheum Dis. 2023;82(9):1218–26.
80. Punnoose A, Claydon-Mueller LS, Weiss O, Zhang J, Rushton A, Khanduja V. Prehabilitation for patients undergoing orthopedic surgery: a systematic review and meta-analysis. JAMA Netw Open. 2023;6(4):e238050.
81. Chalmers PN, Salazar DH, Steger-May K, Chamberlain AM, Stobbs-Cucchi G, Yamaguchi K, et al. Radiographic progression of arthritic changes in shoulders with degenerative rotator cuff tears. J Shoulder Elb Surg. 2016;25(11):1749–55.
82. Vocelle AR, Weidig G, Bush TR. Shoulder structure and function: the impact of osteoarthritis and rehabilitation strategies. J Hand Ther. 2022;35(3):377–87.
83. Dwyer MK, Stafford K, Mattacola CG, Uhl TL, Giordani M. Comparison of gluteus medius muscle activity during functional tasks in individuals with and without osteoarthritis of the hip joint. Clin Biomech. 2013;28(7):757–61.
84. Franssen RF, Janssen-Heijnen ML, Barberan-Garcia A, Vogelaar FJ, Van Meeteren NL, Bongers BC. Moderate-intensity exercise training or high-intensity interval training to improve aerobic fitness during exercise prehabilitation in patients planned for elective abdominal cancer surgery? Eur J Surg Oncol. 2022;48(1):3–13.
85. Marchand A-A, Suitner M, O'Shaughnessy J, Châtillon C-É, Cantin V, Descarreaux M. Feasibility of conducting an active exercise prehabilitation program in patients awaiting spinal stenosis surgery: a randomized pilot study. Sci Rep. 2019;9(1):12257.
86. Fors M, Enthoven P, Abbott A, Öberg B. Effects of pre-surgery physiotherapy on walking ability and lower extremity strength in patients with degenerative lumbar spine disorder: secondary outcomes of the PREPARE randomised controlled trial. BMC Musculoskelet Disord. 2019;20:1–11.
87. Huang A-H, Chou W-H, Wang WT-J, Chen W-Y, Shih Y-F. Effects of early aquatic exercise intervention on trunk strength and functional recovery of patients with lumbar fusion: a randomized controlled trial. Sci Rep. 2023;13(1):10716.
88. Pedrosa GF, Lima FV, Schoenfeld BJ, Lacerda LT, Simões MG, Pereira MR, et al. Partial range of motion training elicits favorable improvements in muscular adaptations when carried out at long muscle lengths. Eur J Sport Sci. 2022;22(8):1250–60.
89. Kay AD, Baxter B, Hill M, Blazevich A. Effects of eccentric resistance training on lower-limb passive joint range of motion: a systematic review and meta-analysis. Med Sci Sports Exerc. 2023;55(4):710–21.
90. Dejaco B, Habets B, van Loon C, van Grinsven S, van Cingel R. Eccentric versus conventional exercise therapy in patients with rotator cuff tendinopathy: a randomized, single blinded, clinical trial. Knee Surg Sports Traumatol Arthrosc. 2017;25:2051–9.

91. Ortega-Castillo M, Medina-Porqueres I. Effectiveness of the eccentric exercise therapy in physically active adults with symptomatic shoulder impingement or lateral epicondylar tendinopathy: a systematic review. J Sci Med Sport. 2016;19(6):438–53.
92. Bobes Álvarez C, Issa-Khozouz Santamaria P, Fernández-Matías R, Pecos-Martín D, Achalandabaso-Ochoa A, Fernández-Carnero S, et al. Comparison of blood flow restriction training versus non-occlusive training in patients with anterior cruciate ligament reconstruction or knee osteoarthritis: a systematic review. J Clin Med. 2020;10(1):68.
93. Kesänen J, Leino-Kilpi H, Lund T, Montin L, Puukka P, Valkeapää K. The Knowledge Test Feedback Intervention (KTFI) increases knowledge level of spinal stenosis patients before operation—a randomized controlled follow-up trial. Patient Educ Couns. 2016;99(12):1984–91.
94. Strøm J, Nielsen CV, Jørgensen LB, Andersen NT, Laursen M. A web-based platform to accommodate symptoms of anxiety and depression by featuring social interaction and animated information in patients undergoing lumbar spine fusion: a randomized clinical trial. Spine J. 2019;19(5):827–39.
95. Gautschi OP, Stienen MN, Hermann C, Cadosch D, Fournier J-Y, Hildebrandt G. Web-based audiovisual patient information system—a study of preoperative patient information in a neurosurgical department. Acta Neurochir. 2010;152:1337–41.
96. Edwards R, Gibson J, Mungin-Jenkins E, Pickford R, Lucas JD, Jones GD. A preoperative spinal education intervention for spinal fusion surgery designed using the rehabilitation treatment specification system is safe and could reduce hospital length of stay, normalize expectations, and reduce anxiety: a prospective cohort study. Bone Joint Open. 2022;3(2):135–44.
97. Huysmans E, Goudman L, Coppieters I, Van Bogaert W, Moens M, Buyl R, et al. Effect of perioperative pain neuroscience education in people undergoing surgery for lumbar radiculopathy: a multicentre randomised controlled trial. Br J Anaesth. 2023;131(3):572–85.
98. Rolving N, Nielsen CV, Christensen FB, Holm R, Bünger CE, Oestergaard LG. Does a preoperative cognitive-behavioral intervention affect disability, pain behavior, pain, and return to work the first year after lumbar spinal fusion surgery? Spine (Phila Pa 1976). 2015;40:593.
99. Rolving N, Nielsen CV, Christensen FB, Holm R, Bünger CE, Oestergaard LG. Preoperative cognitive-behavioural intervention improves in-hospital mobilisation and analgesic use for lumbar spinal fusion patients. BMC Musculoskelet Disord. 2016;17:1–7.
100. Lotzke H, Brisby H, Gutke A, Hägg O, Jakobsson M, Smeets R, et al. A person-centered prehabilitation program based on cognitive-behavioral physical therapy for patients scheduled for lumbar fusion surgery: a randomized controlled trial. Phys Ther. 2019;99(8):1069–88.
101. Buvanendran A, Sremac AC, Merriman PA, Della Valle CJ, Burns JW, McCarthy RJ. Preoperative cognitive–behavioral therapy for reducing pain catastrophizing and improving pain outcomes after total knee replacement: a randomized clinical trial. Reg Anesth Pain Med. 2021;46(4):313–21.
102. Zhang F, Wang L-Y, Chen Z-L, Cao X-Y, Chen B-Y. Cognitive behavioral therapy achieves better benefits in relieving postoperative pain and improving joint function: a systematic review and meta-analysis of randomized controlled trials. J Orthop Sci. 2024;29:681.
103. Armaghani SJ, Lee DS, Bible JE, Archer KR, Shau DN, Kay H, et al. Preoperative opioid use and its association with perioperative opioid demand and postoperative opioid independence in patients undergoing spine surgery. Spine. 2014;39(25):E1524–30.
104. Dunn LK, Durieux ME, Nemergut EC. Non-opioid analgesics: novel approaches to perioperative analgesia for major spine surgery. Best Pract Res Clin Anaesthesiol. 2016;30(1):79–89.
105. Costelloe C, Burns S, Yong RJ, Kaye AD, Urman RD. An analysis of predictors of persistent postoperative pain in spine surgery. Curr Pain Headache Rep. 2020;24:1–6.
106. Santa Mina D, Scheede-Bergdahl C, Gillis C, Carli F. Optimization of surgical outcomes with prehabilitation. Appl Physiol Nutr Metab. 2015;40(9):966–9.
107. Powell R, Scott NW, Manyande A, Bruce J, Vögele C, Byrne-Davis LM, et al. Psychological preparation and postoperative outcomes for adults undergoing surgery under general anaesthesia. Cochrane Database Syst Rev. 2016;(5):CD008646.

108. Aglio LS, Mezzalira E, Mendez-Pino L, Corey SM, Fields KG, Abbakar R, et al. Surgical prehabilitation: strategies and psychological intervention to reduce postoperative pain and opioid use. Anesth Analg. 2022;134(5):1106–11.
109. Jirarattanaphochai K, Jung S. Nonsteroidal antiinflammatory drugs for postoperative pain management after lumbar spine surgery: a meta-analysis of randomized controlled trials. J Neurosurg Spine. 2008;9(1):22–31.
110. De Oliveira Jr GS, Castro-Alves LJ, McCarthy RJ. Single-dose systemic acetaminophen to prevent postoperative pain: a meta-analysis of randomized controlled trials. Clin J Pain. 2015;31(1):86–93.
111. Smith H, Elliott J. Alpha2 receptors and agonists in pain management. Curr Opin Anesthesiol. 2001;14(5):513–8.
112. Mathiesen O, Dahl B, Thomsen BA, Kitter B, Sonne N, Dahl JB, et al. A comprehensive multimodal pain treatment reduces opioid consumption after multilevel spine surgery. Eur Spine J. 2013;22:2089–96.
113. Garcia RM, Cassinelli EH, Messerschmitt PJ, Furey CG, Bohlman HH. A multimodal approach for postoperative pain management after lumbar decompression surgery: a prospective, randomized study. Clin Spine Surg. 2013;26(6):291–7.
114. Kim S-I, Ha K-Y, Oh I-S. Preemptive multimodal analgesia for postoperative pain management after lumbar fusion surgery: a randomized controlled trial. Eur Spine J. 2016;25:1614–9.
115. Matsudaira K, Seichi A, Kunogi J, Yamazaki T, Kobayashi A, Anamizu Y, et al. The efficacy of prostaglandin E1 derivative in patients with lumbar spinal stenosis. Spine (Phila Pa 1976). 2009;34:115.
116. Pereira L, Kerr J, Jolles B. Intra-articular steroid injection for osteoarthritis of the hip prior to total hip arthroplasty: is it safe? A systematic review. Bone Joint J. 2016;98(8):1027–35.
117. Bannuru RR, Natov NS, Obadan IE, Price LL, Schmid CH, McAlindon TE. Therapeutic trajectory of hyaluronic acid versus corticosteroids in the treatment of knee osteoarthritis: a systematic review and meta-analysis. Arthritis Care Res. 2009;61(12):1704–11.
118. Rao NV, Rho JG, Um W, Ek PK, Nguyen VQ, Oh BH, et al. Hyaluronic acid nanoparticles as nanomedicine for treatment of inflammatory diseases. Pharmaceutics. 2020;12(10):931.
119. Wang Q, Yang X, Gu X, Wei F, Cao W, Zheng L, et al. Celecoxib nanocrystal-loaded dissolving microneedles with highly efficient for osteoarthritis treatment. Int J Pharm. 2022;625:122108.
120. Familiari F, Ammendolia A, Rupp MC, Russo R, Pujia A, Montalcini T, et al. Efficacy of intra-articular injections of hyaluronic acid in patients with glenohumeral joint osteoarthritis: a systematic review and meta-analysis. J Orthop Res. 2023;41(11):2345–58.
121. Moreno-Garcia A, Rodriguez-Merchan EC. Orthobiologics: current role in orthopedic surgery and traumatology. Arch Bone Joint Surg. 2022;10(7):536.
122. Muchedzi TA, Roberts SB. A systematic review of the effects of platelet rich plasma on outcomes for patients with knee osteoarthritis and following total knee arthroplasty. Surgeon. 2018;16(4):250–8.
123. Sánchez M, Jorquera C, Sánchez P, Beitia M, García-Cano B, Guadilla J, et al. Platelet-rich plasma injections delay the need for knee arthroplasty: a retrospective study and survival analysis. Int Orthop. 2021;45:401–10.
124. Rosenberg J, Nielsen HJ, Rasmussen V, Hauge C, Pedersen IK, Kehlet H. Effect of preoperative abstinence on poor postoperative outcome in alcohol misusers: randomised controlled trial. BMJ (Clin Res Ed). 1999;318(7194):1311–6.
125. Oppedal K, Møller AM, Pedersen B, Tønnesen H. Preoperative alcohol cessation prior to elective surgery. Cochrane Database Syst Rev. 2012;(7):CD008343.
126. Eliasen M, Grønkjær M, Skov-Ettrup LS, Mikkelsen SS, Becker U, Tolstrup JS, et al. Preoperative alcohol consumption and postoperative complications: a systematic review and meta-analysis. Ann Surg. 2013;258(6):930–42.
127. Jackson KL, Devine JG. The effects of smoking and smoking cessation on spine surgery: a systematic review of the literature. Glob Spine J. 2016;6(7):695–701.

Cancer Prehabilitation

Casey Brown, Romer Orada, and Maryanne Henderson

1 Overview of the Continuum of Cancer Care

The global cancer incidence for all cancers is approximately 19.3 million new cases with ten million deaths, as noted in data from 2020 [1]. Of these, breast cancer is the most common with 2.26 million new cases in 2020 followed by lung cancer at 2.21 million new cases in 2022. Lung cancer is followed by breast cancer for the most deadly malignancies [1, 2].

Cancer diagnoses occur because of screening, incidental findings, or detection following a workup driven by unexplained symptoms. According to the World Health Organization (WHO), screening differs from early diagnosis such that screening tools are applied to asymptomatic individuals without evidence of active disease, in comparison to a symptomatic population [3]. Early detection of cancer remains one of the most critical factors in long-term survival [4, 5] providing patients the best chance for optimal treatment response. According to the *Surveillance, Epidemiology, and End Results* (*SEER*) Program, the incidence of all cancers in adults has gradually been decreasing; however, certain cancers have seen notable increases in diagnosis at earlier ages. For example, colorectal cancer (CRC) is the third most common cause of cancer-related deaths in the United States. Screening for CRC among adults aged 50 and over has dramatically reduced the mortality of CRC in this age group. However, the incidence of early-onset CRC (age

C. Brown
PGY4, University of Pittsburgh Medical Center, Pittsburgh, PA, USA
e-mail: browncc7@upmc.edu

R. Orada (✉)
Miami Cancer Institute, Baptist Health South Florida, Miami, FL, USA

M. Henderson
University of Pittsburgh Medical Center, Pittsburgh, PA, USA
e-mail: hendersonmj@upmc.edu

A. Watson, K. Barr (eds.), *A Prehabilitation Guide for All Providers*,
https://doi.org/10.1007/978-3-031-72862-4_6

less than 50 years) has been rising by 1–2% annually since 2000. As early as 2014, guidelines include recommendations for earlier initial screening between ages 45 and 50 years for high-risk adults such as for individuals with a family history of CRC, inflammatory bowel disease, and Lynch syndrome, amongst other risk factors [6, 7].

Similar to CRC, the populations living with- and surviving breast and prostate cancers are increasing. In the United States, there are four million women living with a history of breast cancer [2], and survival rates for breast cancer have increased to >90% for those diagnosed in the past 10 years [2]. Prostate cancer is the most common cancer in males in the United States and is associated with a 5-year relative survival of >98%.

The National Cancer Institute (NCI) reports as of January 2022 there were an estimated 18.1 million cancer survivors in the United States with a lifetime prevalence in North America of approximately 40% [1, 8]. Due to early detection and treatment people are living longer after cancer diagnosis [8]. The number of cancer survivors is projected to increase to 26 million by 2040 [4]. Cancer is becoming a chronic disease that needs to be managed due to increasing survival rates. As part of the cancer continuum of care, early rehabilitation intervention is increasingly important in the course of patient care and can generate significant improvements in patient outcomes [9].

In cancer rehabilitation, the continuum of care is divided into the following stages: prevention, diagnosis, treatment (which may involve surgery, radiation, chemotherapy, and immunotherapy), and survivorship (Fig. 1) [8]. The Dietz classification of cancer rehabilitation promotes targeted exercise and rehabilitation throughout the continuum. Exercises address physical, psychological, and cognitive impairments to promote independence, improve function, reduce symptoms, and improve quality of life [8]. Dietz classifies cancer rehabilitation into four categories: preventative or prehabilitation, restorative, supportive, and palliative rehabilitation.

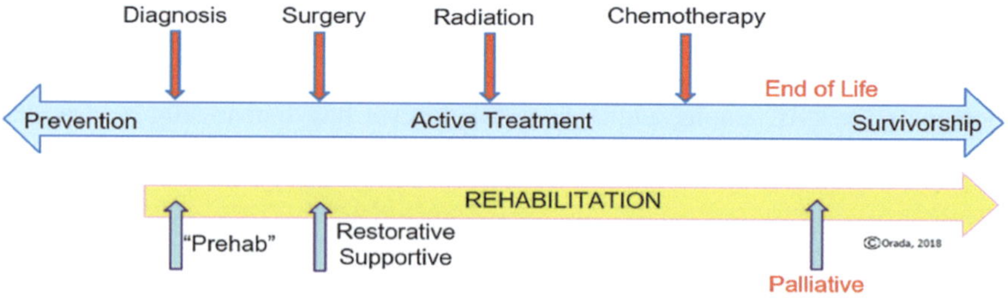

Fig. 1 The cancer rehabilitation continuum diagram with emphasis that rehabilitation starts at cancer diagnosis [10]

2 What Is Cancer Prehabilitation?

Cancer (aka oncologic) prehabilitation is a growing area of focus in healthcare, as it has the potential to significantly improve patient outcomes. Prehabilitation is defined as "[A] process on the cancer continuum of care that occurs between the time of cancer diagnosis and the beginning of acute treatment. It includes physical and psychological assessments that establish a baseline functional level, identify impairments, and provide interventions that promote physical and psychological health to reduce the incidence and/or severity of future impairments" [11]. Oncologic prehabilitation is the systematic process of improving patients' physical, psychosocial, and nutritional status by augmenting the body's ability to manage the physiologic stress of cancer-related therapy [12]. Further, behavioral strategies introduced prior to treatment may result in long-term health and quality of life benefits [12] beyond the primary goal of prehabilitation-reducing the occurrence and severity of oncologic treatment-related side effects [13, 14]. Prehabilitation as an intervention is specific and individualized with special consideration of the patient's functional and psychosocial status, type of cancer, anticipated treatments, and health-impairing habits [12, 14]. As detailed in chapter "Basic Prehabilitation Pillars" (Chap. 2), multimodal prehabilitation programs ideally encompass:

1. cardiopulmonary rehabilitation through aerobic training
2. local/regional resistance training
3. dietary and nutritional interventions to optimize lean body mass and prevent malnutrition
4. psychological interventions to reduce stress
5. cessation of adverse health activities such as alcohol and tobacco use
6. medication optimization [12]

3 Why Cancer Prehabilitation?

Cancer treatments often lead to varying degrees of impairments and disability. In addition to experiencing a high mortality risk, patients with cancer routinely experience anxiety, emotional distress, poor quality of life, anorexia, decreased cardiorespiratory function, cognitive impairment, and locoregional musculoskeletal dysfunction. Prehabilitation can reduce physical, nutritional, and psychological burdens.

These programs prepare the patient for upcoming oncologic treatment and introduce interventions to reduce the risk of cancer progression and recurrence, ultimately improving treatment outcomes [15]. Prehabilitation preparation offers numerous benefits to those undergoing cancer treatment by addressing common risk factors for poor clinical outcomes most notably including physical inactivity, frailty, poor nutrition, poor cardiovascular status, mental health disorders, and metabolic diseases like diabetes mellitus. Patient confidence, caregiver support, psychological factors (depression, anxiety), health literacy, transportation, and safety concerns all impact behavioral change and successful rehabilitation. Supervised programs typically induce a larger physical benefit compared to unsupervised programs. Incorporating other strategies like self-monitoring, goal setting, social support, feedback, and problem-solving further supports behavioral changes to optimize patient outcomes. Therefore, a specialist like an oncologic physiatrist may be essential for facilitating exercise adoption, nutritional support, psychologic intervention, and encouraging lasting behavioral change to improve cancer-related outcomes [15].

4 Physical Function Parameters Correlate with Poor Cancer Outcomes

Cardiorespiratory fitness/aerobic capacity is very important to consider in patients with cancer as it is associated with poor health-related outcomes. Physical inactivity is inversely related to all-cause mortality in lung, colon, urologic, and breast cancers [16]. Cardiorespiratory fitness level at cancer diagnosis is an independent prognostic indicator for post-surgical morbidity and mortality in lung, colon, urologic, esophageal, and breast cancers [15, 17]. Physical inactivity is a modifiable risk factor for breast cancer mortality and recurrence [16]. Aerobic fitness markers such as ventilatory thresholds (VT), peak oxygen uptake (VO_2 peak), and maximal oxygen uptake during maximal exercise (VO_2 max) are gold standard measures and are associated with all-cause, cancer-related, and cardiovascular disease-related mortality. VO_2 peak is difficult to obtain; therefore, the 6-minute walk test (6MWT) is used as an easily measurable physical fitness evaluation. The 6MWT represents patients' functional capacity and positively correlates with overall cancer survival. The 6-minute walk test is an independent prognostic factor for survival postoncologic surgery [18].

Frailty Correlates with Poor Cancer Outcomes

Frailty emerges as a significant prognostic factor impacting cancer survival, including lung, colorectal, prostate, and breast cancer [19–25]. The prevalence of frailty in lung cancer is a striking 45%, which escalates the hazard ratio for mortality by threefold [19]. Similarly, the prevalence of frailty among patients with breast cancer reaches a considerable 43% [21]. Frailty increases the risk of hospitalization, mortality, and falls in patients with breast cancer. With colorectal cancer, patients with frailty face worse overall survival, cancer-specific survival, and recurrence-free survival rates compared to their non-frail counterparts [20, 23]. With hematologic cancer, frailty is associated with poor therapeutic response, increased chemotherapy toxicity, and worse survival. These findings underscore the critical role of assessing frailty in cancer management, elucidating its adverse impact on long-term outcomes.

Integrating frailty assessment into cancer care pathways offers opportunities to tailor interventions based on individual patient vulnerabilities. The Frailty Index based on laboratory tests (FI-lab), incorporates a wide range of health deficits, including comorbidities, laboratory parameters, and functional impairments, providing a quantitative measure of frailty [26, 27]. In prostate cancer, the Geriatric 8 screening tool serves as a valuable indicator of frailty, with lower scores associated with more advanced disease stages and poorer overall survival [24]. However, the Comprehensive Geriatric Assessment (CGA) appears the most reasonable clinical tool for evaluating frailty in patients with cancer [22, 28]. CGA is a multidimensional evaluation encompassing physical, cognitive, psychological, and social domains [22, 28]. Frailty's multifaceted nature, encompassing comorbidities, cognitive decline, and reduced functional status, underscores its significance as a predictor of patient vulnerability and mortality risk.

Sarcopenic Obesity in Cancer Outcomes

Obesity is linked to increased risk for various cancers including breast, colorectal, esophageal, and urologic cancers such as renal cell carcinoma. Overall, obesity is associated with reduced overall and cancer-specific survival and increased recurrence risk [29, 30]. However, the "obesity paradox" suggests that patients with cancer and comorbid obesity may have better outcomes than those with normal weight [31]. Specifically in lung cancer, renal cell carcinoma, and melanoma, obese patients may have better survival outcomes compared to non-obese patients [32]. Although weight loss does reduce cancer incidence, weight loss as an intervention may not be beneficial to cancer survival. Therefore, targeting sarcopenic obesity may result in improved cancer-related outcomes [31–33]. Sarcopenic obesity, characterized by muscle loss and increased fat mass, is associated with poor treatment outcomes, longer hospital stays, and shorter survival [32–34].

Routine computerized tomography (CT) assessing body composition has prognostic indications for patients undergoing oncologic surgery [34, 35]. CT-derived body composition quantitatively analyzes the abominable musculature at L3. This L3 muscle index quantitatively marks sarcopenia. A preoperative CT at L3 during the prehabilitation phase may help identify patients with obesity who have comorbid sarcopenia or myosteatosis [35]. The L3 muscle index may guide protein intake. Interval CT assessments can also monitor treatment effects [35]. In patients with sarcopenic obesity lifestyle interventions targeting increased physical activity rather than weight loss may improve cancer outcomes and quality of life [33].

Nutrition Risk Factor for Poor Clinical Outcomes

Malnourished patients with cancer have increased surgical mortality and postoperative complications [36]. Malnutrition results in weight loss, and decreased muscle mass and subcutaneous fat caused by a nutritional deficit. Nutritional deficiencies are most common in cancer affecting the head, neck, and gastrointestinal system, specifically head and neck, esophageal, gastric, and colorectal cancers [24, 34, 37–41]. Cancer may increase catabolism in addition to mechanically obstructing oral intake. Malnutrition places patients at risk for wound infections, respiratory insufficiency, septicemia, pneumonia, and increased hospital length of stay. Preoperative nutrition improves clinical outcomes and reduces complications. Nutritional deficiencies increase with neoadjuvant cancer treatments and occur stepwise with each treatment [35].

Malnourished patients often innately reduce physical activity as a means of conserving energy. Undernourished patients have a decreased functional capacity, and without correction, experience reduced functional gains with exercise [36]. Specifically in malnourished patients, nutrition is essential and likely synergistic with physical activity outcomes [36]. Appropriate nutrition is an essential pillar that enhances an exercise prehabilitation protocol.

Depression and Anxiety Risk Factors for Poor Cancer Outcomes

Depression and anxiety severity are strongly linked with cancer outcomes [42]. Untreated psychological impairments, like depression, are poor prognostic factors in cancer treatment [43]. Patients with a new cancer diagnosis experience a variety of stressors such as anxiety, depression, sleep changes, fatigue, pain, and impaired quality of life [43, 44]. Specifically, depression and anxiety are associated with increased risk of cancer incidence, as well as cancer-specific and all-cause mortality [42]. Psychological distress results in poor prognosis and cancer survival with specific increased mortality demonstrated in lung, bladder, breast, prostate, head and neck, colorectal, and kidney cancers [26, 42]. Depression is highly prevalent, occurring in up to 40% of patients with breast cancer [45]. In breast cancer, depression and anxiety independently predict breast cancer recurrence and survival [26]. Acute and chronic stress from a new cancer diagnosis reduces quality of life, contributes to a proinflammatory process, increases sympathetic nervous system tone, and induces hypothalamic–pituitary–adrenal axis dysregulation [43, 46]. Specifically, cortisol dysregulation is associated with reduced survival in females with metastatic breast cancer [46]. Depression significantly impacts health-related quality of life—specifically physical, emotional, social, and cognitive function [45].

Like depression, cancer-related fatigue is defined as functionally impairing physical, emotional, and cognitive exhaustion accompanying cancer and its treatment [47]. Cancer-related fatigue significantly impacts quality of life and is a prognostic factor for survival in breast, esophageal, lung, and prostate cancer. Patients with colorectal cancer or endometrial cancer who had comorbid cancer-related fatigue had increased all-cause mortality [47]. Early detection and intervention for patients suffering from cancer-related fatigue may improve clinical outcomes, prognosis, and quality of life [26, 42, 45].

A new cancer diagnosis and impending treatment plan result in stress and psychosocial impairments. Patients report a significant deterioration in their HRQoL from pre-diagnosis to at least eighteen months post-treatment [48, 49]. The deterioration of HRQoL may persist for ten years post-treatment and predominantly affects younger, working-age patients [50]. Confronted with new stressors, patients vary in their psychological responses and recovery which inherently affects Health-related quality of life (HRQoL) [46, 48]. Commonly reported concerns include fear of recurrence, physical damage by adjuvant therapy, premature death, not seeing children grow, and loss of social activities [46]. Stress negatively impacts cancer prognosis, whereas social support positively affects cancer outcomes [43]. Impaired psychological and psychosocial adaptations after diagnosis and through treatment are associated with decreased quality of life during survivorship [46]. HRQoL accurately predicts patients' response to treatment and survival time [48, 49]. Psychological adaptations often require cognitive, behavioral, and social facilitation and support [43, 46]. A multidisciplinary prehabilitation plan may reduce the severity of physical and psychological dysfunction. Cancer diagnosis is a critical juncture for implementing psychosocial interventions and improving quality of life.

Locoregional Dysfunction Pertinent to Treatment-Related Side Effects

Each type of cancer and its associated treatments may result in specific local or regional comorbidities. Locoregional deficits that occur during cancer treatment often impair function, cause pain, and impact a patient's quality of life. Patients are often unable to tolerate continued treatment due to local regional deficits. While resistance training and aerobic exercise improve surgical outcomes, they have no effect on continence for those undergoing colorectal, urological, or gynecological surgeries. Similarly, aerobic exercise has little to no effect on upper limb dysfunction and lymphedema in those with head and neck cancer, breast cancer, leukemia, or lymphoma. Patients may be unable to tolerate beneficial locoregional radiation due to a decreased range of motion and/or pain. Additionally, locoregional deficits may place patients undergoing cancer treatment at risk for poor clinical outcomes. For example, patients are at increased risk for falls due to incontinence, impaired gait speed, and balance deficits from pelvic floor dysfunction or lower extremity lymphedema associated with rectal, urologic, prostate, and gynecological cancers. Identifying impairments present on diagnosis as well as assessing individual risks for locoregional morbidities improves cancer-related outcomes. Additionally, empowering patients with knowledge of mechanisms of morbidity development as well as preventative exercises may result in improved cancer-related outcomes and overall quality of life.

Assess CV Health Before Prescribing Exercise

There is a high incidence of cardiovascular disease in patients with cancer, and cardiovascular disease (CVD), is the second leading cause of mortality and morbidity in cancer survivors after recurrent malignancy in the United States [51, 52]. Cancer and cardiovascular disease have become the two most prevalent diseases on the globe with mounting evidence demonstrating their interconnectedness [53]. In

2020, Helen Strongman and colleagues concluded that "survivors of most site-specific cancers had increased medium-term to long-term risk for one or more cardiovascular diseases compared with that for the general population [54]." Overall, diabetes, age over 65 years, hypertension, hyperlipidemia, smoking, family history, obesity, and peripheral vascular disease are all significant predictors of increased all-cause and CVD-specific mortality in patients with cancer and the presence of these cardiac risk factors should raise the threshold for formal cardiac assessment before prescribing aerobic exercise if symptoms are equivocal [55].

On top of this, many cancer treatments are cardiotoxic and may impact cardiac function and quality of life. Chemotherapy and radiation, specifically, are cardiotoxic and may increase symptomatic cardiovascular disease. Cardiotoxic chemotherapy medications impact cardiac muscle and increase the risk for arrhythmias, congestive heart failure, myocardial infarctions, and even death. Patients should be taught to recognize and report cardiovascular symptoms such as shortness of breath, dyspnea, orthopnea, chest pain, dizziness, syncope, and irregular heartbeats.

Two classes of chemotherapy medications, anthracyclines, and trastuzumab, are frequently implicated in cardiac toxicity [56]. Anthracyclines are essential therapies for hematological malignancies, pediatric cancers, and solid tumors. However, anthracyclines also affect cardiac contractility, reduce blood flow, impair oxygenation, and induce long-term inflammation, arrhythmias, and congestive heart failure. Anthracycline chemotherapy drugs may substantially increase the risk of reduced left ventricular ejection fraction and subsequent clinical heart failure [54, 56]. Trastuzumab, a monoclonal antibody, is an immunotherapy that directly causes cardiac toxicity [57]. This treatment is essential for patients with human epidermal growth factor receptor 2 (HER2) positive breast cancer. Trastuzumab also causes left ventricular dysfunction and is likely to drive part of the observed elevated heart failure risk in patients after breast cancer treatment [54].

Similarly, radiation cardiomyopathy is a heart disease caused by radiation injury to cardiomyocytes [58]. Radiation therapy, the standard of care for many cancer types, is cardiotoxic and increases the risk for cardiomyopathy. Radiation induces oxidative stress in healthy cardiac cells which results in injury and apoptosis. Patients may develop diastolic dysfunction or coronary artery disease, which typically occurs 6–12 months post-radiation [59, 60]. The cardiac impact of radiation therapy directly impacts long-term morbidity as well as cardiovascular function [61].

In the management and treatment of cancer, consideration of the importance of cardiotoxicity is critical as it can have a significant impact on patient quality of life and outcomes. Regular cardiac monitoring including vital signs and baseline echocardiogram is essential for patients undergoing cancer treatment with chest wall radiation or chemotherapy with known cardiotoxicity. Cardiac-specific markers such as cardiac troponin (cTn) and B-type natriuretic peptide (BNP) can detect subclinical cardiotoxicity during antineoplastic treatment [62]. Along with cardiac imaging and functional testing, these cardio-specific biomarkers may predict which patients are at risk of developing cancer-associated treatment cardiotoxicity even before the start of therapy [62] or tracking progression during treatment.

Exercise may play a significant role in managing potential cardiotoxicity by strengthening cardiac muscle and improving overall cardiovascular fitness in cancer survivors. However, patients still need to be closely monitored and have proper guidance from their physicians to ensure safety prior to engaging in any form of exercise program.

5 Exercise Prescriptions for Prehabilitation

Physical exercise is the cornerstone of prehabilitation programs. Exercise improves patients' baseline functional capacity leading to improved cancer-related outcomes [17]. Physical exercise prescriptions are generalized across cancer types; however, most published prehabilitation literature is disproportionately from esophageal, lung, and colon cancer trials (see Table 1, included in the Appendix) [105]. Prehabilitation exercise programs may yield significant improvements in 6MWT, VO_2 peak, VO_2 max, and METS prior to surgery [17]. Exercise interventions in patients with cancer improved mortality rates, hospital lengths of stay, and pulmonary-related complications [106]. Specifically, physical activity of moderate intensity or greater has improved mortality rates in those with comorbid heart failure, chronic kidney disease, and chronic obstructive pulmonary disease [106]. Postoperatively, patients who underwent a prehabilitation exercise program retained an increased 6MWT distance (6MWD) compared to their baseline prior to the prehabilitation program [17]. This prehabilitation-facilitated 6MWD effect lasted beyond 4–8 weeks postoperatively [17, 70, 71].

Targeting aerobic activity with moderate to vigorous intensity may yield the greatest benefits to aerobic fitness. Preoperative physical exercise recommendations are generalized from studies involving patients with esophageal, colorectal, lung, and urologic cancers. Broadly, programs lasting 3–6 weeks demonstrated statistically improved cardiorespiratory fitness measured via 6MWT, VO_2 max, VO_2 peak, and maximal heart rate (HR max); though, program durations under 1 week did not promote statistically significant improvements in cardiorespiratory fitness or postoperative outcomes [71, 79]. Similarly, aerobic exercise training occurring at least three times a week with at least 30 min duration, targeting an intensity of greater than 50% HR max, work rate (WR) at ventilatory threshold (VT), or Borg rating 12–13 improved health-related outcomes and preoperative cardiorespiratory fitness (see Table 1, included in the Appendix). Discussed later, high-intensity interval training occurring greater than twice a week with greater than 30 min duration, targeting greater than 100% peak power output (PPO), 80% HR max, was also associated with improved preoperative cardiorespiratory fitness.

Resistance training is specifically defined as one exercise targeting each major muscle group, 2–4 sets per exercise, and 8–15 repetitions per set to improve pre- and postoperative strength [63, 79, 99]. Although resistance training improves preoperative strength testing, it does not have an apparent impact on cardiorespiratory fitness [63, 79, 99]. Currently under-represented in the literature, preoperatively enhancing strength may reduce falls, reduce sarcopenia, and reduce cancer-related pain [63, 79, 99]. Further research is required to confirm this in the cancer rehabilitation population.

As a method for enhancing aerobic fitness, high-intensity interval training (HIIT) programs are feasible and cardio-metabolically beneficial in the prehabilitation

Table 1 Cancer physical activity prehabilitation studies

Study	Population	Multidisciplinary	Intervention(s)	Outcomes measured	Significant outcomes
Esophagogastric cancer					
Allen et al. [63]	54 participants with esophagogastric cancer undergoing neoadjuvant treatment	Exercise, psychological, nutrition	15-week program, twice weekly supervised cycling 20 min 40–60% HRR, resistance training 6 exercises, 2 sets, 12 repetitions, thrice weekly HEP. Six session psychological coaching. Non-specific needs-based nutrition intervention from the dietician	CPET, skeletal muscle cross-sectional area at L3, QoL questionnaire	Statistically significant attenuated peak VO_2 reductions, skeletal muscle loss, hand grip strength reduction, improved global health status, and improved quality of life post-neoadjuvant therapy in the prehabilitation group compared to usual care group
Minnella et al. [64]	51 participants with esophagogastric cancer	Exercise and nutrition	5-week program, home-based program, thrice weekly, 30 min moderate aerobic exercise (Borg rating 12–13) once a week strength training 30 min, 8 exercises with 3 sets, 8–12 repetitions Daily protein intake 1.2–1.5 g/kg of body weight with whey protein supplementation	6MWT, 30-day postoperative morbidity, Clavien-Dindo classification of complications, CCI, LOS, readmission rate, emergency department visits	Statistically significant improved 6MWT preoperatively and attenuated 6MWT reductions postoperative assessments in the prehabilitation group compared to controls Not statistically significant reductions in Clavien-Dindo classification of complication, CCI, LOS, readmission rate, emergency department visits in the prehabilitation group compared to controls

Sheill et al. [65]	Participants with lung or esophagus cancer post neoadjuvant treatment but preoperatively	Exercise, nutrition	2-week supervised HIIT program 5 days a week on an ergometer cycle, 40 min total, 5-min warm up PPO, 15 second intervals at 100% PPO, 15s recovery, and 3-min cool down Nutritional counseling on dietary energy intake 25–30 kcal/kg/day and protein intake 1.25–1.5 g/kg/day	CPET, short physical performance battery, leg press 1-RM, international physical activity questionnaire, PowerBreath K series, Dietary interview, EORTC-QLQ-C30, Clavien-Dindo score, comprehensive complications index, self-reported functional recovery, postoperative morbidity score	Outcomes not yet completed
Christensen et al. [66]	50 participants with gastroesophageal cancer undergoing neoadjuvant treatment prior to surgery	Exercise only	Average 18 sessions or 9 weeks supervised HIIT program occurring twice weekly for a total of 75 min, 10 min warm up at 50 W, 21–28 min HIIT 4 × 4 min with 3 min low- intensity active recovery Resistance training four exercises for major muscle groups 4 sets of 8–12 repetitions	1-RM, DEXA, Fat mass, bone mass, CPET, FACT-E, CCI, Clavien-Dindo grade, postoperative complications, CTC	Statistically significant improved neoadjuvant treatment tolerability, reduced hospital admissions, reduced rate of treatment postponement, reduced rates of CTC, rates of all postoperative complications in the prehabilitation group compared to controls Statistically significant improvements in emotional wellbeing subscale, FACT-E from baseline compared to preoperatively

(continued)

Table 1 (continued)

Study	Population	Multidisciplinary	Intervention(s)	Outcomes measured	Significant outcomes
Colorectal cancer					
Carli et al. [67]	418 participants with colorectal cancer	Exercise, nutrition, Psychological interventions	4-week supervised program occurring once a week, 30 min of moderate aerobic training and 25-min resistance training. 1.5 g/kg of body weight daily protein intake with whey protein supplementation. Assessment psychology trained nurse and treatment with personalized coping strategies and given an audio track to listen to 3 times per week	CCI, 6MWT, LOS, emergency department visits, readmission rates	Non statistically significant postoperative improvement trends in 6MWT, CCI, 6MWT, LOS, emergency department visits, readmission rates in the prehabilitation group compared to controls
van Rooijen et al. [68]	714 participants with colorectal cancer	Exercise, nutrition, psychological interventions	4-week supervised HIIT program, 28–32 min total with 4 intervals high intensity, lasting 2–3 min with target 85–100% VO_2 peak, and 4 intervals moderate-intensity for 4 min. Resistance training was 2 set with 10 repetitions of 6 exercises. 1.5–1.8 g/kg of body weight daily protein intake with whey protein supplementation Screening with GAD-7 and PHQ-9 and 1.5-h psychological interventions	CPET, CCI, 6MWT, patient-reported outcomes measurements, HRQoL	Ongoing cancer prehabilitation study

Gillis et al. [69]	106 participants with colorectal cancer	Exercise, nutrition, psychological intervention	4-week unsupervised program occurring 3 days per week up to 50 min per session with 20 min of aerobic exercise >40% heart rate reserve and resistance training 20 min with 8 exercises with 8–12 repetitions 1.2 g/kg of body weight with whey protein supplementation 60-min session with a trained psychologist who taught relaxation exercises imagery and visualization	6MWT, HRQoL, postoperative complications rates, LOS, emergency department visits, and 30-day readmission rates, HADS	Statistically significant improvements in 6MWT and functional walking capacity preoperatively and 8 weeks postoperatively in the prehabilitation group compared to controls No statistically significant improvement trends in self-reported physical activity, perioperative outcomes, LOS, emergency department visits, and 30-day readmission rates, self-reported measure of physical functioning, bodily pain, vitality, social functioning, mental health, anxiety, depression in the prehabilitation group compared to controls
Carli et al. [70]	112 participants with colorectal cancer	Exercise only but compared to a light exercise program of walking for 30 min a day	4-week unsupervised program with aerobic exercise (cycling) lasting 20–30 min per day targeting >50% maximal heart rate 3–5 days per week and weight training exercises (pushups, sit-ups, lunges) 12 repetitions 10–15 min per day, 3 times a week	6MWT, CPET, HADS, Clavien-Dindo classification	Statistically significant improvements in peak VO_2 max 4 weeks postoperatively No statistically significant improvements in 6MWT, and depression

(continued)

Table 1 (continued)

Study	Population	Multidisciplinary	Intervention(s)	Outcomes measured	Significant outcomes
Li et al. [71] RCT	87 participants with colorectal cancer	Exercise, nutrition, psychological intervention	1-week, HEP aerobic exercise 30 min, 3 times a week with 50% maximal heart rate Nutrition: 1-h nutritionist visit and identification of modifiable dietary behaviors excessive alcohol intake, fat intake. protein intake of 1.2 g/kg body weight Psychological: 90-min visit with a trained psychologist focusing on anxiety reduction techniques (breathing and relaxation exercises). Patients were given a compact disk to take home	6MWT, functional walking capacity, CHAMPS questionnaire, SF-36, HADS	Statistically significant improvements in preoperative functional walking capacity, 6MWT, self-reported physical activity, depression, and improved functional walking capacity 8 weeks postoperatively in the prehabilitation group compared to controls Non-statistically significant improvements in HRQoL, perioperative complications
Dronkers et al. [72]	42 participants with colorectal cancer	Exercise only	2–4 weeks supervised program twice a week aerobic training (50–75% maximal heart rate) 20–30 min and resistance training one set 8–15 repetitions Inspiratory muscle training against 60% of maximal inspiratory pressure for 15 min a day HEP encouraged to exercise 30 min per day	Steps per day, TUG, chair rise time, maximal inspiratory pressure, respiratory muscle analyzer, LAPAQ, physical activity questionnaire, physical work capacity, abbreviated fatigue questionnaire, QoL questionnaires, postoperative complications, pneumonia, LOS	Statistically significant reduction in postoperative pulmonary complications with patients >4000 steps per day compared to <4000 steps per day Non-statistically significant improvement trends in hospital length of stay, TUG, LAPAQ, Respiratory Muscle Energy Analyzer, physical work capacity, and quality of life questionnaires

Kim et al. [73]	21 participants with colorectal surgery	Exercise	4 weeks of supervised daily aerobic cycling training target 40–65% HR max for 30 min per day	VO_2 max, PPO, VT, HR peak, 6MWT, Respiratory exchange ratio	Statistically significant difference in HR peak, VT, PPO compared to the control group
West et al. [74]	39 participants with rectal cancer	Exercise only	6-week supervised paired partner exercise training program with 3 sessions per week of HIIT with 40 min total of interval training on a braked cycle. 10 min of combined warm up and cool down and 4–6 sets of high intensity (VO_2 max 80%) for 2–3 min alternating moderate intensity (VO_2 50%) for 3–2 min	VO_2 uptake at lactate threshold, VO_2 peak, average number of steps	Statistically significant difference in VO_2 uptake at lactate threshold, VO_2 peak at 6 weeks post neoadjuvant chemoradiotherapy as well as average number of steps between baseline and pre-neoadjuvant chemoradiotherapy in the exercise group versus control
Chen et al. [75]	116 participants with colorectal cancer	Exercise, nutrition, psychological interventions	4-week HEP, 3 times a week of 20 min aerobic exercise targeting 50% maximal heart rate and 20 min resistance exercise with 8–12 repetitions targeting major muscle groups A registered dietician evaluated daily 1.2 g/kg of body weight with whey protein supplementation A 60-min session with a trained psychologist on relaxation and breathing techniques to reduce anxiety	3-day dietary recall, CHAMPS, 6MWT, WC classifying if patients met 150 min of moderate-intensity or 75 min of vigorous intensity exercise a week as recommended by the American Cancer Society	The prehabilitation group statistically significantly met ACS exercise guidelines compared to the control group. The prehabilitation group statistically improved their 6MWT and WC prior to surgery compared to baseline

(continued)

Table 1 (continued)

Study	Population	Multidisciplinary	Intervention(s)	Outcomes measured	Significant outcomes
Dunne et al. [76]	38 participants with metastatic colon cancer to the liver	Exercise only	A 4-week program with 12 interval exercise sessions lasting for 30 min on a recumbent bike alternating between above 90% VO_2 peak and below 60% VO_2 peak	Cardiopulmonary exercise test (VO_2 at anaerobic threshold, VO_2 peak, oxygen pulse at anaerobic threshold, oxygen pulse peak, peak work rate, heart rate reserved, SF-36	Statistically significant improvements in VO_2 anaerobic threshold, VO_2 peak, oxygen pulse at anaerobic threshold, peak work rate, and improved QoL and mental health in the prehabilitation group pre-operatively compared to baseline
Singh et al. [77]	12 participants with rectal cancer recurrence	Exercise only concurrent neoadjuvant chemoradiation	16-week supervised twice weekly 60-min aerobic exercise 20 min with 60–80% of maximal heart rate and resistance training targeting major muscle groups (chest press, seated row, latissimus pull down, leg extension, leg curl, and leg press) 6–12 repetitions with 2–4 sets. HEP twice a week for 15 min	Maximal number of repetitions at 70% of 1 repetition maximum baseline, 6MWT, 6-min backward walk, 400 m walk, repeated chair rise, total body composition, EORTC-QLQ C30, Leisure Score Index of Godin, Leisure time Exercise Questionnaire, SF-36	Statistically significant improvements in 6M backward walk test, 400 m walk test from baseline to preoperative testing. Statistically significant improvements in chest press, seated row, leg press, leg extension, lean body mass, and total body fat mass preoperatively compared to post-operatively

Berkel et al. [78]	57 patients with colorectal cancer	Exercise	3-week supervised program with aerobic exercise consisting of 7 min warm up at 50% work rate at ventilatory threshold, 30 min HIIT 6 × 5 min intervals 120–160 s at 120% and 180–140 s rest at 50% WR at VAT as well as a 20 min resistance 3 sets of 8 repetitions for all major muscle groups at 70–80 s 1-RM	CPET, MET, VAT, postoperative complication rate, hospital readmission rates	Statistically significant reductions in overall postoperative complications on Charlson score, improvements to VO_2 at the ventilatory anaerobic threshold and VO_2 peak in the prehabilitation group versus control Statistically significant short nutritional assessment questionnaire and hemoglobin levels were associated with reduced postoperative complications
Peng et al. [79]	240 participants with colorectal cancer	Exercise and nutrition	Day of surgery, preoperative exercises hand squeeze, biceps flexion, shoulder abduction, ankle rotation, quadriceps contraction, deep inhalation slow exhalation, deep inhalation with gentle cough, abdominal curl, pelvic muscle contraction, lumbar extension, and relaxation Preoperative nutrition, preoperative fasting 6–8 h solid fluids, 200–400 mL carbohydrate drink 2–3 h prior	I-FEED scoring for GI classification, pre- and postoperative quality of life, non-bowel adverse events	Statistically significant preoperative and postoperative hand grip strength in the prehabilitation group

(continued)

Table 1 (continued)

Study	Population	Multidisciplinary	Intervention(s)	Outcomes measured	Significant outcomes
Bousquet-Dion et al. [80]	80 participants with colorectal cancer	Exercise, nutrition, and psychological intervention	3-week mixed home 3–4 days per week and once a week supervised exercise program. 3–4 days per week aerobic exercise targeting 60–70% HR max, walking, cycling, or jogging. 3–4 days per week 8 resistance exercises targeting core, upper and lower limbs, 2 sets 8–15 repetitions Protein requirement 0.8 g/kg/day and provided whey supplementation. 60-min session with trained psychologist who taught visualization techniques and breathing exercises and a home audio track with instructions	Anthropometric measurements, functional tests, 6MWT, QoL questionnaires, HADS, SF-36, ED-SD, CHAMPS NRS2002, SGA, 3-day food diary	Statistically significant improvements in number of patients meeting ACS physical activity recommendations, and moderate to vigorous exercise per week. Statistically significant difference in 6MWT between those who met ACS guidelines and those who did not at the preoperative, 4 weeks, and 8 weeks assessments. Inactive patients were more likely to improve functional capacity with supervision

Lung cancer					
Ferreira et al. [81] RCT	95 participants with non-small cell lung cancer	Exercise, nutrition, psychological intervention	4-week supervised program 3 days per week with moderate-vigorous intensity aerobic training 30 min and resistance training 2 sets, 10 exercises, 8–12 repetitions 1.5 g/kg ideal body weight protein intake with whey protein supplementation One hour psychologist session teaching relaxation exercises and deep breathing. Encouraged 2–3 times per week audio with relaxation exercises	6MWT, HRQoL, FACT-L, HADS, LOS, CCI	Statistically significant improvements 6MWT at 4 weeks postoperative visit, improved general health, mental health, physical function, social function in prehabilitation group Non statistically significant improvement trends in LOS, emergency room visits, readmissions, Clavien-Dindo grade, and CCI in prehabilitation group

(continued)

Table 1 (continued)

Study	Population	Multidisciplinary	Intervention(s)	Outcomes measured	Significant outcomes
Quist et al. [82]	114 participants with advanced-stage lung cancer	Exercise only	6-week supervised exercise training program with groups of 10–12 participants twice weekly lasting 1.5 h 10-min aerobic warm up targeting 60–90% maximal heart rate, 10–15 min of high intensity interval cycling targeting 85–95% maximal heart rate. Strength training using 6 machines completing 3 rounds with 5–8 repetitions each targeting 70–90% one repetition maximum. 10 min of stretching and 15–20 min of progressive relaxation	VO_2 peak, one repetition maximum test, 6MWT, HRQoL, Functional assessment of Cancer Therapy- Lung (FACT-L) scale, Hospital Anxiety and Depression Scale, FEV1 lung capacity	Statistically significant improvement in VO_2 peak and 6MWT, one repetition maximum, reduction in anxiety (HADS-A), and improved social and emotional wellbeing in prehabilitation group Not statistically significant improvements in depression (HADS-D), functional wellbeing, and FEV1 lung capacity
Licker et al. [83] RCT	151 participants with lung cancer	Exercise only	2–3 weeks of a HIIT program 2–3 times a week. 5-min warm up 50% maximal HR, two 10-min series of 15-s sprint intervals at 80–100% peak work rate with 15 s pauses, 4-min rest between 2 series, and a 5-min cool down 30% maximal HR	6MWT, peak heart rate, peak VO_2, peak WR, 30-day postoperative morbidity, length of stay in PACU, rate of admissions to the ICU	Statistically significant increase in VO_2 peak, peak WR, 6MWT, distance preoperatively, reduced postoperative pulmonary complications, rates of atelectasis, and length of PACU stays in the prehabilitation group versus the control group. Preoperative peak VO_2 and COPD were predictors of postoperative pulmonary complications

Lai et al. [84] RCT	48 participants with lung cancer	Exercise, respiratory specific exercises, and medical pharmacotherapy intervention	One-week supervised training program, daily 15–20-min aerobic recumbent cycling and 15–30 min of stair climbing with a targeted BORG score 5–7 Lung exercises: 15–30 min of diaphragmatic breathing with prolonged inhalation, exhalation, and breath holds. Incentive spirometry every 2 h, 12–20 times per set. Medical intervention: aerosol inhalation of bronchodilators and glucocorticoids (Bricanyl 2 mL + Pulmicort Respirin 4 mL twice daily) Mucosolvan injection 30 mg twice daily	Postoperative length of stay, duration of antibiotic use, peak expiratory flow, 6MWD, energy expenditure, pulmonary complications, total hospital costs, medicine cost, material cost, European Organization of Research and Treatment of Cancer-Quality of Life Questionnaire-Lung Cancer	Statistically significant improvements in postoperative LOS, duration of antibiotic use, peak expiratory flow, 6MWD, increased energy expenditure, and reduced pulmonary complications and dyspnea scores in the prehabilitation group
Lai et al. [85] RCT	60 participants with lung cancer	Exercise and respiratory specific exercises	One week supervised aerobic daily 30-min aerobic recumbent cycling Lung exercises: diaphragmatic breathing twice a day for 15–20 min with prolonged inhalation, exhalation, and breath holds. Incentive spirometry every 2–3 times per day for 20 min	6MWD, pulmonary function tests, HRQoL	Statistically significant improvements in the 6MWD, pulmonary exhalation function test in the prehabilitation group pre-operatively compared to baseline, reduced postoperative length of stay, total hospital length of stay, and postoperative pulmonary complications

(continued)

Table 1 (continued)

Study	Population	Multidisciplinary	Intervention(s)	Outcomes measured	Significant outcomes
Bobbio et al. [86]	12 participants with non-small cell lung cancer	Exercise and respiratory- specific exercises	A 4-week supervised program, 5 days a week, 40-min aerobic recumbent cycling targeting 50–80% maximal work rate and resistance training of the upper extremity and trunk Patient taught incentive spirometry exercise to repeat twice daily at home	Pulmonary function tests, CPET, VO_2 max	Statistically significant improved VO_2 max, workload capacity, and oxygen pulse in the prehabilitation group pre-operatively compared to baseline
Stefanelli et al. [87]	40 participants with non-small cell lung cancer	Exercise and respiratory- specific exercises	3 weeks supervised HIIT with 15 sessions over 3 weeks, 3 h in duration, targeting 70% of maximal workload. Non-specific respiratory breathing exercises	CPET, PFT, Borg scale	Statistically significant improvements in VO_2 predicted, Borg grades, DLCO, FEV1 baseline versus preoperative testing in the prehabilitation group
Bhatia and Kayser [88]	151 participants with lung cancer	Exercise only	25 days with 8 supervised HIIT sessions 2–3×/week, 2 × 10 min cycling at peak power 15 s with 15 s rest	CPEP, 6MWT	Statistically significant improvements in PPO, VO_2 peak, WR peak, HR during training, resting HR, and 6MWT between usual care and prehabilitation groups at preoperative testing
Egegaard et al. [89]	15 participants with lung cancer pre-radiotherapy	Exercise only	7 weeks, supervised training sessions times a week, 5-min warm up targeting 50% work peak, two sets of 5 × 30 s intervals at 80–95% peak power with 30 s rest, continuous cycling at 80% peak power between HIIT sets	CPET, VO_2 peak, 6MWD, PFT, FACT-L, HADS	Due to low power no statistically significant outcomes Trends in improved mental and treatment-related fatigue

Sheill et al. [65]	Participants with lung or esophagus cancer preoperative post-neoadjuvant treatment	Exercise, nutrition	2-week supervised HIIT program 5 days a week on an ergometer cycle lasting 40 min total with a 5-min warm up PPO, 15 s intervals at 100% PPO, 15 s recovery, and 3-min cool down Nutritional counseling on dietary energy intake 25–30 kcal/kg/day and protein intake 1.25–1.5g/kg/day	CPET, short physical performance battery, leg press 1-RM, international physical activity questionnaire, PowerBreath K series, Dietary interview, EORTC-QLQ-C30, Clavien-Dindo score, comprehensive complications index, self-reported functional recovery, post-operative morbidity score	Outcomes not yet completed
Pehlivan et al. [90]	60 participants with lung cancer	Exercise and respiratory- specific exercises	1 week preoperatively 3 times per day treadmill walking each session lasting 10–30 min Breathing exercises included diaphragmatic, pursed lip, segmental breathing exercise, insensitive spirometry, coughing exercises	CPET, PFT, DLCO, V/Q distributions, DEXA	Statistically significant improvements in VC, FEV1, PaO_2, $PaCO_2$, DLCO, maximum HR, maximum speed, distance covered, contralateral V/Q distribution and reduced pulmonary complications in the prehabilitation group compared to the control group

(continued)

Table 1 (continued)

Study	Population	Multidisciplinary	Intervention(s)	Outcomes measured	Significant outcomes
Karenovics et al. [91]	151 participants with lung cancer	Exercise only	2–4-week supervised program with 3 times a week HIIT sessions using a cycle ergometer. Two 10-min sessions with 15s sprints with all out WR, 15s pauses with 4 min of rests between sessions	CPET, PFTs, carbon monoxide transfer factor tested preoperatively and 1 year post-operatively	Statistically significant preoperative improvements CPET % predicted, mean VO_2 peak, WR peak baseline compared to preoperative testing and prehabilitation group versus usual care group Statistically significant reduced in hospital pulmonary complications, and short LOS in the prehab versus control group No statistically significant long-term improvements
Sebio et al. [92]	40 participants with lung cancer	Exercise and respiratory- specific exercises	7-week supervised program 3–5 times a week, 30 min interval training targeting 80% W peak for 1 min with 4 min active rest at 50% W peak on a cycle ergometer and 6 resistance exercises targeting the main muscle groups for three sets 15 repetitions with 45s rest between sets Home breathing exercises were performed twice daily at home using an incentive spirometer with 30 s sustained inspiration at maximal vital capacity and end inspiratory hold 2–3 s	CPET, SF-36, postoperative outcomes Melbourne group scale, 6MWT, Colinet Comorbidity score	Statistically significant improvements in exercise tolerance, the physical summary complaint of SF-36, muscle strength, constant cycling endurance test, number of repetitions of arm curls, chair-to-stand from baseline to preoperative assessment

Gravier et al. [93]	50 participants with non-small cell lung cancer	Exercise and respiratory specific exercises	6 weeks, 3–5 times a week of aerobic training with 5-min warm up and cool down and 20–35 min at ventilatory threshold. Resistance training targeted quadriceps press, whole leg extension, upper limb pull down at 60–70% 1-RM, 3 sets of 12 15 min daily inspiratory muscle strengthening 30% maximum inspiratory pressure	CPET, VE/VCO$_2$ slope, number of training sessions to obtain physiologic effect	Statistically significant improvements in VO$_2$ peak, W peak, Wvt, VO$_2$vt/VO$_2$peak, VE/VCO$_2$ slope and VO$_2$ peak after 15 prehabilitation sessions compared to baseline
Urologic cancer					
Jensen et al. [94]	158 participants with bladder cancer	Exercise intervention with the control group receiving nutritional intervention as well	2-week supervised daily home therapy aerobic exercise program twice a day for 30 min with a step trainer Nutrition screening and counseling on cessation of alcohol and smoking with targeted minimum energy intake of 6300 kJ (1500 kcal) per day and 1.2 g/kg of protein per day	Pain VAS-1, Comorbidity Index score, Nutritional Risk Screening tool (NRS-2002), Nutritional intake energy and protein, length of hospital stay, 90-day mortality, readmission rate, Bristol bowel function score	Statistically significant first 7 days postoperatively increased walking distance in the prehabilitation exercise group versus control Non-significant trends in improved pain scores (VAS 1–10), improved Nutritional Risk Score, improved bowel function (Bristol 1–6)

(continued)

Table 1 (continued)

Study	Population	Multidisciplinary	Intervention(s)	Outcomes measured	Significant outcomes
Santa Mina et al. [95]	86 participants with prostate cancer	Exercise only	Unsupervised, home-based, 60-min moderate-intensity exercise program 3–4 days a week Education through a manual, online videos and logbook adherence	6MWT, grip strength, maximal isometric strength for elbow flexion and extension, body composition body fat percentage, waist circumference, BMI, HRQoL measure through functional Assessment of Cancer Therapy-Prostate, fatigue through FACT-F, HADS, Pain Disability Index, International Prostate Symptom Score, International Index of Erectile Function, Community Health Activities Model Program for Seniors, CHAMPS	Statistically significant return to baseline 6MWT 4 weeks postoperatively return to baseline grip strength at 12–26 weeks postoperatively in the prehabilitation group. Preoperatively, 4 weeks, and 12 weeks postoperatively reduced body fat percentage in the prehabilitation group. Improved HADS-anxiety score at 26 weeks postoperatively Non-significant trends in reduced intraoperative complications as well as partial and complete nerve-sparing
Banerjee et al. [96]	60 participants with bladder cancer post-neoadjuvant treatment	Exercise only	3–6-week supervised HIIT cycle ergometer program occurring twice a week with 5–10 min warm-up at 50 W, 6 × 5 min intervals 2.5 min rests against 50W resistance at targeting Borg ratings of 13–15 or 70–85% predicted HR max	CPET, postoperative recovery outcomes	Statistically significant improvements in preoperative VO_2 peak, PPO, minute ventilation, anaerobic threshold and reductions in length of stay in the high dependency units, and LOS of stay in the prehabilitation group

Blackwell et al. [97]	40 patients with urologic cancer (bladder, prostate, kidney cancers)	Exercise only	4-week supervised HIIT program 3–4 times per week with a 2-min warm-up, 5 × 1 min high intensity 100–115% of maximal load and a 2-min active recovery	CPET, Dukes Activity Status Index, EuroQol group 5-Level, Warwick Edinburgh Mental wellbeing Scale, DEXA scan	Statistically significant improvements in CPET, VO_2 at anaerobic threshold, VO_2 peak, resting systolic and diastolic blood pressure, resting MAP, cancer-related fatigue
Schulz et al. [98]	20 participants with prostate cancer		8–12 week supervised twice weekly program with aerobic exercise on ergometer 15–30 min 50–75% HRR and 6–8 resistance exercises 1–2 sets, 10–12 repetitions at 50–75% 1-RM as well as HEP 2–3 days/week aerobic exercise	Godin Leisure time physical activity questionnaire, functional assessment of cancer therapy-prostate instrument, Center for Epidemiologic Studies-Depression scale, international prostate symptom score,	Statistically significant improvements in self-reported Godin Score, number of chair stands, self-reported wellbeing 6-month pre and postoperatively compared to control and baseline Trends in improvements in QoL and psychosocial outcomes
Breast cancer					
Mijwel et al. [99]	240 participants with breast cancer during chemotherapy prior to surgery	Exercise only	16 weeks supervised HIIT with either resistance training or moderate intensity aerobic training, twice a week 60-min session 3 × 3 min of high-intensity intervals with 1 min active recovery targeting 16–18 on BORG scale Either resistance training high-load exercises targeting major muscle groups 2–3 sets with 8–12 repetitions at 70% 1-RM or aerobic training 20 min moderate-intensity continuous exercise prior to HIIT	HRQoL, CRF, muscle strength (mid-thigh pull and hand grip), return to work, cardiorespiratory fitness, body mass, Piper Fatigue Scale, EORTC-QLQ, Memorial Symptom Assessment scale	Statistically significant reductions in cancer-related fatigue, total symptoms, increase in hand grip and lower extremity strength in both exercise groups Aerobic training + HIIT significantly reduced body mass, improved quality of life in role, emotional functioning, and return to work

(continued)

Table 1 (continued)

Study	Population	Multidisciplinary	Intervention(s)	Outcomes measured	Significant outcomes
Knoerl et al. [100]	47 participants with breast cancer	Exercise only versus Exercise with Mind-body intervention	Twice a week 60–90-min supervised session with 30–45-min aerobic moderate-intensity exercise and 20 min strength training, 6 exercises as well as HEP targeting 180 min aerobic 40 min resistance exercise goal each week Mind-body intervention: twice daily listening to relaxation audio guide, book *Prepare for Surgery, Heal Faster*	EORTC-QLQ-C-30, Perceived stress scale, HADS, 7-day physical activity interview, daily mind-body log	Statistically significant improvements in cognitive function, fatigue, pain, stress and anxiety with both intervention groups Mind-body group-specific statistically significant improvements in insomnia, depression, anxiety, physical function, role function, global health status, and quality of life
Heiman et al. [101]	370 participants with breast cancer	Exercise only	2-week HEP with 30 min medium intensity aerobic exercise	Postoperative 4 weeks after surgery self-reported mental recovery, LOS, unplanned reoperations, unplanned readmissions, CCI	No statistically significant trends in improved physical and mental recovery and reduced 30-day CCI
Pancreatic cancer					
Mikami et al. [102]	26 patients with pancreatic preoperatively during chemotherapy	Exercise	12 days supervised in the hospital program prior to surgery Muscle strengthening squatting, heel raising, step ups, 100 times a day each Aerobic exercise: cycle ergometry 30 min per day, treadmill walking 20 min per day, hand grip ergometry 20 min per day each targeting 11–13 on the Borg scale	CPET, 6MWT, FIM Score, adverse events, peak oxygen uptake, post-operative complications	Statistically significant improvements in peak VO_2, peak HR, peak WR, 6MWT, preoperatively compared to baseline No postoperative wound infections, delirium, deep vein thrombosis

Hematologic cancer					
McCourt et al. [103]	50 participants with myeloma	Exercise	5-week supervised program 3 times a week; aerobic treadmill, walking, cycling 15–40 min targeting 60–80% HR reserve and resistance training targeting shoulder press, bench press, squat, seated row, lunge, step ups, bridge, scissors, hip twist with 10 repetitions each	Feasibility, recruitment rate, adherence rates, EORTC C30, FACT-BMT, EQ5D, FACIT-F, 6MWT, time sit to stand, hand grip strength, self-reported physical activity	Improved QoL, fatigue, functional capacity, and physical activity in the prehabilitation group compared to controls. Limited statistical significance due to small sample size trends in improvement in functional measures pre-autologous stem cell transplant
Mawson et al. [104]	23 participants with myeloma	Exercise	6-week supervised program, aerobic treadmill, bike, seated rowing machine training (non-specific recommendations) and upper and lower limb strengthening exercises, core stability and balance exercises	Feasibility, recruitment rate, adherence rates, 6MWT, FACT-MM, Warwick-Edinburgh mental wellbeing score, international physical activity questionnaire	Statistically significant increase in 6MWT 74.9% of participants attended scheduled sessions, retention rate of 57%

Note. List of randomized clinical trials evaluating the role of aerobic and resistance exercise preoperatively to improve clinical outcomes in patients with cancer. Abbreviations. *CPET* cardiopulmonary exercise testing, VO_2 *max* maximum rate of oxygen consumption, VO_2 *peak* peak oxygen uptake, *HEP* home exercise program, *6MWT* 6 minute walk test, *QoL* quality of life, *HRQoL* health care related quality of life, *HRR* heart rate reserve, *CCI* comprehensive complication index, *LOS* length of hospital stay, *HIIT* high intensity interval training, *PPO* peak power output, *1-RM* 1 repetition maximum, *W* work, *EORTC-QLQ-C30* European Organization for the Research and Treatment of Cancer Quality of Life Questionnaire, *DEXA* dual x-ray absorptiometry, *FACT-E, -L, -F -MM* functional assessment of cancer therapy, -esophageal, -lung, -fatigue, -multiple myeloma, *CTC* common toxicity criteria, *HRQoL* health related quality of life, *HADS* Hospital Anxiety and Depression Scale, *CHAMPS* Community Health Activities Model Program for Seniors, *TUG* timed up and go, *LAPAQ* LASA Physical Activity Questionnaire, *VT* ventilatory threshold, *WC* work capacity, *m* meter, *WR* work rate, *VAT* ventilation at anaerobic threshold, *MET* metabolic equivalents, *NRS2002* nutrition risk screening 2002, *SGA*, Subjective Global Assessment, *ACS* American Cancer Society, *FEV1* forced expiratory volume in 1 second, *PACU* post anesthesia care unit, *ICU* intensive care unit, *COPD* chronic obstructive pulmonary disease, *DLCO* diffusing capacity of the lungs for carbon monoxide, *PFT* pulmonary function test, *V/Q* ventilation perfusion ratio, *VC* vital capacity, PaO_2 partial pressure of arterial oxygen, $PaCO_2$ partial pressure of arterial carbon monoxide, *SF-36* short form survey for quality of life outcomes, VE/VCO_2 ventilatory equivalent of carbon monoxide, *VAS-1* Visual Analogue Scale-1, *BMI* body mass index, *HRR* heart rate reserve, *FIM* functional independence measure period of cancer treatment. HIIT involves sequential short periods of strenuous aerobic exercise punctuated with low-intensity, active recovery periods. The total time spent in vigorous exercise is cumulatively more aerobically strenuous compared to continuous exercise at moderate intensity. Due to the short timeline between diagnosis and treatment, high-intensity interval training (HIIT) may have a role in optimizing aerobic fitness in a limited available period [107]. Extensive research has suggested preoperative benefits of HIIT in patients with esophagogastric, colorectal, lung, bladder, kidney, prostate, and breast cancer as well as in patients with multiple myeloma receiving pre-autologous stem cell transplant (ASCT) [65, 66, 82, 83, 87–89, 97, 99, 102–104]. Palma et al. [107] conducted a systematic review and meta-analysis of studies evaluating the benefits of HIIT in prehabilitation [107]. Descriptive data analysis demonstrates that supervised HIIT programs in patients cleared for activity are medically safe with a low risk of major adverse events. HIIT more quickly increases functional capacity measurements, with statistical benefits in patients' 6MWT, VO_2 max, and lean body mass while reducing body fat, both predictors of cancer-related mortality. Despite the increase in physical capacity, there has been only one study in participants with lung cancer that demonstrated a pulmonary benefit [87]. However, the pulmonary benefit may be due to diaphragmatic breathing exercises rather than the HIIT program alone. Despite the lack of evidence of directly improving pulmonary function tests (PFTs), HIIT reduces post-operative pulmonary-specific complications in patients with lung cancer [83, 91].

Several RCTs show other benefits from HIIT including the potential to reduce cancer-related fatigue, insomnia, depression, anxiety, and improve physical functioning, role function, and overall quality of life in patients with breast, and lung cancers [82, 89, 99]. Patients undergoing neoadjuvant treatment prior to surgery may especially benefit from HIIT, specifically those with breast, colorectal, bladder, and esophagogastric cancers [63, 65, 66, 77, 96, 99, 102]. Christensen et al. [66] demonstrated that HIIT can reduce cardiac toxicities of neoadjuvant treatment. A typical HIIT prehabilitation program lasts 2–4 weeks, 2–4 times a week for 20–40 min with vigorous intervals targeting 100% WR, 80% VO_2 max, >70–80 W peak, or 80–100% peak power. Most intervals are interspersed with rest breaks approximately equal in duration to the vigorous intervals. Overall, HIIT is a feasible therapy in prehabilitation that can effectively improve functional capacity preoperatively and attenuate toxicities associated with neoadjuvant therapy.

When utilized, patients receive neoadjuvant therapy preoperatively to reduce tumor burden or size. Neoadjuvant chemotherapies and immunotherapies have many potential side effects such as impairing cardiometabolic function, cancer-related fatigue, anorexia, reduced quality of life, and sarcopenia. Therefore, initiation of a prehabilitation exercise program before and during neoadjuvant treatment may improve or prevent the deterioration of patients' cardiometabolic profile prior to surgery [63, 65, 66, 74, 77, 96, 108–113]. Current evidence supports that exercise before, during, and after neoadjuvant therapies is both safe and feasible in trials of patients with colorectal, esophagogastric, bladder, breast, pancreatic, and ovarian cancer. However, most available data regarding prehabilitation and neoadjuvant therapy is from those with rectal, pancreatic, and esophageal cancer [63, 65, 66, 74, 77, 108, 111–114]. Patients in these trials significantly improved or attenuated the loss of their VO_2 peak or 6MWT, improved their quality of life, improved neoadjuvant treatment tolerability, and reduced hospital admissions, rate of treatment postponement, rates of common toxicities, and rates of overall postoperative complications [66, 108, 109, 111, 114]. However, personalized therapy guidelines for those undergoing neoadjuvant therapy for any specific cancer are uncertain currently due to limited clinical data. Despite the paucity of evidence, at least 30 min of moderate to vigorous aerobic exercise (> 60% HRR, HR max) or HIIT programs at least 2–3 days a week appear efficacious for attenuating neoadjuvant toxicities [63, 66, 74, 77, 96, 113, 114]. However, intensity and frequency are likely inversely related such that lighter intensity requires greater frequency, ie daily, compared to 2–3 days per week of HIIT, to improve patients' 6MWT or VO_2 peak. However, if tolerated, HIIT currently has the strongest evidence for attenuating cardiometabolic toxicities of neoadjuvant therapies.

Lung Cancer

Prehabilitation exercise programs are strongly beneficial to the cardiometabolic health of patients with lung cancer (see Table 1, included in the Appendix) [81–85, 87–89]. Several studies have demonstrated that a one-week prehabilitation program consisting of daily 40–60 min of aerobic exercise at a Borg score of 4–7 significantly improved participants' 6MWT, PFT, and reduced postoperative length of stay and postoperative pulmonary complications [84, 85, 90]. Note, that the exercise program was augmented by daily respiratory training exercises for 15–60 min including diaphragmatic breathing, breath holds, incentive spirometry, and intentional coughing. In this population, most prehabilitation programs that significantly benefit VO_2 peak, WR peak, HR max, are 4–6 weeks in duration, 3 or more sessions per week, 20–30 min moderate-vigorous intensity aerobic exercise, >50% HRmax, with and without resistance training with 4–6 major muscle group exercises, 2–4 sets with 6–12 repetitions [82, 86, 92, 93]. Participants treated with prehabilitation also demonstrated an improvement in the HRQoL, Functional Assessment of Cancer Therapy-Lung scale, and Hospital Anxiety and Depression scale.

HIIT programs have demonstrated a strong and feasible benefit to the cardiometabolic capacity of patients with lung cancer. As demonstrated in with other malignancies, HIIT programs specifically improved cardiometabolic outcomes, exercise tolerance, muscle strength, endurance, peak power output, VO_2 peak, WR peak, HR rate during training, resting HR, VO_2 predicted, 6MWT, Borg score, and PFTs preoperatively [65, 74, 78, 81, 87–89, 91, 92]. However, prehabilitation HIIT programs primarily demonstrate a preoperative cardiometabolic benefit rather than a sustained 1-year physical improvement [91]. Notably, Stefanelli et al. [87] proposed the only HIIT program to demonstrate improvements in pulmonary function specifically DLCO and FEV1 preoperatively [87]. They demonstrated that pulmonary benefit may be due to the augmentation of the HIIT program with diaphragmatic breathing exercises. Discussed further in the local regional exercise sections, breathing exercises such as deep breathing and breath holds as well as incentive spirometry may improve the lung function of patients with lung cancer rather than aerobic exercise alone.

Esophageal Cancer

Prehabilitation exercise programs for esophageal cancer typically occur preoperatively during neoadjuvant chemotherapy courses [71, 74, 87, 99]. Neoadjuvant chemotherapy is cardiotoxic, causing reductions in VO_2 peak, VO_2 max, 6MWT (see Table 1, included in the Appendix). Allen et al. [63], Minnella et al. [64], and Christensen et al. [66] demonstrate that aerobic prehabilitation programs during neoadjuvant chemotherapy attenuate VO_2 peak and 6MWT reductions induced by neoadjuvant chemotherapy [71, 74, 99]. Allen et al. [63] and Minnella et al. [64] demonstrated a feasible aerobic exercise program occurring 2–3 weekly for 20–30 min, a program targeting 40–60% HRR or Borg rating 12–13 during neoadjuvant therapy. Allen et al. [63] and Minnella et al. [64], Christensen et al. [66] demonstrated feasibility of 1–2 times a week resistance exercise program of 2–3 sets of 4–8 exercises with 8–12 repetitions during neoadjuvant therapy. However, Christensen et al. [66], who specifically tested a HIIT prehabilitation program demonstrated statistically reduced postoperative complications in the prehabilitation group compared to controls. Prehabilitation aerobic and resistance training attenuated the effects of neoadjuvant chemotherapy on VO_2 peak reductions, skeletal muscle loss, hand grip strength reductions, 6MWT reductions and improved neoadjuvant treatment tolerability, reduced hospital admissions, reduced rate of treatment postponement, and reduced rates of common toxicities compared to those who did not undergo a rehabilitation program. Ameliorated cardiorespiratory fitness implies improved postoperative outcomes for patients with esophagogastric cancers.

Inspiratory Muscle Strengthening Benefits Patients with Esophageal and Lung Cancer

Postoperative pulmonary complications frequently result in morbidity and mortality in patients with lung and esophageal cancer as well as increased hospital length of stay and length of stay in the intensive care unit [90, 115–119]. The prolonged length of stay from postoperative pulmonary complications results in increased healthcare costs as well as increased hospital-acquired debility. Therefore, optimizing patients' preoperative lung function is essential to obtaining the best postoperative outcomes. Current evidence supports inspiratory muscle strengthening and breathing exercises for improving pulmonary lung function as well as reducing postoperative pulmonary complications specifically in patients with lung and esophageal cancer.

In the existing literature, pulmonary rehabilitation with incentive spirometry and inspiratory muscle training improved pulmonary lung function and decreased postoperative pulmonary complications in participants with lung and esophageal cancer (see Table 2, included in the Appendix) [90, 115–119]. Inspiratory muscle strengthening involves either incentive spirometry or an inspiratory threshold loading device varying from 20 to 60% maximal inspiratory pressure with 30–60 breaths one to four times a day or exercises lasting 10–30 min a day [116–118]. Pulmonary

Table 2 Respiratory and inspiratory muscle strengthening locoregional prehabilitation

Study	Population	Intervention(s)	Outcomes measured	Outcomes
Barassi et al. [115]	32 participants with lung cancer and actively smoking	7-day treatment, yoga breathing diaphragmatic breathing with 12 s breathing cycle 4 s inspiration, 4 s air retention, 8 s of exhalation, 3 sets of 10 yoga breaths with 30–60 s pauses repeated 30 times a day compared to standard deep slow breathing 3 sets of 10 deep breaths	CPET, PFT, HR, SpO_2	Statistically significant improvements in FVC, FEV1, Tiffeneau-Pinelli index, peak inspiratory flow, peak expiratory flow, HR, and SpO_2 from baseline compared to preoperative testing in the yoga breathing group. Statistically significant improvements in SpO_2 in the yoga group compared to the standard breathing
Bobbio et al. [86]	12 participants with non-small cell lung cancer	4-week supervised program, 5 days a week for 40 min of aerobic recumbent cycling targeting 50–80% maximal work rate and resistance training of the upper extremity and incentive spirometry exercises twice daily at home	PFT, CPET, VO_2 max	Statistically significant improved VO_2 max, workload capacity, and oxygen pulse in the prehabilitation group pre-operatively compared to baseline
Gravier et al. [93]	50 participants with non-small cell lung cancer	6 weeks, 3–5 times per week aerobic training 5 min warm up and cool down, 20–35 min at the ventilatory threshold and resistance training targeting quadriceps press, whole leg extension, upper limb pull down at 60–70% 1RM, 3 sets of 12 as well as 15 min daily inspiratory muscle strengthening 30% maximum inspiratory pressure	CPET, VE/VCO_2 slope, number of training sessions to obtain physiologic effect	Statistically significant improvements in VO_2 peak, W peak, Wvt, VO_2vt/VO_2 peak Statistically significant changes in VE/VCO_2 slope and VO_2 peak after 15 prehabilitation sessions compared to baseline

(continued)

Table 2 (continued)

Study	Population	Intervention(s)	Outcomes measured	Outcomes
Lai et al. [84]	48 participants with lung cancer	One-week supervised training program, daily 15–20 min aerobic recumbent cycling and 15–30 min of stair climbing with a targeted Borg score 5–7. 15–30 min of diaphragmatic breathing with prolong inhalation, exhalation, and breath holds and incentive spirometry use every 2 h with 12–20 times per set Medical intervention: aerosol inhalation of bronchodilators and glucocorticoids (Bricanyl 2 mL + Pulmicort Respirin 4 mL twice daily) Mucosolvan injection 30 mg twice daily	Postoperative length of stay, duration of antibiotic use, peak expiratory flow, 6MWT, energy expenditure, pulmonary complications, total hospital costs, medicine cost, material cost, European Organization of Research and Treatment of Cancer-Quality of Life Questionnaire-Lung Cancer	Statistically significant improvements in postoperative length of stay, duration of antibiotic use, peak expiratory flow, 6MWT, increased energy expenditure, and reduced pulmonary complications and dyspnea scores in the prehabilitation group
Lai et al. [85]	60 participants with lung cancer	One week supervised aerobic daily 30-min aerobic recumbent cycling combined with diaphragmatic breathing twice a day for 15–20 min with prolonged inhalation, exhalation, and breath holds and incentive spirometry use every 2–3 times per day for 20 min	6MWD, pulmonary function tests, HRQoL	Statistically significant improvements in the 6MWD, pulmonary exhalation function test in the prehabilitation group preoperatively compared to baseline and reduced postoperative length of stay, total hospital length of stay, and postoperative pulmonary complications in the prehabilitation group

Sebio et al. [92]	40 participants with lung cancer	7-week supervised program 3–5 times per week with 30 min HIIT targeting 80% W peak for 1 min with 4 min active rests 50% W peak on a cycle ergometer and 6 resistance exercises targeting the main muscle groups for three sets of 15 repetitions with 45s rest between sets Home breathing exercises twice daily using an incentive spirometer with 30 sustained inspirations at maximal vital capacity and end inspiratory hold 2–3 s	CPET, SF-36, postoperative outcomes Melbourne group scale, 6MWT, Colinet Comorbidity score	Statistically significant improvements in exercise tolerance, the physical summary complaint of SF-36, muscle strength, constant cycling endurance test, number of repetitions of arm curls, chair-to-stand from baseline to preoperative assessment
Pehlivan et al. [90]	60 participants with lung cancer	1 week preoperatively, 3 times a day treadmill walking and diaphragmatic, coughing, pursed lip, segmental breathing exercises and insensitive spirometry use	CPET, PFT, DLCO, V/Q distributions, DEXA	Statistically significant improvements in VC, FEV1, PaO_2, $PaCO_2$, DLCO, maximum heart rate, maximum speed, distance covered, contralateral V/Q distribution and reduced pulmonary complications in the prehabilitation group compared to the control group
Stefanelli et al. [87]	40 participants with non-small cell lung cancer	3 weeks supervised HIIT with 15 sessions over 3 weeks for 3 h on the ergometer rowing and bicycle targeting 70% of maximal workload. Non-specific respiratory breathing exercises	CPET, PFT, Borg scale	Statistically significant improvements in VO_2 predicted, Borg grades, DLCO, FEV1 baseline versus preoperative testing in the prehabilitation group

(continued)

Table 2 (continued)

Study	Population	Intervention(s)	Outcomes measured	Outcomes
van Adrichem et al. [116]	39 participants with esophageal cancer	3 weeks, 3 times a week supervised consisting of 6 by 6 inspiratory maneuvers on inspiratory threshold loading device Resting time decreased 60s down to 5 s over time	Postoperative pulmonary complications, hospital length of stay, duration of mechanical ventilation, reintubations, maximal inspiratory pressure, PFT	Statistically significant improvements in postoperative pulmonary complications, length of stay, reintubations compared to controls, peak inspiratory flow, maximal inspiratory pressure in the inspiratory training group compared to controls
Valkenet et al. [117]	120 patients with esophageal cancer	2-week home program of 30 breaths twice a day on a flow resistive inspiratory loading device at 60% of maximum inspiratory pressure	Postoperative pulmonary complications, inspiratory muscle function, PFT, postoperative complications, duration of mechanical ventilation, length of hospital stay	Statistically significant improvements mean maximal inspiratory muscle strength, preoperative inspiratory muscle endurance in the intervention group compared to baseline
Morano et al. [118]	24 participants with lung cancer	4 weeks, 5 times per week to daily aerobic exercise for 30 min at 80% WR max and inspiratory muscle training using threshold inspiratory muscle trainer 10–30 min day 20–60% maximal inspiratory pressure	PFT, postoperative respiratory morbidity, hospital length of stay, duration of chest tube	Statistically significant improvements in FVC, predicted FVC, 6MWT, maximal inspiratory pressure, maximal expiratory pressure, postoperative morbidity, length of stay, duration of chest tube

Benzo et al. [119]	19 participants with lung cancer and COPD	4 weeks of 10 supervised preoperative exercise sessions lasting 15–20 min daily using inspiratory muscle training threshold with an inspiratory muscle trainer at "somewhat hard" perceived exertion and slowed breathing with respiratory rate <10 breaths per minute	Hospital length of stay, postoperative pulmonary complications, duration of mechanical ventilation, duration of chest tubes	Statistically significant improvements in hospital length of stay and reduced time requiring a chest tube compared to controls

Note. List of randomized clinical trials evaluating the role of respiratory exercises and inspiratory muscle training preoperatively to improve clinical outcomes in patients with cancer. Abbreviations. *s* seconds, *CPET* cardiopulmonary exercise testing, *PFT* pulmonary function test, *HR* heart rate, *HIIT* high intensity interval training, SpO_2 blood oxygen saturation, *FVC* forced vital capacity, *FEV1* forced expiratory volume 1 second, VO_2 *max* maximum volume of oxygen consumption, *1RM* 1 repetition maximum, VE/VCO_2 minute ventilation/carbon dioxide production, VO_2 *peak* peak oxygen consumption at maximum exercise, *W* work, *Wvt* work at anaerobic threshold, VO_2vt oxygen consumption at ventilatory threshold, *6MWD* 6 minute walk test, *HRQoL* healthcare related quality of life, *SF-36* short form 36, *VC* vital capacity, PaO_2 arterial partial pressure of oxygen, $PaCO_2$ arterial partial pressure of carbon dioxide, *DLCO* diffusing capacity for carbon monoxide, *V/Q* ventilation/perfusion, *DEXA* dual x-ray absorptiometry, *WR max* maximum work rate rehabilitation programs vary in duration from 1 to 4 weeks, and frequency from daily to three times a week with statistically significant improvements in pulmonary function tests [90, 115–119]. However, the type of additional breathing exercise varied from deep, slow breathing over 12 s for 3 sets of 10 breaths to inspiration at maximal vital capacity with end-inspiratory breath holds. Yoga breathing and standard deep inspiratory breathing both improved pulmonary lung function test values of FVC, FEV1, peak inspiratory and expiratory flow, as well as resting heart rate [115]. However, patients who performed yoga breathing significantly improved their oxygen saturation (SpO_2) compared to the standard breathing group. Yoga breathing was characterized by diaphragmatic or abdomen breathing with a 16-s breathing cycle 4 s of inspiration, 4 se of air retention, and 8 s of exhalation for 3 sets of 10 yoga breaths with 30–60 s pauses repeated 30 times a day. Participants with COPD and those who are actively smoking or completing neoadjuvant therapies all benefited from inspiratory muscle strengthening [115–117, 119].

Breathing exercises safely augment cardiopulmonary exercise prehabilitation regardless of the intensity [84–87, 92, 93]. Unlike breathing exercises, however, aerobic exercise has not demonstrated an impact on pulmonary function. Breathing exercises are feasible to combine with moderate to vigorous intensity aerobic exercise or even HIIT prescriptions. Both individually and when combined with an aerobic exercise program, breathing exercises improve pulmonary function tests and improve postoperative outcomes. Unfortunately, it is unclear if breathing exercises and an aerobic prehabilitation program are synergistic regarding improving cardiopulmonary function and postoperative outcomes.

Colorectal Cancer

Colorectal prehabilitation exercise recommendations typically target improved cardiorespiratory fitness to improve postoperative outcomes. A 4–week, ≥3 days per week 30-min aerobic exercise program targeting >50% HR max resulted in cardiometabolic enhancements (see Table 1, included in the Appendix) [62, 81, 100, 114]. Additionally, resistance training with 4–8 exercises, 8–12 repetitions three times a week may contribute to the prehabilitation cardiometabolic benefits specifically, pre-and postoperative 6MWT, VO_2 peak, and VO_2 max up to 4 weeks postoperatively [81, 100, 114]. Li et al. [71] demonstrated a 1-week aerobic exercise program three times a week targeting 50% HR max was sufficient to improve cardiometabolic parameters such as 6MWT, and functional walking capacity pre- and postoperatively. Peng et al. [79] demonstrated that preoperative exercises on the day of surgery including hand squeezes statistically improve pre and postoperative hand grip strength; however, the clinical benefits are unclear regarding this improvement. Carli et al. [67] did not demonstrate cardiometabolic benefits in participants who exercised 1 day a week for 30 min at moderate-intensity aerobic training combined with 25 min of resistance training [84]. Uniquely, Dronkers et al. [72] demonstrated greater than 4000 steps daily for 2–4 weeks preoperatively statistically reduced postoperative pulmonary complications [70]. Therefore, overall preoperative physical activity benefits postoperative physical fitness, however aerobic frequency of greater than three times a week may be necessary for cardiometabolic benefits.

Preoperative HIIT training can attenuate neoadjuvant chemotherapy's effect on cardiopulmonary fitness in patients undergoing treatment for colorectal cancer. Berkel et al. [78] demonstrated a HIIT exercise program can statistically reduce postoperative complications on Charlson score in addition to statistically improving VO_2 VT and VO_2 peak. West et al. [74] demonstrated a HIIT program preserved VO_2 uptake at the lactate threshold, and VO_2 peak at 6 weeks post neoadjuvant chemoradiotherapy. Berkel et al. [78] and West et al. [74]) demonstrated a 3–6 week supervised HIIT program three times a week for 30 min with 4–6 sets of 2–3 min intervals targeting 100–120% WR at VT or 80% VO_2 max and rests targeting 50% VO_2 max or WR at VT effectively enhanced participants cardiometabolic abilities. In addition to HIIT, neoadjuvant chemotherapeutic cardiac effects are also attenuated by moderate-vigorous intensity exercises [77]. Patients with rectal cancer recurrence undergoing neoadjuvant chemotherapy demonstrate cardiometabolic preservation with prehabilitation [77].

Urologic Cancer

Specifically for participants with bladder cancer, Jensen et al. [94] demonstrated that as little as 2 weeks of preoperative aerobic prehabilitation is effective in improving postoperative physical fitness if completed daily for 60 min. In participants with prostate cancer, Santa Mina et al. [95] demonstrated a 10-week prehabilitation, 3–4 days a week of aerobic moderate-intensity exercise lasting for 60 min was effective in improving participants' 6MWT. Blackwell et al. [97] demonstrated that a 20-min HIIT program occurring 3–4 times a week improves cardiometabolic markers in 4 weeks in participants with bladder, prostate, and kidney cancers [97]. In addition to cardiometabolic improvements, participants with bladder cancer post neoadjuvant chemotherapy who completed prehabilitation have statistically reduced overall hospital lengths of stay as well as stay in high-dependency units [96]. A preoperative aerobic exercise program concurring with neoadjuvant treatment, specifically HIIT for patients with urological cancer can improve their physical and clinical outcomes.

Pelvic Floor Dysfunction as Sequelae of Colorectal, Urologic, and Gynecological Cancer

Urinary and bowel incontinence is common after any surgery that disrupts the pelvic floor [120–123]. Radical prostatectomy for prostate cancer, hysterectomy and trachelectomy for gynecological cancers, proctocolectomy for colorectal cancers, and cystectomy for bladder cancers alter the pelvic floor and place the patient at risk for incontinence induced by postoperative intrinsic sphincter deficiency. Urinary incontinence dramatically impacts a patient's quality of life as well as places them at increased risk for falls and skin breakdown. Physical activity in the form of aerobic exercise or resistance training appears to have little or no effect on continence [98]. Current evidence for patients with prostate cancer undergoing radical prostatectomy demonstrates preoperative pelvic floor muscle exercises improve urinary incontinence [121–123]. However, there is limited evidence on preoperative pelvic floor muscle exercises benefiting patients with rectal cancer undergoing anus-preserving surgery [120].

A pelvic floor prehabilitation program focusing on improving pelvic musculature contraction strength and endurance improves urinary continence and ultimately quality of life in patients with prostate and rectal cancer (see Table 3, included in the Appendix) [98, 120, 122, 124–126]. Frequency, duration, and supervision of the pelvic floor program appear to affect treatment outcomes. Most supervised pelvic floor programs last 1 month, occur between 3 times per week and daily, and last 10–30 min per session [122, 124, 125]. Milios et al. [122] indicate that 120 contractions daily result in statistically significant improvements in continence post-radical prostatectomy. Wu et al. [120] demonstrated that pelvic floor muscle therapy benefits patients with rectal cancer demonstrating statistically significant improvements in rectal tone, pressure, and compliance up to 6 months postoperatively. Unfortunately, the direct benefit to continence and quality needs further elucidation in patients with rectal cancer. Of note, the quality of the contractions appears essential in ultimately improving continence. Home pelvic floor muscle therapy programs yield less significant results compared to a supervised program with constant appraisal and feedback regarding contraction technique [123, 125]. Pelvic floor prehabilitation programs enhance postoperative quality of life by improving continence [122, 124], and improvements in healthcare-related quality of life may last up to 3 months postoperatively. Pelvic floor functional improvements are directly affected by the quantity, duration, frequency, and quality of pelvic floor exercises.

Lower Extremity Lymphedema Sequelae of Colorectal, Urologic, and Gynecological Cancer

Lower extremity lymphedema is a common comorbidity affecting those with gynecological cancer [127], specifically due to surgical disruption in pelvic drainage. Evidence supports complex decongestive therapy and specific exercises benefit patients with upper extremity lymphedema from breast cancer. However, evidence is limited on the benefit of locoregional-specific exercises and complex decongestive therapy for lower extremity lymphedema. Currently, a study by Wu et al. [120] is the only randomized clinical trial addressing the prevention of lower extremity lymphedema specifically in patients with gynecologic cancer [127]. In this study, a total of 109 patients with cervical, endometrial, or ovarian cancer received lower extremity exercises and manual lymphatic drainage techniques up to 40 days preoperatively. Patients performed 15–20 repetitions twice a day of exercises that targeted the full range of motion of the hip, knee, and ankle in all mechanically applicable planes. Participants taught the leg exercises and manual lymphatic drainage had a statistically significant reduction in lymphedema free time postoperatively. This

Table 3 Pelvic floor locoregional prehabilitation

Study	Population	Intervention(s)	Outcomes measured	Outcomes
Centemero et al. [124]	143 men with prostate cancer	1 month supervised intensive PFME for 30 min. Twice a week 30 min, HEP, patients altered between maximal and submaximal contractions with feedback regarding endurances and contraction quality, breathing coordination, typifying muscle contraction as tonic, and modifying incorrect physical attitudes	Continence at 1, 3, months postoperatively, quality of life, Continence Society male short form	Statically significant improvements in continence and improvements International Continence Society male short form (testing QoL) postoperatively at 1 months, and 3 months in the prehabilitation group compared to controls
Milios et al. [122]	97 men with prostate cancer	5-week supervised PFME with 6 sets with 10 slow (1 s duration) contractions and 10 fast contractions (10 s duration) for a total of 120 contractions per day Usual care was daily 3 sets with 10 contractions of PFME per day	Continence 24 h postoperatively by pad weight, rapid response test using ultrasound to measure pelvic floor muscle contraction and sustained endurance test for sustained pelvic contraction	Statistically significant improvements in continence 24 h postoperatively at 2, 6, and 12 weeks postoperatively, improvements in speed and duration of a rapid and sustained contraction, respectively Statistically significant improvements in continence score international prostate symptom score at 2 and 6 weeks postoperatively, respectively in the prehabilitation group compared to controls
Anan et al. [125]	70 patients with prostate cancer	1-month HEP with 3 min of PFME 3 times a day	Self-reported continence postoperatively, incontinence questionnaire short form score	Statistically significant improvements in continence 3 months postoperatively with improvement trends 3 days, 1 month postoperatively in the prehabilitation group compared to controls
Dijkstra et al. [121]	122 participants with prostate cancer	4 weeks, once a week PMFE with biofeedback 10 maximum voluntary contractions lasting 3 s, 3 maximum endurance contractions lasting 30 s, and a Valsalva maneuver	Stress urinary incontinence, QoL, Pelvic floor Inventories, King's Health Questionnaire, International Prostate Symptom Score, bladder diary, 24-h pad test at 1-year follow-up	No statistical difference at 1 year postoperatively with trends in improvements 6 weeks, 3, 6, and 9 months postoperatively in the prehabilitation group compared to controls

(continued)

Table 3 (continued)

Study	Population	Intervention(s)	Outcomes measured	Outcomes
Goode et al. [123]	245 participants with prostate cancer	1–4 weeks, HEP with online video 5–10 min each 45 PFME per day 15 sets, 3 times per day with 1 s contraction increasing to 10 s contraction	International Consultation on Incontinence Questionnaire Short Form, Urinary Incontinence Subscale of Expanded Prostate Cancer Index Composite, International Prostate Symptom Score QoL question and Global Perception of Improvement	No statistical difference between men completing >80% of sessions compared to those completing <80% of sessions
Ocampo et al. [126]	16 participants with prostate cancer	4-weeks supervised PFME three times a day	Muscle function of the external urethral sphincter, contraction pressure of the levator ani, urinary incontinence, and HRQoL	Statistically significant improvements in the cross-sectional area of the external urethral sphincter, higher pressure contraction of the levator ani, preoperatively and improved continence postoperatively after foley removal in the prehabilitation group compared to controls
Wu et al. [120]	126 patients with rectal cancer	4 weeks daily HEP with videos, PFME maintain contraction 5–10 s, relax 10 s, 10 time a session, 5 sessions per day. PFME with biofeedback sensor, 3 times a week for 20 min	High-resolution anorectal manometry, Intestinal Function Questionnaire	Statistically significant improvements in anal resting pressure, rectal resting pressure, anal maximum systolic pressure, anal maximum systolic time, initial rectal volume, rectal fecal sensory capacity, rectal maximum tolerance capacity, rectal compliance, anorectal hypertensive zone and total score of intestinal function at 1, 3, and 6 months postoperatively in the prehabilitation group compared to controls

Note. List of randomized clinical trials evaluating the role of pelvic floor muscle training preoperatively to improve clinical outcomes in patients with cancer. Abbreviations. *HEP* home exercise program, *QoL* quality of life, *PFME* pelvic floor muscle exercises, *s* seconds, *HRQoL* healthcare-related quality of life, *HRR* heart rate reserve, *1RM* one repetition maximum suggests that dedicated lower extremity techniques reduce the incidence of lymphedema in participants with gynecological cancer. Although the data is limited, the current evidence positively supports the benefit of early education and treatment with locoregional therapy for patients with gynecologic cancer in a low-risk intervention.

Breast Cancer

Prehabilitation programs' effect on the cardiometabolic profile of patients with breast cancer is limited by the amount of current evidence (see Table 1, included in the Appendix). The current literature supports the positive impact of physical activity on mental health and cancer-related fatigue. Mijwel et al. [99] and Knoerl et al. [100] both demonstrate preoperative aerobic programs statistically improve cognitive function, cancer-related fatigue, stress, anxiety, and total cancer symptoms pre- and postoperatively [99, 100]. Although the studies are limited on the benefits of exercise prehabilitation programs benefits on cardiometabolic fitness in patients with breast cancer, there is evidence that exercise prehabilitation programs benefit these patients' emotional quality of life, cognitive function, and reduce fatigue.

Upper Limb Lymphedema Sequelae of Breast and Head and Neck Cancer

Upper limb dysfunction and lymphedema are common sequelae of breast cancer and treatment, but may also occur in the treatment of head and neck cancers and lymphoma [128, 129]. Upper limb dysfunction is characterized by reduced range of motion, shoulder pain, and muscle dysfunction. Cancerous tumors, chest irradiation, and surgical treatments disrupt the lymphatic system, nerves, soft tissue, and musculature leading to lymphedema and/or upper limb dysfunction. Upper limb pain questionnaires, subjective perception of postoperative functional impairment of the arm (SPOFIA), and disabilities of the arm, shoulder, and hand (DASH) scores increase after breast cancer treatment [128, 129]. Ten to forty percent of patients undergoing radiation therapy and approximately 50% of patients undergoing standard lymph node dissection develop lymphedema. Many patients develop upper limb pathology regardless of prior symptoms and muscle dysfunction best predicts the severity of arm pain more than risk factors like advanced age or time since surgery treatment [128, 129]. Current data support preoperative evaluation and targeted locoregional prehabilitation to reduce the development of upper quadrant dysfunction and lymphedema from breast cancer treatments (see Table 4, included in the Appendix) [129–137].

Upper extremity prehabilitation identifies and treats current dysfunction to prevent further progression. Physical therapy treats the potential causes of pain and dysfunction such as muscle shortening (contracture), reduced range of motion, loss of muscle activity, scarring, and fibrosis. Prehabilitation education on upper limb

Table 4 Upper extremity disfunction and lymphedema locoregional prehabilitation

Study	Population	Intervention(s)	Outcomes measured	Outcomes
Baima et al. [129]	60 participants with breast cancer	Non-specific supervised with HEP brochure and videos	Exercise compliance, shoulder pain, shoulder abduction ROM, seroma formation	Statistically significant improvements in pain 1 month postoperatively in the prehabilitation group compared to controls
Springer et al. [130]	94 participants with breast cancer	Non-specific supervised preoperative shoulder assessment with individualized postoperative rehabilitation program	Shoulder ROM, manual muscle test, pain, upper arm volume, upper limb disability questionnaire	Statistically significant improved ROM 1, 3, 6 months and pain scores postoperatively in the prehabilitation group compared to controls
Nilsson et al. [131]	180 participants with breast cancer 14	Preoperative fitness was evaluated	Physical activity level preoperatively, self-assessed physical and mental recovery, hospital length of stay	Statistically significant preoperative physical fitness was associated with increased return to baseline fitness
Singh et al. [132]	73 participants with breast cancer	Non-specific supervised exercise education shoulder ROM, strength, and upper limb girth assessment	Shoulder ROM, upper limb strength, upper limb girth, functional and QoL	Significant improvements in flexion ROM with trends in improvement in limb strength, girth, function, and QoL in the prehabilitation group compared to controls
Smoot et al. [133]	396 participants with breast cancer	Preoperative ROM, grip strength, pain, functional status questionnaires	ROM, grip strength	Preoperative shoulder flexion and abduction ROM was a strong predictor of 1-month postoperative ROM, preoperative grip strength predictor postoperative grip strength and preoperative exercise increase shoulder flexion subclinical importance at 1 month

(continued)

Table 4 (continued)

Study	Population	Intervention(s)	Outcomes measured	Outcomes
Byun et al. [134]	61 participants	Non-specific preoperative education with a physical therapist	Passive shoulder ROM, VAS, short DASH, SPADI, and arm circumference preoperatively	Statistically significant improvements in arm abduction, flexion 6 months postoperatively, improvements in VAS, DASH, and SPADI scores at 1 month postoperatively compared to controls
Sato et al. [135]	149 participants with breast cancer	1-week preoperative education and monitoring arm function program with exercises that prevent shoulder dysfunction and lymphedema	Arm girth, shoulder ROM, grip strength, SPOFIA, DASH score	Statistically significant improvements in SPOFIA and grip strength with preoperative education at 1 and 3 months postoperatively in the prehabilitation group compared to controls
Sato et al. [136]	67 participants with breast cancer	Preoperative education on lymphedema and arm dysfunction with emphasis on prevention exercises, arm monitoring for function changes, (ROM, identifying numbness and pain, arm girth)	ROM, arm girth, grip strength, SPOFIA, DASH, SF-36, health-related quality of life	Statistically significant improvements in SPOFIA, Grip strength, and horizontal arm extension at 1 week and 12 months postoperatively in the prehabilitation group compared to controls
Temur and Kapucu [137]	108 participants with breast cancer	Preoperative education regarding self-management of lymphedema (symptoms and signs, development mechanisms, skin care, protecting the arm, exercising) however exercise intervention commenced postoperatively	DASH, upper extremity circumference measurement, EORTC QLQ-30	Statistically significantly reduced lymphedema and quality of life in the intervention group

Note. List of randomized clinical trials evaluating the role of arm range of motion and exercises preoperatively on clinical outcomes in patients with cancer. Abbreviations: *HEP* home exercise program, *QoL* quality of life, *ROM* range of motion, *VAS* visual analog scale, *DASH* disability of arm, shoulder, and hand, *SPADI* shoulder pain and disability index, *SPOFIA* Subjective Perception of Post-Operative Functional Impairment of the Arm, *EORTC QLQ-30* European Organization for the Research and Treatment of Cancer Quality of Life Questionnaire, *SF-36* short form-36 dysfunction and lymphedema (including the pathophysiology, techniques for monitoring dysfunction, shoulder ROM, strengthening, and stretching exercises) empowers patients with the ability to treat and prevent breast cancer sequalae. Prior research identified that patients who participated in prehabilitation programs demonstrated improved arm range of motion (ROM), arm circumference, grip strength and SPOFIA, pain scores via the visual analog score (VAS), reduced arm swelling, and overall quality of life postoperatively compared to controls who participated in a postoperative rehabilitation program [130]. Unfortunately, specifics regarding shoulder strengthening and range of motion exercises were not specified.

Temur and Kapucu [137] and Dönmez and Kapucu [138] demonstrated specific therapeutic exercises to treat upper limb dysfunction and lymphedema [137, 138]. However, despite the preoperative evaluation and education, the studies focused on *postoperative* rehabilitation. Patients were given 12 active and passive stretching exercises for which they gradually increased from 6 to −10 times a day, lasting from 30 to 60 min. These exercises consisted of shoulder shrugs, large and small shoulder circles, arm circles, wall pushups, weightless overhead presses, and moving the shoulder through full abduction, adduction, flexion, and extension [137]. Dönmez and Kapucu [138] confirmed that a physical exercise program consisting of ball squeezing and hand opening and closing exercises lasting 3–5 min, twice daily aided in the prevention of lymphedema.

Current data support the benefit of locoregional prehabilitation to improve arm ROM, postoperative pain scores, quality of life, grip strength, and reduce postoperative lymphedema. However, a critical portion of the current prehabilitation data is preoperative education as preventative care. The postoperative period may be the wrong time to initiate education on arm function and dysfunction as patients may be preoccupied with pain, function, recovery, and managing medications. Evaluating and empowering a patient for their own recovery prior to surgery appears critical to reducing upper limb dysfunction and lymphedema. In the presurgical phase, early rehabilitation and functional education may make patients more aware of their affected arm and how to improve its function to foster improved postoperative rehabilitation. Preoperative education appears critical in improving postoperative outcomes and quality of life in patients at risk for developing lymphedema [129–137].

Hematologic Cancer

Bone marrow transplants are a potentially life-saving procedure for individuals with certain types of cancer and/or blood disorders such as leukemia, lymphoma, and multiple myeloma. The purpose of treatment is to replace damaged or diseased bone marrow cells with healthy cells from either an existing donor, known as an allogeneic transplant, or the patient's own marrow or stem cells through autologous transplantation. Despite the potential to cure life-threatening diseases, there are several risks and complications associated with this type of cancer treatment. The most serious complication is graft-versus-host disease (GvHD), which occurs when the transplanted immune cells attack the patient's own healthy and normal body tissues.

Other side effects include organ damage from chemotherapy used to prepare for the transplant; infection due to immunosuppression; inability for cure by one transplant; and death due to complications of the procedure itself.

Chimeric antigen receptor T cell (CAR-T cell) therapy is a revolutionary type of immunotherapy, a new treatment arm developed for certain cancers. It is applied in clinical practice for hematological malignancies including leukemia, lymphoma, and multiple myeloma [139]. This form of cancer treatment takes advantage of the body's own immune cells—T cells—to specifically target and attack cancer cells. CAR (chimeric antigen receptors) are engineered molecules embedded onto the surface of T cells to recognize the antigens on cancer cells. Once these receptors bind to the antigens, they signal the T cells to destroy the cancer cells. The process starts with the collection of some of a patient's own T cells from their blood and sending them off for laboratory processing. A specialized gene editing technique is used to insert new genetic material that codes for an antigen receptor into these collected T cells in order for them to recognize and bind to tumor antigens.

While CAR-T cell therapies are associated with promising results with high rates of survival, they can also come with potentially life-threatening side effects. Common side effects can range from minor symptoms such as headache, fever, nausea, and vomiting to more severe complications like immune effector cell-associated neurotoxicity syndrome (ICANS) and cytokine release syndrome (CRS). CRS is often considered a hallmark of CAR-T therapy as it occurs in up to 90% of patients and is caused by an excessive release of cytokines when CAR-T Cells bind to their targets, resulting in high fever, chills, nausea, and other flu-like symptoms. The severity can range from mild to life-threatening; however, most cases can be managed with medication or supportive therapies such as intravenous fluids or steroids.

Prehabilitation potentially has benefits for patients about to undergo transplants. Ideally, the prehabilitation program starts at diagnosis in preparation for cancer-directed treatment and eventual transplantation. These include physical conditioning, nutritional counseling, and psychological guidance. The comprehensive approach allows patients to tolerate the rigorous treatments associated with the transplant process. The physical component of prehabilitation includes engaging in low-impact exercises such as walking and resistance exercise training to maintain muscle mass throughout chemotherapy and/or radiation therapy—which are essential parts of the treatment regimen prior to harvesting stem cells for reinfusion during the transplant procedure.

Currently, there are limited studies evaluating the effect of physical exercise prior to autologous stem cell transplant for patients with multiple myeloma (see Table 1, included in the Appendix) [103, 104]. McCourt et al. [103] and Mawson et al. [104] indicate that physical activity is feasible prior to autologous stem cell transplant (ASCT) and may convey cardiometabolic benefits. The supervised prehabilitation programs are 5–6 weeks, 3 times per week targeting 15–40 min of aerobic exercise at 60–80% of heart rate reserve and resistance training of up to 9 exercises with 10 repetitions. Participants experienced improved quality of life, cancer-related fatigue, functional capacity, 6MWT, and physical activity prior to ASCT. Although the data is limited, prehabilitation exercise programs appear beneficial to patients with hematologic cancers requiring ASCT.

There are no data available yet on prehabilitation before chimeric antigen receptor T cell therapy. However, according to Iukuridze et al. [140], sarcopenia is an important and independent predictor of outcomes after CAR-T, including the increased burden of acute toxicities (59.1% sarcopenic patients developed CRS, 30.1% developed ICANS—immune effector cell-associated neurotoxicity syndrome) and prolonged length of hospitalization (25.6 vs 21.9 days) [140]. A follow-up study by Lee et al. [40, 141] demonstrated patients with abnormally low skeletal muscle mass at baseline were at greatest risk of ICANS (HR, 1.74; 95% CI, 1.05–2.87) and had a longer length of hospitalization (mean 27.7 vs 22.9 days; $P < 0.05$) compared with those with normal muscle mass [141]. In addition, the same group identified abnormal skeletal muscle mass was independently associated with risk of disease progression (HR, 1.70; 95% CI, 1.11–2.57) and worse survival (HR, 2.44; 95% CI, 1.49–4.00) at 1 year compared with normal skeletal muscle. The research concludes that baseline anthropomorphic/functional data gathered before treatment may inform risk stratification prior to CAR T-cell therapy or prompt initiation of prehabilitation and nutritional optimization before lymphodepletion. It includes activities such as diet modifications and exercise routines tailored specifically to improve the strength and endurance of an individual patient prior to beginning therapy.

As with other cancer diagnoses, rehabilitation of patients with hematological malignancies presenting with functional impairments and limitations can be very beneficial. In general, these patients present with cognitive impairment, muscle weakness, reduced exercise capacity, neuropathy, cancer-related fatigue, and reduced physical activity. Patients receiving CAR T cell therapy may present with general deconditioning and neurological complications which translate to neuromuscular and cognitive impairments that benefit from multidisciplinary rehabilitation intervention prior to, during, and after treatment, although the research data is limited [142].

6 Nutritional Intervention

Regardless of cancer type and anticipated treatment, all patients should have a nutrition screen early to determine their risk for malnutrition [143]. As a key component of a prehabilitation program, early nutrition interventions can improve patient outcomes [143]. The European Society for Clinical Nutrition in Surgery and Enhanced Recovery after Surgery (ERAS) have set protocols with improved 5-year survival post-oncologic surgery [35]. ERAS emphasizes the importance of early and integrated nutritional care into the overall management of the patient [35]. The nutrition care process model described a four-step process nutritional assessment, diagnosis, intervention, monitoring, and evaluation [143].

The first step is identifying malnutrition and quantifying the severity. There are several assessments specifically used for oncologic patients with unintentional weight loss. The subjective global assessment (SGA) and patient-generated subjective global assessment (PG-SA) are the most validated tools used to diagnose malnutrition in oncologic patients. Other validated assessments are the Royal Marsden Nutrition Screening Tool, Abridged patient-generated subjective global assessment, NUTRISCORE, Bach Mai Boston Tool, and Malnutrition screening tool for cancer [143]. The NUTRISCORE appears the most sensitive (97.3%) and specific (95.9%) for correctly identifying malnourished patients with cancer [143]. Failing to correctly diagnose malnutrition may hinder a patient's functional gains from other multimodal prehabilitation domains like exercise [36]. The National Institute of Health Research Cancer and Nutrition Collaboration suggests using the severity of malnutrition to target nutrition care. Those with severe (SGA C, PG-SGA >8) or moderate (SGA B, PG-SGA 4–8) malnutrition require a registered dietician guiding nutritional intervention. Therefore, nutrition assessment guides the individualized nutritional care plan and support [36]. Early nutritional intervention is paramount as soon as nutritional risks become apparent [35].

A registered dietician (RD) should evaluate patients identified with malnutrition [143]. RDs complete comprehensive interventions, including collecting a thorough nutritional history and biochemical data and intervening on behavioral, social, and environmental factors that affect nutritional status [143]. The European Society for Clinical Nutrition and Metabolism (formerly European Society for Parenteral and Enteral Nutrition- ESPEN) guidelines indicate the following are indicators for risk of severe malnutrition:

- weight loss >10–15% within 6 months,
- body mass index <18.5 kg/m^2,
- Subjective Global Assessment Grade C or NRS ≥5.
- preoperative serum albumin <30 g/L without hepatic or renal dysfunction [35].

Those with severe malnutrition require RD-guided nutritional interventions as well as close nutrition monitoring [143]. Food records and 24-h dietary food recalls (possibly involving mobile apps) both assess nutrition history and offer patients a way to monitor and meet estimated protein and calorie requirements [143]. Those not at malnutrition risk should at a minimum receive "usual care" regarding nutrition, such as a hand-out emphasizing a balanced diet with protein, fruits, and vegetables.

Although non-diagnostic, biochemical data are useful to evaluate and monitor a patient's nutrition status. Some data suggest preoperative serum albumin is a prognostic indicator for postoperative complications [35]. Traditionally, albumin is a predictor of nutrition status [35]; however, albumin is a negative acute phase reactant such that inflammation may cause hypoalbuminemia rather than being the result of protein insufficiency [35]. Prealbumin has a shorter half-life compared to albumin and acute changes in serum levels may be a stronger predictor of adequate nutritional intervention [143], but prealbumin is also a negative acute phase reactant. Therefore C-reactive protein is reviewed in conjunction with prealbumin to determine inflammation-induced depression in prealbumin [144]. Finally, elevated hemoglobin A1c and blood glucose levels may predict an increased risk for surgical complications, and improvements in blood glucose control may enhance oncologic surgical outcomes [35]. Additionally, due to perioperative rates of morbidity and mortality, iron deficiency anemia should be treated during the prehabilitation phase [145]. Therefore, iron repletion is the standard of care for preoperative medical optimization [145].

In order to improve postoperative outcomes, nutritional prehabilitation must occur at least 7–14 days prior to oncologic surgery [143]. Patients should avoid long periods of preoperative fasting and reduce factors that exacerbate stress-related catabolism and impair gastrointestinal function [35]. Most clinical organizations like ESPEN, the Clinical Oncology Society of Australia, the Enhanced Recovery After Surgery Society, and the European Society of Surgical Oncology indicate most patients require 25–30 kcal/kg/day [143] and 1.5/kg/day of ideal body weight. Additionally, ESPEN guidelines indicate that the estimated protein needs of patients are between 1.2 and 2.0 g/kg/day. Enhanced recovery after surgery (ERAS) guidelines emphasize early exercise to facilitate protein synthesis; however, this requires appropriate nutritional support [35] to maximize benefits and support recovery from exercise.

In non-frail patients, diet impacts cancer outcome rather than caloric intake. In animal models, low carbohydrate, ketogenic diet, calorie restriction, and intermittent fasting resulted in improved insulin levels and inhibition of metastasis [146, 147]. Clinical studies demonstrate these diets are safe and feasible, and improve metabolic parameters, such as fasting insulin, body weight, and fat mass [146, 147]. Although the data is limited, intermittent fasting in non-cachectic or sarcopenic patients may improve chemotherapy efficacy with an increased rate of complete or partial radiological response [148].

With regards to supplementation, a variety and combination of protein, vitamin, mineral, and high-calorie supplements [36] may prove beneficial. Whey protein supplementation is the most common protein supplement used in the literature [36]. The nutrition assessment directs specialized oral nutritional care with the addition of a supplement, like protein or a supplemental dose of vitamins or minerals [36, 149]. The nutritional assessment also informs clinical decision-making regarding enteral and parenteral nutrition. Alternative nutrition support is indicated for patients whose intake is below 50% of predicted values for more than 7 days or is expected to have no intake for 5 days perioperatively [35, 149]. However, the typical instructions regarding nutrition include the following: increasing protein intake, consuming balanced meals, and consuming protein supplements or snacks post-exercise [36]. Unfortunately, a set of core outcome measures has not been standardized. Due to the heterogeneity of the nutritional data and standardized monitoring measurements described in systematic reviews and meta-analyses, more precise nutritional interventions are inconclusive [36].

"Immunonutrition" is the concept of stimulating the immune system with the appropriate nutrition [149–151]. Current data suggests that L-arginine supplementation may stimulate T-cell antitumor response [150], and L-arginine may improve T-cell survival, enhance memory T-cell formation, and improve anti-tumor responses [150]. Preoperative immunonutrition intervention with omega-3 fatty acids, arginine, and nucleotides has limited data showing improved patient outcomes [151]. Specifically, patients pretreated with immunonutrition prior to gastrointestinal cancer surgery had reduced infections, surgical complications, and hospital length of stays compared to patients consuming a regular diet [151]. More research is required prior to making recommendations supporting this intervention; though, the risk of harm is likely very low.

7 Psychosocial Intervention as a Pillar of Prehabilitation

Emotional distress, physical symptoms, health-related behaviors, caregiver fatigue, spiritual care, and assistance with practical social problems are all avenues for psychosocial interventions [43]. Emotional problems consist of adjustment disorders, generalized anxiety, anxiety regarding medical care, and depression [43]. Patients with premorbid psychiatric conditions prior to cancer diagnosis have a poor prognosis [43]. Screening tools such as the emotional thermometer, Patient-Reported Outcomes *Measurement* Information System, Patient Health Questionnaire (PHQ-9), and Generalized Anxiety Disorder (GAD-7) can be used clinically to identify depression and anxiety quickly and efficiently in patients with cancer [152–154]. Treatments for depression in patients with cancer do not differ from the standard treatments of depression including combined medical management and therapies like cognitive behavioral therapy [43]. However, medical management needs special consideration due to the interactions of antidepressants, antipsychotics, and cancer treatments [43]. Of note, cancer and depressive symptoms are similar; therefore, mindfulness and care are needed in the diagnostic process. The psychological intervention of a mind-body audio relaxation guide on preparing for surgery and healing, listened to twice daily, statistically improved the amount of vigorous intensity activity performed by participants. The mind-body intervention improved self-reports of insomnia, depression, anxiety, physical and role function, and overall quality of life 1 month postoperatively.

Physical symptoms of mood disorder consist of pain, fatigue, sexual or reproductive dysfunction, insomnia, and cognitive dysfunction [43]. Practical social problems often involve returning to work, finding childcare, financial insecurity, and housing assistance. Spiritual aspects involve religious considerations, finding/maintaining meaning and purpose, mortality, and bereavement. Identifying and intervening on emotional disorders like anxiety, depression, or social dysfunction is critical for quality of life. Interventions such as improving interpersonal communication and strengthening the patient's social support network are essential to promote emotional well-being and reduce anxiety and depression [43, 46]. Psychosocial support groups for patients with breast cancer may result in reduced cortisol levels, regulation of proinflammatory cytokines, alteration of metastasis-related genes, and increased type I interferon response genes [43]. Stress management skills such as relaxation techniques and coping strategies decrease cancer-related distress and improve quality of life.

Pain and fatigue are common causes of cancer-related distress. Invasive tumor growth, immobility, operations, chemotherapy, and radiation therapy contribute to both pain and fatigue [43]. Emotional disturbances like depression, anxiety, uncertainty, and hopelessness augment the perception of pain and fatigue. The National Cancer Institute's (NCI) Symptom Management and Quality of Life Steering Committee recommends screening for fatigue using the patient reported outcomes measurement information system (PROMIS) fatigue scale or the 10-item Edmonton symptom assessment system (ESAS) [152]. PROMIS and ESAS are both broad psychological screens that include questions on fatigue. Interventions such as cognitive behavioral therapy, psychoeducation, hypnosis, relaxation techniques, yoga, and exercise improve mood as well as pain and fatigue. These techniques enhance coping skills, acceptance patterns, and self-autonomy, as well as reduce catastrophic thought and malicious thought patterns. Cancer-related fatigue impairs quality of life and causes significant psychosocial distress. Interventions such as education, physical exercise, and energy expenditure planning treat symptomatic fatigue. Pharmacologic treatment with stimulants such as modafinil and methylphenidate is controversial with regard to efficacy and the impact of side effects like anorexia. Energy expenditure planning is a personalized intervention regulating a patient's activity level to their daily needs. Energy planning prioritizes activities of most importance and timing high energy expending activities in coordination with patients' predicted energy levels. Additionally, rest, reducing/coping with stress, and participating in enjoyable activities may improve symptomatic fatigue.

Employment is also a significant concern for patients treated for cancer. For example, in the United States, 1.3 million people with breast cancer are under the age of 65 and potentially employable [2]. Over 80% of women returning to work experience increased sick absences [155]. Return to work after cancer-related sick leave is challenging and failure to do so can result in social isolation, financial losses, reduced self-esteem [155, 156], even leaving patients vulnerable to bankruptcy [156, 157]. Patients who were encouraged to work before and during treatment had reduced sickness-related absences and improved physical work capacity [158]. Overall, patients' support, quality of life, and health-related well-being improve patients' work-related outcomes and may help maintain feelings of normalcy and social participation [155–157]. As such, occupational-related therapy is a critical consideration in the continuum of cancer prehabilitation and rehabilitation during/after treatment.

Sexual dysfunction negatively impacts the quality of life. Prostate, bladder, and gynecological cancers directly affect sexual and reproductive health [43]. Cancer treatments such as operations, chemotherapy, and radiation therapy may directly harm sexual and reproductive structures. Hormonal changes from operative stress and chemotherapeutics induce generalized sexual dysfunction due to cancer-related fatigue, pain, impaired self-esteem, impaired body image, and strained relationships. Patient's psychological response varies in regard to sexual health; however, discussion of fertility and family planning prior to oncologic intervention is essential to sexual health. For some, sexuality can seem unimportant in comparison to a life-threatening disease. For others, sexuality emphasizes emotional bonding, vitality, and pleasure.

Chemotherapy and radiation therapy directly impair reproduction [43]. Therefore, family and fertility planning are essential during the prehabilitation phase prior to treatment. Men may freeze sperm to maintain fertility, while women's reproductive health requires more intensive treatment such as ovarian transposition prior to pelvic radiation or cryopreservation of fertilized ova. These decisions regarding fertility potentiate the emotional and financial burden concerning a new cancer diagnosis and impending treatment. Therefore, information and consultation with reproductive specialists may be essential for certain patients' care during the pretreatment phase.

Exercise Benefits for Depression and Anxiety

Exercise has demonstrated a positive impact on symptoms of depression and anxiety in patients with cancer. Resistance training often includes one exercise targeting each major muscle group with two sets per exercise, and 8–15 repetitions per set [15]. Supported by strong evidence, this specific amount of this type of physical activity reduces anxiety, depression, and fatigue, and improves quality of life as well as perceived physical function [15]. Physical activity improves sleep quality and bone health specifically for osteoporosis prevention [15].

In addition to improving physical fitness, exercise has a positive impact on other cancer mortality-related risk factors and other health-related outcomes, such as quality of life [105]. Exercise significantly improves anxiety, depression and cancer-related fatigue symptoms experienced by patients with breast, prostate, colorectal, gynecological, ovarian, endometrial, cervical, head and neck, lung, and hematological cancer [105]. Specifically, moderate to vigorous intensity aerobic exercise 3 times a week for 12 weeks, or twice weekly aerobic exercise combined with twice-weekly resistance training for 6–12 weeks improves anxiety, depression, and fatigue. Resistance training alone may not impact anxiety, depression nor fatigue. Similarly, there is insufficient evidence that exercise intensity has a dose–response relationship with anxiety, depression, or fatigue symptoms [105]. However, exercise programs with durations beyond 30 min and lengths beyond 12 weeks had improved outcomes on anxiety, depression, and fatigue symptoms [105]. As a specific exercise modality, HIIT has demonstrated improved cognitive health, specifically improved mood, reduced cancer-related fatigue, reduced emotional and physical pain, and improved health-related quality of life [105]. Aerobic exercise moderately improves sleep through increased total sleep time, reduced onset latency, and improved sleep efficiency [105]. Moderate to vigorous aerobic exercise 3–4 times a week for 30–40 min over 12 weeks improves sleep in populations without cancer. Walking specifically as an aerobic exercise demonstrates a positive impact on sleep in those with cancer. Education regarding exercise as part of the multidisciplinary treatment is essential for those with cancer experiencing mood symptoms.

Summary table of risk factors, identification, and intervention

Risk factor	Identification of risk factors	Intervention(s)
Physical deconditioning	6-min Walk Test VO_2 Peak HR Max	Aerobic exercise 3–6 weeks >3×/week, > 30 min duration, >50% HR max, WR at VT, or Borg rating 12–13. HIIT program 2–4 weeks, 2–4×/week for 20–40 min with intervals targeting 100% WR, 80% VO_2 max, >70–80 W peak, or 80–100% peak power
Chemotherapy	Planned presurgical chemotherapy	Aerobic exercise (>60% HRR, HR max) or HIIT program (as above), ≥2–3 days per week
Poor pulmonary function	Pulmonary function tests, FVC, FEV1	Incentive spirometry 20–60% maximal inspiratory pressure, 30–60 breaths 1–4×/day or 10–30 min duration/day. 16 s breathing cycle 4 s inspiration, 4 s air retention, 8 s of exhalation. 3 sets of 10 breaths with 30–60 s pauses repeated 30×/day
Incontinence/ pelvic floor disruption	Incontinence or planned gynecological, colorectal, and urological oncologic surgery disrupts the pelvic floor	>1 month, > 3×/week, 10–30 min per supervised session > 120 contractions daily
Lower extremity lymphedema	Current lymphedema or planned gynecological, colorectal, and urological oncologic surgery	>1 month, 2× per day, 15–20 repetitions exercises targeting a full range of motion of the hip, knee, and ankle
Upper extremity dysfunction and lymphedema	Arm ROM and circumference, grip strength, SPOFIA, DASH, VAS	12 active and passive shoulder stretching exercises, 6–10×/day, for 30–60 min
Poor nutrition	Weight loss >10–15% within 6 months body mass index <18.5 kg/m² SGA Grade C or NRS ≥5 preoperative serum albumin <30 g/L without hepatic or renal dysfunction	Registered dietician referral for comprehensive nutritional intervention
Depression/ anxiety	HADS, PROMIS, PHQ-9, GAD-7	Referral to a mental health professional
Cancer-related fatigue	PROMIS ESAS	Referral for cognitive behavioral therapy, psychoeducation relaxation techniques, yoga, and exercise (as above)

Risk factor	Identification of risk factors	Intervention(s)
Frailty	CGA, FI-LAB Geriatric 8 Screening	Patient-centered exercise and nutrition as above
Sarcopenic obesity	CT L3 muscle index	Resistance training >2–4 weeks, >3×/week, 1 exercise/ major muscle group, 2–4 sets/exercise, 8–15 repetitions/set or 25–30 min duration

Abbreviations: work rate (WR), ventilatory threshold (VT), high-intensity interval training (HIIT), the highest amount of oxygen consumed at peak exercise (VO_2 Peak), subjective global assessment (SGA), heart rate reserve (HRR), Heart Rate Maximum (HR max) Comprehensive Geriatric Assessment (CGA), Frailty Index (FI-LAB), Hospital Anxiety and Depression Scale (HADS), Patient-Reported Outcomes *Measurement* Information System (PROMIS), Patient Health Questionnaire (PHQ-9), Generalized Anxiety Disorder (GAD-7), Edmonton Symptom Assessment System (ESAS), Forced Vital Capacity (FVC), Forced Expiratory Volume in 1 second (FEV1), range of motion (ROM), Subjective Perception of Postoperative Functional Impairment of the Arm (SPOFIA), Disabilities of the Arm, Shoulder, and Hand (DASH), Visual Analogue Score (VAS)

8 Conclusion: The Promise of Cancer Prehabilitation

Multidisciplinary treatment with nutrition, exercise, and psychosocial intervention at cancer diagnosis has promising results impacting patients' clinical outcomes as they experience the cancer continuum. The prehabilitation phase offers a unique opportunity to augment a patient's physical fitness, nutrition, and psychological well-being starting with a cancer diagnosis.

Exercise is essential in the treatment of all patients, but especially those with cancer. Prehabilitation improves a patient's functional status from cardiometabolic capacity to specific locoregional dysfunction. Early initiation of a comprehensive exercise prescription has the potential to mitigate the side effects of cancer treatment and for patients to have improved outcomes. Prehabilitation may potentially reduce cancer-related morbidity and mortality, but more immediately it may improve patients' quality of life as they begin to navigate the cancer continuum. Specific exercises can improve cardiovascular fitness to improve neoadjuvant and postoperative outcomes. Targeted locoregional exercises in the prehabilitation phase can improve pulmonary outcomes in lung and esophageal cancer, continence and reduce lower extremity lymphedema in urologic, colorectal, and gynecological cancers, reduce upper extremity dysfunction and lymphedema in breast cancer. Additionally, exercise can reduce pain, cancer-related fatigue, and anxiety centered around cancer diagnosis and treatment.

Patients often report a significant deterioration in their health-related quality of life at diagnosis and up to 10 years post-treatment. Psychosocial support addressing emotional distress, physical symptoms, social challenges, and spiritual concerns results in improved healthcare quality of life in patients with cancer. PROMIS, PHQ-9, GAD-7, and ESAS identify depression, anxiety, and fatigue quickly and efficiently in patients with cancer. Timely cognitive behavioral therapy and mind-body interventions may improve cancer outcomes in those with emotional disorders, such as anxiety and depression. Early treatment of pain and fatigue management strategies encompass cognitive behavioral therapy, psychoeducation, and physical exercises. Addressing cancer-related sexual dysfunction prior to treatment improves patients' psychological sexual health.

Nutritional interventions start with early screening to identify malnutrition risks, utilizing validated tools like the subjective global assessment (SGA) and Patient-Generated Subjective Global Assessment (PG-SA). Severe cases necessitate registered dietitian (RD)-guided interventions. Monitoring and evaluation are integral parts of the process. Preoperative nutrition optimization, including protein and calorie intake, reduces a patient's frailty and sarcopenia, resulting in enhanced oncologic outcomes. However, standardized outcome measures are lacking, and further research is needed.

Prehabilitation intervenes by optimizing exercise, nutrition, and psychosocial factors that may improve a patient's ability to tolerate the physical and psychosocial challenges of cancer treatment. The early intervention augments post-interventional rehabilitation and leads to improved outcomes. The promise of prehabilitation is to intervene early and to reduce the severity of physical and psychological symptoms, reduce cancer treatment comorbidities, as well as reduce morbidity and mortality. Therefore, prehabilitation is essential to supporting and improving patients' health care-related quality of life and clinical outcomes as they navigate the cancer continuum.

Action Points

1. Exercise interventions should focus on global conditioning, resistance training for supporting skeletal muscle, and locoregional targeted therapies specific to the patient's cancer type and expected treatment impacts such as for cardiopulmonary outcomes after thoracic procedures, pelvic floor/continence after gynecologic/urologic and colorectal treatments, or lymphedema in treating head and neck, breast, gynecologic/urologic, and colorectal cancers.
2. Screen patients early and intervene quickly for developing psychiatric/spiritual distress. Addressing contributing factors like pain, sexual dysfunction, or fatigue may improve the outcomes of direct psychological therapies.
3. Screen for malnutrition and involve registered dieticians to ensure appropriate macronutrient composition—adequate protein, calorie-controlled, etc.—will ensure weight maintenance with improving body composition for optimized outcomes. Both frailty and obesity confer greater risk and, often, weight loss even for patients with obesity may worsen outcomes.
4. Cancer prehabilitation should be well integrated into the cancer care continuum as it provides an opportunity to improve the quality of life before, during, and after cancer therapies. These improvements in nutrition, physical function through exercise, and psychiatric illness may reduce cancer morbidity/mortality and cancer recurrence and its severity, positively impacting overall survival.

References

1. Ferlay J, Colombet M, Soerjomataram I, Parkin DM, Pineros M, Znaor A, et al. Cancer statistics for the year 2020: an overview. Int J Cancer. 2021;149(4):778–89.
2. Miller KD, Nogueira L, Devasia T, Mariotto AB, Yabroff KR, Jemal A, et al. Cancer treatment and survivorship statistics, 2022. CA Cancer J Clin. 2022;72(5):409–36.
3. Europe WHO. Increase effectiveness, maximize benefits and minimize harm. Copenhagen: WHO Regional Office for Europe; 2020.
4. Cronin KA, Scott S, Firth AU, Sung H, Henley SJ, Sherman RL, et al. Annual report to the nation on the status of cancer, part 1: National Cancer Statistics. Cancer. 2022;128(24):4251–84.
5. Shah MS, DeSantis TZ, Weinmaier T, McMurdie PJ, Cope JL, Altrichter A, et al. Leveraging sequence-based faecal microbial community survey data to identify a composite biomarker for colorectal cancer. Gut. 2018;67(5):882–91.
6. Cooper CP, Gelb CA. Opportunities to expand colorectal cancer screening participation. J Womens Health (Larchmt). 2016;25(10):990–5.
7. Ahnen DJ, Wade SW, Jones WF, Sifri R, Mendoza Silveiras J, Greenamyer J, et al. The increasing incidence of young-onset colorectal cancer: a call to action. Mayo Clin Proc. 2014;89(2):216–24.
8. Chowdhury RA, Brennan FP, Gardiner MD. Cancer rehabilitation and palliative care-exploring the synergies. J Pain Symptom Manag. 2020;60(6):1239–52.
9. Silver JK. Cancer prehabilitation and its role in improving health outcomes and reducing health care costs. Semin Oncol Nurs. 2015;31(1):13–30.
10. Watson AG, Orada RB. An overview of the epidemiology, types of lung cancer, staging, and rehabilitation continuum of care. Lung Cancer Rehab. 2023:1–21.
11. Silver JK, Baima J, Mayer RS. Impairment-driven cancer rehabilitation: an essential component of quality care and survivorship. CA Cancer J Clin. 2013;63(5):295–317.
12. Santa Mina D, van Rooijen SJ, Minnella EM, Alibhai SMH, Brahmbhatt P, Dalton SO, et al. Multiphasic prehabilitation across the cancer continuum: a narrative review and conceptual framework. Front Oncol. 2020;10:598425.
13. Silver JK, Baima J. Cancer prehabilitation: an opportunity to decrease treatment-related morbidity, increase cancer treatment options, and improve physical and psychological health outcomes. Am J Phys Med Rehabil. 2013;92(8):715–27.
14. Carli F, Silver JK, Feldman LS, McKee A, Gilman S, Gillis C, et al. Surgical prehabilitation in patients with cancer: state-of-the-science and recommendations for future research from a panel of subject matter experts. Phys Med Rehabil Clin N Am. 2017;28(1):49–64.
15. Schmitz KH, Campbell AM, Stuiver MM, Pinto BM, Schwartz AL, Morris GS, et al. Exercise is medicine in oncology: engaging clinicians to help patients move through cancer. CA Cancer J Clin. 2019;69(6):468–84.
16. Kashyap D, Pal D, Sharma R, Garg VK, Goel N, Koundal D, et al. Global increase in breast cancer incidence: risk factors and preventive measures. Biomed Res Int. 2022;2022:9605439.
17. Michael CM, Lehrer EJ, Schmitz KH, Zaorsky NG. Prehabilitation exercise therapy for cancer: a systematic review and meta-analysis. Cancer Med. 2021;10(13):4195–205.
18. Marjanski T, Badocha M, Wnuk D, Dziedzic R, Ostrowski M, Sawicka W, et al. Result of the 6-min walk test is an independent prognostic factor of surgically treated non-small-cell lung cancer. Interact Cardiovasc Thorac Surg. 2019;28(3):368–74.
19. Komici K, Bencivenga L, Navani N, D'Agnano V, Guerra G, Bianco A, et al. Frailty in patients with lung cancer: a systematic review and meta-analysis. Chest. 2022;162(2):485–97.
20. Chen S, Ma T, Cui W, Li T, Liu D, Chen L, et al. Frailty and long-term survival of patients with colorectal cancer: a meta-analysis. Aging Clin Exp Res. 2022;34(7):1485–94.
21. Jauhari Y, Gannon MR, Dodwell D, Horgan K, Tsang C, Clements K, et al. Addressing frailty in patients with breast cancer: a review of the literature. Eur J Surg Oncol. 2020;46(1):24–32.
22. Overcash J. Frailty in older adults: assessment, support, and treatment implications in patients with cancer. Clin J Oncol Nurs. 2018;22(6):8–18.

23. Davey MG, Joyce WP. Impact of frailty on oncological outcomes in patients undergoing surgery for colorectal cancer—a systematic review and meta-analysis. Surgeon. 2023;21(3):173–80.
24. Masaki Momota et al.. Geriatric 8 screening of frailty in patients with prostate cancer. Int J Urol 2020;27(8):642–648.
25. Wang K, She Q, Li M, Zhao H, Zhao W, Chen B, et al. Prognostic significance of frailty status in patients with primary lung cancer. BMC Geriatr. 2023;23(1):46.
26. Wang X, Wang N, Zhong L, Wang S, Zheng Y, Yang B, et al. Prognostic value of depression and anxiety on breast cancer recurrence and mortality: a systematic review and meta-analysis of 282,203 patients. Mol Psychiatry. 2020a;25(12):3186–97.
27. Searle SD, Mitnitski A, Gahbauer EA, Gill TM, Rockwood K. A standard procedure for creating a frailty index. BMC Geriatr. 2008;8:1–10.
28. Abel GA, Klepin HD. Frailty and the management of hematologic malignancies. Blood. 2018;131(5):515–24.
29. Petrelli F, Cortellini A, Indini A, Tomasello G, Ghidini M, Nigro O, et al. Association of obesity with survival outcomes in patients with cancer: a systematic review and meta-analysis. JAMA Netw Open. 2021;4(3):e213520.
30. Picon-Ruiz M, Morata-Tarifa C, Valle-Goffin JJ, Friedman ER, Slingerland JM. Obesity and adverse breast cancer risk and outcome: mechanistic insights and strategies for intervention. CA Cancer J Clin. 2017;67(5):378–97.
31. Strulov Shachar S, Williams GR. The obesity paradox in cancer—moving beyond BMI. Cancer Epidemiol Biomarkers Prev. 2017;26(1):13–6.
32. Jurdana M, Cemazar M. Sarcopenic obesity in cancer. Radiol Oncol. 2024;58(1):1–8.
33. Friedenreich CM, Ryder-Burbidge C, McNeil J. Physical activity, obesity and sedentary behavior in cancer etiology: epidemiologic evidence and biologic mechanisms. Mol Oncol. 2021;15(3):790–800.
34. Lopez-Rodriguez-Arias F, Sanchez-Guillen L, Lillo-Garcia C, Aranaz-Ostariz V, Alcaide MJ, Soler-Silva A, et al. Assessment of body composition as an indicator of early peripheral parenteral nutrition therapy in patients undergoing colorectal cancer surgery in an enhanced recovery program. Nutrients. 2021;13(9)
35. Weimann A. Is there a rationale for perioperative nutrition therapy in the times of ERAS? Innov Surg Sci. 2019;4(4):152–7.
36. Gillis C, Davies SJ, Carli F, Wischmeyer PE, Wootton SA, Jackson AA, et al. Current landscape of nutrition within prehabilitation oncology research: a scoping review. Front Nutr. 2021a;8:644723.
37. Mueller SA, Mayer C, Bojaxhiu B, Aeberhard C, Schuetz P, Stanga Z, et al. Effect of preoperative immunonutrition on complications after salvage surgery in head and neck cancer. J Otolaryngol Head Neck Surg. 2019;48(1):25.
38. Mudge LA, Watson DI, Smithers BM, Isenring EA, Smith L, Jamieson GG, et al. Multicentre factorial randomized clinical trial of perioperative immunonutrition versus standard nutrition for patients undergoing surgical resection of oesophageal cancer. Br J Surg. 2018;105(10):1262–72.
39. Ma C, Tsai H, Su W, Sun L, Shih Y, Wang J. Combination of arginine, glutamine, and omega-3 fatty acid supplements for perioperative enteral nutrition in surgical patients with gastric adenocarcinoma or gastrointestinal stromal tumor (GIST): a prospective, randomized, double-blind study. J Postgrad Med. 2018;64(3):155–63.
40. Lee SY, Lee J, Park HM, Kim CH, Kim HR. Impact of preoperative immunonutrition on the outcomes of colon cancer surgery: results from a randomized controlled trial. Ann Surg. 2023a;277(3):381–6.
41. Sittitrai P, Ruenmarkkaew D, Booyaprapa S, Kasempitakpong B. Effect of a perioperative immune-enhancing diet in clean-contaminated head and neck cancer surgery: a randomized controlled trial. Int J Surg. 2021;93:106051.

42. Wang YH, Li JQ, Shi JF, Que JY, Liu JJ, Lappin JM, et al. Depression and anxiety in relation to cancer incidence and mortality: a systematic review and meta-analysis of cohort studies. Mol Psychiatry. 2020b;25(7):1487–99.
43. Lang-Rollin I, Berberich G. Psycho-oncology. Dialogues Clin Neurosci. 2018;20(1):13–22.
44. Satin JR, Linden W, Phillips MJ. Depression as a predictor of disease progression and mortality in cancer patients: a meta-analysis. Cancer. 2009;115(22):5349–61.
45. Calderon C, Carmona-Bayonas A, Hernandez R, Ghanem I, Castelo B, Martinez de Castro E, et al. Effects of pessimism, depression, fatigue, and pain on functional health-related quality of life in patients with resected non-advanced breast cancer. Breast. 2019;44:108–12.
46. Antoni MH. Psychosocial intervention effects on adaptation, disease course and biobehavioral processes in cancer. Brain Behav Immun. 2013;30:S88–98.
47. Adam S, van de Poll-Franse LV, Mols F, Ezendam NPM, de Hingh I, Arndt V, et al. The association of cancer-related fatigue with all-cause mortality of colorectal and endometrial cancer survivors: Results from the population-based PROFILES registry. Cancer Med. 2019;8(6):3227–36.
48. Montazeri A. Health-related quality of life in breast cancer patients: a bibliographic review of the literature from 1974 to 2007. J Exp Clin Cancer Res. 2008;27(1):32.
49. Neyt M, Albrecht J. The long-term evolution of quality of life for disease-free breast cancer survivors: a comparative study in Belgium. J Psychosoc Oncol. 2006;24(3):89–123.
50. Koch L, Jansen L, Herrmann A, Stegmaier C, Holleczek B, Singer S, et al. Quality of life in long-term breast cancer survivors—a 10-year longitudinal population-based study. Acta Oncol. 2013;52(6):1119–28.
51. Hou Y, Zhou Y, Hussain M, Budd GT, Tang WHW, Abraham J, et al. Cardiac risk stratification in cancer patients: a longitudinal patient-patient network analysis. PLoS Med. 2021;18(8):e1003736.
52. Murphy S, Kochanek K, Xu J, Arias E. Mortality in the United States, 2020. NCHS data brief, no 427. National Center for Health Statistics; 2021. p. 10.
53. Curigliano G, Lenihan D, Fradley M, Ganatra S, Barac A, Blaes A, et al. Management of cardiac disease in cancer patients throughout oncological treatment: ESMO consensus recommendations. Ann Oncol. 2020;31(2):171–90.
54. Strongman H, Gadd S, Matthews A, Mansfield KE, Stanway S, Lyon AR, et al. Medium and long-term risks of specific cardiovascular diseases in survivors of 20 adult cancers: a population-based cohort study using multiple linked UK electronic health records databases. Lancet. 2019;394(10203):1041–54.
55. Finke D, Heckmann MB, Wilhelm S, Entenmann L, Hund H, Bougatf N, et al. Coronary artery disease, left ventricular function and cardiac biomarkers determine all-cause mortality in cancer patients-a large monocenter cohort study. Clin Res Cardiol. 2023;112(2):203–14.
56. Screever EM, Meijers WC, Moslehi JJ. Age-related considerations in cardio-oncology. J Cardiovasc Pharmacol Ther. 2021;26(2):103–13.
57. Koulaouzidis G, Yung AE, Yung DE, Skonieczna-Zydecka K, Marlicz W, Koulaouzidis A, et al. Conventional cardiac risk factors associated with trastuzumab-induced cardiotoxicity in breast cancer: systematic review and meta-analysis. Curr Probl Cancer. 2021;45(5):100723.
58. Bovelli D, Plataniotis G, Roila F, Group EGW. Cardiotoxicity of chemotherapeutic agents and radiotherapy-related heart disease: ESMO Clinical Practice Guidelines. Ann Oncol. 2010;21(Suppl. 5):v277–82.
59. Darby SC, Ewertz M, McGale P, Bennet AM, Blom-Goldman U, Bronnum D, et al. Risk of ischemic heart disease in women after radiotherapy for breast cancer. N Engl J Med. 2013;368(11):987–98.
60. Maltser S, Cristian A, Silver JK, Morris GS, Stout NL. A focused review of safety considerations in cancer rehabilitation. PM R. 2017;9(9S2):S415–S28.
61. Harris EE, Correa C, Hwang WT, Liao J, Litt HI, Ferrari VA, et al. Late cardiac mortality and morbidity in early-stage breast cancer patients after breast-conservation treatment. J Clin Oncol. 2006;24(25):4100–6.

62. Bracun V, Aboumsallem JP, van der Meer P, de Boer RA. Cardiac biomarkers in patients with cancer: considerations, clinical implications, and future avenues. Curr Oncol Rep. 2020;22(7):67.
63. Allen SK, Brown V, White D, King D, Hunt J, Wainwright J, et al. Multimodal prehabilitation during neoadjuvant therapy prior to esophagogastric cancer resection: effect on cardiopulmonary exercise test performance, muscle mass and quality of life-a pilot randomized clinical trial. Ann Surg Oncol. 2022;29(3):1839–50.
64. Minnella EM, Awasthi R, Loiselle SE, Agnihotram RV, Ferri LE, Carli F. Effect of Exercise and nutrition prehabilitation on functional capacity in esophagogastric cancer surgery: a randomized clinical trial. JAMA Surg. 2018;153(12):1081–9. https://doi.org/10.1001/jamasurg.2018.1645.
65. Sheill G, Guinan E, O'Neill L, Normand C, Doyle SL, Moore S, et al. Preoperative exercise to improve fitness in patients undergoing complex surgery for cancer of the lung or oesophagus (PRE-HIIT): protocol for a randomized controlled trial. BMC Cancer. 2020;20(1):321.
66. Christensen JF, Simonsen C, Banck-Petersen A, Thorsen-Streit S, Herrstedt A, Djurhuus SS, et al. Safety and feasibility of preoperative exercise training during neoadjuvant treatment before surgery for adenocarcinoma of the gastro-oesophageal junction. BJS Open. 2019;3(1):74–84.
67. Carli F, Bousquet-Dion G, Awasthi R, Elsherbini N, Liberman S, Boutros M, Stein B, Charlebois P, Ghitulescu G, Morin N, Jagoe T, Scheede-Bergdahl C, Minnella EM, Fiore JF Jr. Effect of multimodal prehabilitation vs postoperative rehabilitation on 30-day postoperative complications for frail patients undergoing resection of colorectal cancer: a randomized clinical trial. JAMA Surg. 2020;155(3):233–42. https://doi.org/10.1001/jamasurg.2019.5474.
68. van Rooijen S, Carli F, Dalton S, Thomas G, Bojesen R, Le Guen M, Barizien N, Awasthi R, Minnella E, Beijer S, Martinez-Palli G, van Lieshout R, Gogenur I, Feo C, Johansen C, Scheede-Bergdahl C, Roumen R, Schep G, Slooter G. Multimodal prehabilitation in colorectal cancer patients to improve functional capacity and reduce postoperative complications: the first international randomized controlled trial for multimodal prehabilitation. BMC Cancer. 2019;19(1):98. https://doi.org/10.1186/s12885-018-5232-6.
69. Gillis C, Li C, Lee L, Awasthi R, Augustin B, Gamsa A, Liberman AS, Stein B, Charlebois P, Feldman LS, Carli F. Prehabilitation versus rehabilitation: a randomized control trial in patients undergoing colorectal resection for cancer. Anesthesiology. 2014;121(5):937–47. https://doi.org/10.1097/ALN.0000000000000393.
70. Carli F, Charlebois P, Stein B, Feldman L, Zavorsky G, Kim DJ, et al. Randomized clinical trial of prehabilitation in colorectal surgery. Br J Surg. 2010;97(8):1187–97.
71. Li C, Carli F, Lee L, Charlebois P, Stein B, Liberman AS, et al. Impact of a trimodal prehabilitation program on functional recovery after colorectal cancer surgery: a pilot study. Surg Endosc. 2013;27(4):1072–82.
72. Dronkers JJ, Lamberts H, Reutelingsperger IM, Naber RH, Dronkers-Landman CM, Veldman A, van Meeteren NL. Preoperative therapeutic programme for elderly patients scheduled for elective abdominal oncological surgery: a randomized controlled pilot study. Clin Rehabil. 2010;24(7):614–22. https://doi.org/10.1177/0269215509358941.
73. Kim DJ, Mayo NE, Carli F, Montgomery DL, Zavorsky GS. Responsive measures to prehabilitation in patients undergoing bowel resection surgery. Tohoku J Exp Med. 2009;217(2):109–15. https://doi.org/10.1620/tjem.217.109.
74. West MA, Loughney L, Lythgoe D, Barben CP, Sripadam R, Kemp GJ, et al. Effect of prehabilitation on objectively measured physical fitness after neoadjuvant treatment in preoperative rectal cancer patients: a blinded interventional pilot study. Br J Anaesth. 2015;114(2):244–51.
75. Chen BP, Awasthi R, Sweet SN, Minnella EM, Bergdahl A, Santa Mina D, Carli F, Scheede-Bergdahl C. Four-week prehabilitation program is sufficient to modify exercise behaviors and improve preoperative functional walking capacity in patients with colorectal cancer. Support Care Cancer. 2017;25(1):33–40. https://doi.org/10.1007/s00520-016-3379-8.

76. Dunne DF, Jack S, Jones RP, Jones L, Lythgoe DT, Malik HZ, Poston GJ, Palmer DH, Fenwick SW. Randomized clinical trial of prehabilitation before planned liver resection. Br J Surg. 2016;103(5):504–12. https://doi.org/10.1002/bjs.10096.
77. Singh F, Newton RU, Baker MK, Spry NA, Taaffe DR, Galvao DA. Feasibility and efficacy of presurgical exercise in survivors of rectal cancer scheduled to receive curative resection. Clin Colorectal Cancer. 2017;16(4):358–65.
78. Berkel AEM, Bongers BC, Kotte H, Weltevreden P, de Jongh FHC, Eijsvogel MMM, et al. Effects of community-based exercise prehabilitation for patients scheduled for colorectal surgery with high risk for postoperative complications: results of a randomized clinical trial. Ann Surg. 2022;275(2):e299–306.
79. Peng LH, Wang WJ, Chen J, Jin JY, Min S, Qin PP. Implementation of the pre-operative rehabilitation recovery protocol and its effect on the quality of recovery after colorectal surgeries. Chin Med J. 2021;134(23):2865–73.
80. Bousquet-Dion G, Awasthi R, Loiselle SE, Minnella EM, Agnihotram RV, Bergdahl A, Carli F, Scheede-Bergdahl C. Evaluation of supervised multimodal prehabilitation programme in cancer patients undergoing colorectal resection: a randomized control trial. Acta Oncol. 2018;57(6):849–59. https://doi.org/10.1080/0284186X.2017.1423180.
81. Ferreira BFA, Preti RC, Schmidt MB, Zacharias LC, Takahashi WY, Monteiro MLR. Multimodal imaging of focal choroidal excavation complicated by choroidal neovascularization in a patient with angioid streaks and pseudoxanthoma elasticum. Retin Cases Brief Rep. 2021;15(2):155–62.
82. Quist M, Adamsen L, Rorth M, Laursen JH, Christensen KB, Langer SW. The impact of a multidimensional exercise intervention on physical and functional capacity, anxiety, and depression in patients with advanced-stage lung cancer undergoing chemotherapy. Integr Cancer Ther. 2015;14(4):341–9.
83. Licker M, Karenovics W, Diaper J, Fresard I, Triponez F, Ellenberger C, et al. Short-term preoperative high-intensity interval training in patients awaiting lung cancer surgery: a randomized controlled trial. J Thorac Oncol. 2017;12(2):323–33.
84. Lai Y, Su J, Yang M, Zhou K, Che G. Impact and effect of preoperative short-term pulmonary rehabilitation training on lung cancer patients with mild to moderate chronic obstructive pulmonary disease: a randomized trial. Zhongguo Fei Ai Za Zhi. 2016;19(11):746–53.
85. Lai Y, Huang J, Yang M, Su J, Liu J, Che G. Seven-day intensive preoperative rehabilitation for elderly patients with lung cancer: a randomized controlled trial. J Surg Res. 2017;209:30–6.
86. Bobbio A, Chetta A, Ampollini L, Primomo GL, Internullo E, Carbognani P, et al. Preoperative pulmonary rehabilitation in patients undergoing lung resection for non-small cell lung cancer. Eur J Cardiothorac Surg. 2008;33(1):95–8.
87. Stefanelli F, Meoli I, Cobuccio R, Curcio C, Amore D, Casazza D, et al. High-intensity training and cardiopulmonary exercise testing in patients with chronic obstructive pulmonary disease and non-small-cell lung cancer undergoing lobectomy. Eur J Cardiothorac Surg. 2013;44(4):e260–5.
88. Bhatia C, Kayser B. Preoperative high-intensity interval training is effective and safe in deconditioned patients with lung cancer: a randomized clinical trial. J Rehabil Med. 2019;51(9):712–8.
89. Egegaard T, Rohold J, Lillelund C, Persson G, Quist M. Pre-radiotherapy daily exercise training in non-small cell lung cancer: a feasibility study. Rep Pract Oncol Radiother. 2019;24(4):375–82.
90. Pehlivan E, Turna A, Gurses A, Gurses HN. The effects of preoperative short-term intense physical therapy in lung cancer patients: a randomized controlled trial. Ann Thorac Cardiovasc Surg. 2011;17(5):461–8.
91. Karenovics W, Licker M, Ellenberger C, Christodoulou M, Diaper J, Bhatia C, et al. Short-term preoperative exercise therapy does not improve long-term outcome after lung cancer surgery: a randomized controlled study. Eur J Cardiothorac Surg. 2017;52(1):47–54.

92. Sebio Garcia R, Yanez-Brage MI, Gimenez Moolhuyzen E, Salorio Riobo M, Lista Paz A, Borro Mate JM. Preoperative exercise training prevents functional decline after lung resection surgery: a randomized, single-blind controlled trial. Clin Rehabil. 2017;31(8):1057–67.
93. Gravier FE, Smondack P, Boujibar F, Prieur G, Medrinal C, Combret Y, et al. Prehabilitation sessions can be provided more frequently in a shortened regimen with similar or better efficacy in people with non-small cell lung cancer: a randomised trial. J Physiother. 2022;68(1):43–50.
94. Jensen BT, Petersen AK, Jensen JB, Laustsen S, Borre M. Efficacy of a multiprofessional rehabilitation programme in radical cystectomy pathways: a prospective randomized controlled trial. Scand J Urol. 2015;49(2):133–41. https://doi.org/10.3109/21681805.2014.967810.
95. Santa Mina D, Hilton WJ, Matthew AG, Awasthi R, Bousquet-Dion G, Alibhai SMH, Au D, Fleshner NE, Finelli A, Clarke H, Aprikian A, Tanguay S, Carli F. Prehabilitation for radical prostatectomy: a multicentre randomized controlled trial. Surg Oncol. 2018;27(2):289–98. https://doi.org/10.1016/j.suronc.2018.05.010.
96. Banerjee S, Manley K, Shaw B, Lewis L, Cucato G, Mills R, et al. Vigorous intensity aerobic interval exercise in bladder cancer patients prior to radical cystectomy: a feasibility randomised controlled trial. Support Care Cancer. 2018;26(5):1515–23.
97. Blackwell JEM, Doleman B, Boereboom CL, Morton A, Williams S, Atherton P, et al. High-intensity interval training produces a significant improvement in fitness in less than 31 days before surgery for urological cancer: a randomised control trial. Prostate Cancer Prostatic Dis. 2020;23(4):696–704.
98. Schulz GB, Locke JA, Campbell KL, Bland KA, Van Patten CL, Black PC, et al. Taking advantage of the teachable moment at initial diagnosis of prostate cancer-results of a pilot randomized controlled trial of supervised exercise training. Cancer Nurs. 2022;45(3):E680–8.
99. Mijwel S, Jervaeus A, Bolam KA, Norrbom J, Bergh J, Rundqvist H, et al. High-intensity exercise during chemotherapy induces beneficial effects 12 months into breast cancer survivorship. J Cancer Surviv. 2019;13(2):244–56.
100. Knoerl R, Giobbie-Hurder A, Sannes TS, Chagpar AB, Dillon D, Dominici LS, et al. Exploring the impact of exercise and mind-body prehabilitation interventions on physical and psychological outcomes in women undergoing breast cancer surgery. Support Care Cancer. 2022;30(3):2027–36.
101. Heiman J, Onerup A, Wessman C, Haglind E, Olofsson Bagge R. Recovery after breast cancer surgery following recommended pre and postoperative physical activity: (PhysSURG-B) randomized clinical trial. Br J Surg. 2021;108(1):32–9. https://doi.org/10.1093/bjs/znaa007.
102. Mikami Y, Kouda K, Kawasaki S, Okada KI, Kawai M, Kitahata Y, et al. Preoperative in-hospital rehabilitation improves physical function in patients with pancreatic cancer scheduled for surgery. Tohoku J Exp Med. 2020;251(4):279–85.
103. McCourt O, Fisher A, Ramdharry G, Land J, Roberts AL, Rabin N, et al. Exercise prehabilitation for people with myeloma undergoing autologous stem cell transplantation: results from PERCEPT pilot randomised controlled trial. Acta Oncol. 2023:1–10.
104. Mawson S, Keen C, Skilbeck J, Ross H, Smith L, Dixey J, et al. Feasibility and benefits of a structured prehabilitation programme prior to autologous stem cell transplantation (ASCT) in patients with myeloma; a prospective feasibility study. Physiotherapy. 2021;113:88–99.
105. Campbell KL, Winters-Stone KM, Wiskemann J, May AM, Schwartz AL, Courneya KS, et al. Exercise guidelines for cancer survivors: consensus statement from international multidisciplinary roundtable. Med Sci Sports Exerc. 2019;51(11):2375–90.
106. Morishita S, Hamaue Y, Fukushima T, Tanaka T, Fu JB, Nakano J. Effect of exercise on mortality and recurrence in patients with cancer: a systematic review and meta-analysis. Integr Cancer Ther. 2020;19:1534735420917462.
107. Palma S, Hasenoehrl T, Jordakieva G, Ramazanova D, Crevenna R. High-intensity interval training in the prehabilitation of cancer patients—a systematic review and meta-analysis. Support Care Cancer. 2021;29(4):1781–94.

108. Alejo LB, Pagola-Aldazabal I, Fiuza-Luces C, Huerga D, de Torres MV, Verdugo AS, et al. Exercise prehabilitation program for patients under neoadjuvant treatment for rectal cancer: a pilot study. J Cancer Res Ther. 2019;15(1):20–5.
109. Cornette T, Vincent F, Mandigout S, Antonini MT, Leobon S, Labrunie A, et al. Effects of home-based exercise training on VO2 in breast cancer patients under adjuvant or neoadjuvant chemotherapy (SAPA): a randomized controlled trial. Eur J Phys Rehabil Med. 2016;52(2):223–32.
110. Demmelmaier I, Brooke HL, Henriksson A, Mazzoni AS, Bjorke ACH, Igelstrom H, et al. Does exercise intensity matter for fatigue during (neo-)adjuvant cancer treatment? The Phys-Can randomized clinical trial. Scand J Med Sci Sports. 2021;31(5):1144–59.
111. Morielli AR, Usmani N, Boule NG, Severin D, Tankel K, Joseph K, et al. Feasibility, safety, and preliminary efficacy of exercise during and after neoadjuvant rectal cancer treatment: a phase II randomized controlled trial. Clin Colorectal Cancer. 2021;20(3):216–26.
112. Morielli AR, Usmani N, Boule NG, Tankel K, Severin D, Nijjar T, et al. A phase I study examining the feasibility and safety of an aerobic exercise intervention in patients with rectal cancer during and after neoadjuvant chemoradiotherapy. Oncol Nurs Forum. 2016;43(3):352–62.
113. Singh F, Galvao DA, Newton RU, Spry NA, Baker MK, Taaffe DR. Feasibility and preliminary efficacy of a 10-week resistance and aerobic exercise intervention during neoadjuvant chemoradiation treatment in rectal cancer patients. Integr Cancer Ther. 2018;17(3):952–9.
114. Maurer T, Belau MH, von Grundherr J, Schlemmer Z, Patra S, Becher H, et al. Randomised controlled trial testing the feasibility of an exercise and nutrition intervention for patients with ovarian cancer during and after first-line chemotherapy (BENITA-study). BMJ Open. 2022;12(2):e054091.
115. Barassi G, Bellomo RG, Di Iulio A, Lococo A, Porreca A, Di Felice PA, et al. Preoperative rehabilitation in lung cancer patients: Yoga approach. Adv Exp Med Biol. 2018;1096:19–29.
116. van Adrichem EJ, Meulenbroek RL, Plukker JT, Groen H, van Weert E. Comparison of two preoperative inspiratory muscle training programs to prevent pulmonary complications in patients undergoing esophagectomy: a randomized controlled pilot study. Ann Surg Oncol. 2014;21(7):2353–60.
117. Valkenet K, Trappenburg JCA, Ruurda JP, Guinan EM, Reynolds JV, Nafteux P, et al. Multicentre randomized clinical trial of inspiratory muscle training versus usual care before surgery for oesophageal cancer. Br J Surg. 2018;105(5):502–11.
118. Morano MT, Araujo AS, Nascimento FB, da Silva GF, Mesquita R, Pinto JS, et al. Preoperative pulmonary rehabilitation versus chest physical therapy in patients undergoing lung cancer resection: a pilot randomized controlled trial. Arch Phys Med Rehabil. 2013;94(1):53–8.
119. Benzo R, Wigle D, Novotny P, Wetzstein M, Nichols F, Shen RK, et al. Preoperative pulmonary rehabilitation before lung cancer resection: results from two randomized studies. Lung Cancer. 2011;74(3):441–5.
120. Wu XD, Fu CF, Chen YL, Kong LH, Pan ZZ, Zheng MC. Intervention effect of biofeedback combined with pelvic floor muscle exercise on low anterior resection syndrome in patients with low anus-preserving rectal cancer. Zhonghua Yi Xue Za Zhi. 2019;99(30):2337–43.
121. Dijkstra-Eshuis J, Van den Bos TW, Splinter R, Bevers RF, Zonneveld WC, Putter H, et al. Effect of preoperative pelvic floor muscle therapy with biofeedback versus standard care on stress urinary incontinence and quality of life in men undergoing laparoscopic radical prostatectomy: a randomised control trial. Neurourol Urodyn. 2015;34(2):144–50.
122. Milios JE, Ackland TR, Green DJ. Pelvic floor muscle training in radical prostatectomy: a randomized controlled trial of the impacts on pelvic floor muscle function and urinary incontinence. BMC Urol. 2019;19(1):116.
123. Goode PS, Johnson TM 2nd, Newman DK, Vaughan CP, Echt KV, Markland AD, et al. Perioperative mobile telehealth program for post-prostatectomy incontinence: a randomized clinical trial. J Urol. 2022;208(2):379–87.
124. Centemero A, Rigatti L, Giraudo D, Lazzeri M, Lughezzani G, Zugna D, et al. Preoperative pelvic floor muscle exercise for early continence after radical prostatectomy: a randomised controlled study. Eur Urol. 2010;57(6):1039–43.

125. Anan G, Kaiho Y, Iwamura H, Ito J, Kohada Y, Mikami J, et al. Preoperative pelvic floor muscle exercise for early continence after holmium laser enucleation of the prostate: a randomized controlled study. BMC Urol. 2020;20(1):3.
126. Ocampo-Trujillo A, Carbonell-Gonzalez J, Martinez-Blanco A, Diaz-Hung A, Munoz CA, Ramirez-Velez R. Pre-operative training induces changes in the histomorphometry and muscle function of the pelvic floor in patients with indication of radical prostatectomy. Actas Urol Esp. 2014;38(6):378–84.
127. Wu X, Liu Y, Zhu D, Wang F, Ji J, Yan H. Early prevention of complex decongestive therapy and rehabilitation exercise for prevention of lower extremity lymphedema after operation of gynecologic cancer. Asian J Surg. 2021;44(1):111–5.
128. Toohey K, Hunter M, McKinnon K, Casey T, Turner M, Taylor S, et al. A systematic review of multimodal prehabilitation in breast cancer. Breast Cancer Res Treat. 2023;197(1):1–37.
129. Baima J, Reynolds SG, Edmiston K, Larkin A, Ward BM, O'Connor A. Teaching of independent exercises for prehabilitation in breast cancer. J Cancer Educ. 2017;32(2):252–6.
130. Springer BA, Levy E, McGarvey C, Pfalzer LA, Stout NL, Gerber LH, et al. Pre-operative assessment enables early diagnosis and recovery of shoulder function in patients with breast cancer. Breast Cancer Res Treat. 2010;120(1):135–47.
131. Nilsson H, Angeras U, Bock D, Borjesson M, Onerup A, Fagevik Olsen M, et al. Is preoperative physical activity related to post-surgery recovery? A cohort study of patients with breast cancer. BMJ Open. 2016;6(1):e007997.
132. Singh C, De Vera M, Campbell KL. The effect of prospective monitoring and early physiotherapy intervention on arm morbidity following surgery for breast cancer: a pilot study. Physiother Can. 2013;65(2):183–91.
133. Smoot B, Paul SM, Aouizerat BE, Elboim C, Levine JD, Abrams G, et al. Side of cancer does not influence limb volumes in women prior to breast cancer surgery. Lymphat Res Biol. 2014;12(3):189–93.
134. Byun H, Jang Y, Kim JY, Kim JM, Lee CH. Effects of preoperative personal education on shoulder function and lymphedema in patients with breast cancer: A consort. Medicine (Baltimore). 2022;101(38):e30810.
135. Sato F, Ishida T, Ohuchi N. The perioperative educational program for improving upper arm dysfunction in patients with breast cancer: a controlled trial. Tohoku J Exp Med. 2014;232(2):115–22.
136. Sato F, Arinaga Y, Sato N, Ishida T, Ohuchi N. The perioperative educational program for improving upper arm dysfunction in patients with breast cancer at 1-year follow-up: a prospective, controlled trial. Tohoku J Exp Med. 2016;238(3):229–36.
137. Temur K, Kapucu S. The effectiveness of lymphedema self-management in the prevention of breast cancer-related lymphedema and quality of life: A randomized controlled trial. Eur J Oncol Nurs. 2019;40:22–35.
138. Donmez AA, Kapucu S. The effectiveness of a clinical and home-based physical activity program and simple lymphatic drainage in the prevention of breast cancer-related lymphedema: A prospective randomized controlled study. Eur J Oncol Nurs. 2017;31:12–21.
139. Fujiwara Y, Kato T, Hasegawa F, Sunahara M, Tsurumaki Y. The past, present, and future of clinically applied chimeric antigen receptor-T-cell therapy. Pharmaceuticals (Basel). 2022;15(2)
140. Iukuridze A, Berano Teh J, Ramos J, Vera TC, Lee K, Bhandari R, et al. Sarcopenia is a clinically relevant and independent predictor of health outcomes after chimeric antigen receptor T-cell therapy for lymphoma. Blood. 2021;138(Suppl. 1):2502.
141. Lee K, Iukuridze A, He T, Bosworth A, Lindenfeld L, Teh JB, et al. Association between pretreatment skeletal muscle and outcomes after CAR T-cell therapy. J Natl Compr Cancer Netw. 2023b;21(4):373–82.e1.
142. Obaisi O, Fontillas RC, Patel K, Ngo-Huang A. Rehabilitation needs for patients undergoing CAR T-cell therapy. Curr Oncol Rep. 2022;24(6):741–9.
143. Gillis C, Hasil L, Kasvis P, Bibby N, Davies SJ, Prado CM, et al. Nutrition care process model approach to surgical prehabilitation in oncology. Front Nutr. 2021b;8:644706.

144. Shrotriya S, Walsh D, Bennani-Baiti N, Thomas S, Lorton C. C-Reactive protein is an important biomarker for prognosis tumor recurrence and treatment response in adult solid tumors: a systematic review. PLoS One. 2015;10(12):e0143080.
145. Carli F, Awasthi R, Gillis C, Baldini G, Bessissow A, Liberman AS, et al. Integrating prehabilitation in the preoperative clinic: a paradigm shift in perioperative care. Anesth Analg. 2021;132(5):1494–500.
146. Shen S, Iyengar NM. Insulin-lowering diets in metastatic cancer. Nutrients. 2022;14(17):3542.
147. Zhao H, Jin H, Xian J, Zhang Z, Shi J, Bai X. Effect of ketogenic diets on body composition and metabolic parameters of cancer patients: a systematic review and meta-analysis. Nutrients. 2022;14(19):4192.
148. Gabel K, Cares K, Varady K, Gadi V, Tussing-Humphreys L. Current evidence and directions for intermittent fasting during cancer chemotherapy. Adv Nutr. 2022;13(2):667–80.
149. Weimann A, Braga M, Carli F, Higashiguchi T, Hubner M, Klek S, et al. ESPEN guideline: Clinical nutrition in surgery. Clin Nutr. 2017;36(3):623–50.
150. Geiger R, Rieckmann JC, Wolf T, Basso C, Feng Y, Fuhrer T, et al. L-Arginine modulates t cell metabolism and enhances survival and anti-tumor activity. Cell. 2016;167(3):829–42 e13.
151. Adiamah A, Skorepa P, Weimann A, Lobo DN. The impact of preoperative immune modulating nutrition on outcomes in patients undergoing surgery for gastrointestinal cancer: a systematic review and meta-analysis. Ann Surg. 2019;270(2):247–56.
152. Berger AM, Mitchell SA, Jacobsen PB, Pirl WF. Screening, evaluation, and management of cancer-related fatigue: ready for implementation to practice? CA Cancer J Clin. 2015;65(3):190–211.
153. Yang Y, Sun H, Luo X, Li W, Yang F, Xu W, et al. Network connectivity between fear of cancer recurrence, anxiety, and depression in breast cancer patients. J Affect Disord. 2022;309:358–67.
154. Licková K, Čoček A, Ambruš M, Soumarová R, Vránová J, Klézl P, et al. Rapid screening of depression and anxiety in cancer patients: interview validation of emotion thermometers. Asian J Psychiatr. 2021;65:102827.
155. Soderman M, Friberg E, Alexanderson K, Wennman-Larsen A. Women's experiences of encounters with healthcare professionals' regarding work after breast-cancer surgery and associations with sickness absence: a 2-year follow-up cohort study. Support Care Cancer. 2019;27(4):1197–206.
156. Jagsi R, Ward KC, Abrahamse PH, Wallner LP, Kurian AW, Hamilton AS, et al. Unmet need for clinician engagement regarding financial toxicity after diagnosis of breast cancer. Cancer. 2018;124(18):3668–76.
157. Rosenzweig M, West M, Matthews J, Stokan M, Yoojin Kook YK, Gallups S, et al. Financial toxicity among women with metastatic breast cancer. Oncol Nurs Forum. 2019;46(1):83–91.
158. Bondesson T, Petersson LM, Wennman-Larsen A, Alexanderson K, Kjeldgard L, Nilsson MI. A study to examine the influence of health professionals' advice and support on work capacity and sick leave after breast cancer surgery. Support Care Cancer. 2016;24(10):4141–8.

Bariatric Surgery Prehabilitation

Alexander Watson and Caitlin Halbert

1 Overview: The Continuum of Care in Bariatric Surgery

This is a general sequence of the different steps through which a patient will transition from initially considering bariatric surgery through the postoperative recovery period.

- Lifestyle modifications and non-specialist care: Initial meetings with a general practitioner for guidance on lifestyle modifications for weight loss or participation in nonmedical, commercial weight loss programs.
- Referral to a bariatric surgery program: Consultation with a bariatric surgeon and a multidisciplinary team evaluation that will include a nutritionist or dietitian and behavioral health specialist.
- Patient education: The patient will undergo education surrounding lifestyle, dietary, and other topics related to surgery in preparation.
- Preoperative testing: The multidisciplinary team may require certain tests and studies that include but are not limited to bloodwork, electrocardiogram, barium swallow, upper endoscopy, sleep study, etc. in preparation for surgery.
- Bariatric surgery.
- Immediate postoperative care and food reintroduction: The period after surgery when the diet progresses from liquids and limited foods to the new standard diet of frequent small meals and supplements.
- Maintenance of long-term lifestyle changes: Patients are supported in their weight loss/weight loss maintenance with attention to nutritional supplements with exact composition depending on surgery type, ongoing exercise, and diet

A. Watson
Admire Medical, Middletown, DE, USA
e-mail: alexander@admiremedical.com

C. Halbert (✉)
Christiana Care Health System, Wilmington, DE, USA

A. Watson, K. Barr (eds.), *A Prehabilitation Guide for All Providers*,
https://doi.org/10.1007/978-3-031-72862-4_7

prescriptions to support excess body weight loss (EBWL) while minimizing muscle mass loss.

2 Specialized Treatment Team

- The bariatric surgeon performs an initial consultation and evaluation. If the patient is deemed an acceptable candidate, the surgeon will recommend proceeding with evaluation by the multidisciplinary team. Relative contraindications for surgery include but are not limited to unstable cardiac disease, active mental illness or substance use disorder, active malignancy, or other acute conditions.
- A registered dietitian provides nutritional education in the context of personal preferences and restrictions and assists with translating education into practice for the patient.
- A behavioral health provider assesses the risk of psychosocial impact on surgical outcomes, quality of support network, and risk for disordered eating, substance use disorder, and other high-risk behaviors.
- Medical specialists evaluate and optimize the bariatric patient for general anesthesia. Specialists include but are not limited to providers from internal medicine, anesthesiology, cardiology, pulmonology and sleep medicine, endocrine and obesity medicine.

For patients with chronic pain and functional limitations, physical therapists, physical medicine and rehabilitation (PM&R), and pain management specialists may design plans to optimize physical functioning and maximize physical activity prior to surgery.

3 Defining the Problem in the Prehabilitation Phase: The Medical Necessity of Weight Loss and Bariatric Surgery

Weight loss in patients with obesity is critical and should not be viewed as cosmetic, even for those individuals presently without comorbidities. While any individuals who are diagnosed with overweight or obesity have a component of metabolic diseases, such as hypertension, insulin resistance, diabetes mellitus, and dyslipidemia, significant proportion (10% to nearly 50%) do not have any metabolic comorbidities [1]. Prevalence estimates vary due to inconsistent inclusion criteria, gender, and ethnicity distributions in study sample populations. However, these individuals are typically younger females and carry excess adipose tissue subcutaneously on their hips and buttocks ("gynoid") instead of in/around the abdomen ("android"). As a result, this adipose tissue is less likely to be "adiposopathic," a term for secreting inflammatory cytokines that promote metabolic dysfunction manifesting in elevated LDL cholesterol/LDL particle number (LDL-c/LDL-p), triglycerides, blood pressure, and insulin resistance. Instead, individuals with the metabolically healthy obesity (MHO) phenotype are more likely in the short term to maintain a lower risk of cardiovascular disease, diabetes, and other obesity-associated comorbidities versus other phenotypes [2].

Comorbidities in this MHO phenotype population are more limited to the mechanical impact of excess bodyweight (i.e. "fat *mass* disease") [3]. These individuals may experience complications directly from carrying excess bodyweight such as obstructive sleep apnea (OSA), joint stress/damage [3], and, relative to the heightened risk from metabolic disease, only modestly elevated cancer risk. Hypertension could be considered a fat mass-associated disease as the effects of OSA, renal artery compression by perinephric fat, and perivascular adipose tissue compressing blood vessels, outside of adiposopathic hormonal and metabolic effects [4]. For these reasons, even in the absence of metabolic syndrome, healthcare professionals should treat individuals with obesity using a comprehensive approach and treatments that are standard in pre-surgical preparation.

Patients with MHO can progress to develop metabolic syndrome. Without intervention, adipocytes develop a "sick fat" phenotype, whereby insulin resistance develops. This creates the positive feedback loop of metabolic syndrome and weight gain. Research suggests this turning point likely occurs with the development of metabolic-associated fatty liver disease (MAFLD, formerly described as non-alcoholic fatty liver disease or NAFLD) [5].

The relevance of obesity-associated comorbidities in the context of prehabilitation is that they are presumably more difficult to treat or reverse than they are to prevent. This increased difficulty is partially due to the circular effect of intramuscular fat worsening insulin resistance which promotes further visceral and hepatic fat accrual [6]. Liver fibrosis develops as MAFLD progresses to an inflammatory state, and, once established, further worsens insulin resistance [7]. One study by Tutunchi et al. suggested greater odds of progressively worsening MAFLD fibrosis scores in patients with metabolic syndrome than in individuals who were otherwise metabolically healthy with the same BMI [8].

Further, some comorbidities are risk factors for surgical complications and portend worse response to bariatric surgery.

Table 1 shows a non-exhaustive list of common obesity-related comorbidities, how these are traditionally evaluated, and the implications each has with regard to bariatric surgery outcomes. These risk factors also serve as the modifiable targets for interventions included in the following section. This table (and chapter) should serve as a reference for non-obesity medicine specialists to kickstart pre-surgical optimization by screening for less intuitive comorbidities prior to referral. A primary care physician, physiatrist, orthopedist, etc. who is treating a patient for one obesity-associated comorbidity can initiate early workup and recommendations while the patient is waiting to even be seen by medical/surgical obesity medicine specialists.

Table 1 Risk factors and associated complications

Risk factor	How risk factor has been measured	Known negative effects of risk factor
Sarcopenia/ sarcopenic obesity	DEXA, biometric impedance, CT/ MRI	Gastric leak [9], post-op worsening of sarcopenia/frailty, cancer [10]
Obstructive sleep apnea	Screening with STOP-BANG or Berlin Questionnaire, polysomnography for confirmation	Intraoperative (arrhythmia, hypoxia) and postoperative (infection, ICU transfer, increased LOS) complications [11]
Depression	PHQ-9	Less weight loss after surgery [12, 13] and higher risk for self-harm [14]
Binge eating disorder/bulimia nervosa	BEDS-7, EDDS	Postoperative weight regain [15]; SUD [16]
Dysglycemia	HbA1C, fasting glucose/insulin, or OGTT	Reduced postoperative weight loss [17], increased mortality and complications [18]
Substance use disorder [19]	DAST-10, urine drug screen	Higher incidence of SUD [19, 20]

DEXA dual X-ray absorptiometry, *ICU* intensive care unit, *LOS* length of stay, *PHQ* patient health questionnaire, *BEDS* binge eating disorder screener, *EDDS* eating disorder diagnostic scale, *SUD* substance use disorder, *HbA1C* hemoglobin A1C, *OGTT* oral glucose tolerance test, *DAST* drug abuse screening test

4 Prehabilitation Pillars

Bariatric Surgery-Specific Enhanced Recovery After Surgery (ERAS) Recommendations

There is growing support for prehabilitation prior to bariatric surgery, although official societal guidelines are often not focused on this subject matter. The 2021 ERAS Society update for bariatric surgery notes "prehabilitation and exercise" lack sufficient data for a recommendation; however, the panel recommends with "strong" grades preoperative weight loss and smoking/alcohol cessation—two important components of a multimodal preparatory plan [21]. The 2021 update of the ASMBS position on prehabilitation [22] is similarly agnostic due to the absence of bariatric surgery-specific prehabilitation programs; although, the report cites data supporting the benefit of preoperative exercise and pulmonary training in patients undergoing major abdominal surgery.

Some insurance plans have idiosyncratic requirements prior to authorizations, with some requiring preoperative weight loss using justification that this minimizes complications and predicts the patient's compliance with postoperative recommendations. Research suggests that preoperative weight loss may improve the technical ease of the procedure by reducing visceral organ size [23] and total complications [24]. These results are inconsistent, and studies involving mandatory weight loss often have substantially higher drop-out rates in the intervention group, showing the policy's efficacy as a gatekeeper as much as a means of ensuring optimal postoperative outcomes [25]. Thankfully, many carriers are moving away from this requirement.

Exercise Evidence

The goals of exercise before bariatric surgery are threefold. First, any form of exercise in an untrained individual supports building or maintaining lean mass while losing excess body weight [26–28]. This muscle provides "reserves" to offset the inevitable postoperative loss. Second, for patients with dysglycemia, exercise (particularly combined resistance and aerobic programs) accelerates the insulin-sensitizing process synergistically with caloric/carbohydrate restriction, as noted in chapter "Basic Prehabilitation Pillars." Finally, exercise may improve musculoskeletal pain, independent of total body weight loss. With reduced pain and increased energy levels, patients can continue exercising and implementing the other components of a multimodal prehabilitation program.

Exercise recommendations must conform to the patient's comorbidities, preferences, and activity tolerance; even with similar goals, any two patients may have vastly different exercise prescriptions. Broadly, variety in training style (aerobic, resistance, high-intensity intervals, flexibility, etc.) and in the targeted muscle groups offer benefits of accelerated improvements in body composition [29] and physical resilience, while reducing the risk of overtraining and injury [30]. For motivated individuals, exercise prescriptions should maximize the frequency of training, provided the patient has adequate nutrition and sleep to facilitate recovery.

Data regarding the "ideal" exercise prescription prior to bariatric surgery does not currently exist. However, the present literature offers insights into exercise regimens that exert the fastest improvements in body composition and metabolic metrics. A recent network meta-analysis by O'Donoghue et al. assessed the efficacy of different exercise types in individuals with obesity [31]. This analysis determined that a combination of high-load resistance training with high-intensity aerobic exercise is the most effective style for improving body fat percentage, total body weight, and overall cardiorespiratory fitness (as assessed by VO_{2max}). This regimen may appear ambitious for an untrained individual, but "high load" and "high intensity" are relative measures. In the network meta-analysis described earlier, authors defined "high load" resistance training as training with intensity >75% of the calculated 1 repetition maximum (1RM) in a program with three sessions per week lasting 30–60 min. Similarly, "high intensity" or "vigorous" aerobic training describes regimens of any aerobic-only exercise (running, cycling, swimming, etc.) at an intensity exceeding 65% VO_{2max}, >75% HR_{max}, or >65% heart rate reserve (HRR). There are multiple published formulas for estimating 1RM from lower load/higher repetition sets [32]. Based on how the study defined "high intensity" and "high load," untrained individuals can achieve the requisite level of exertion with effort proportional to their level of conditioning.

Waist circumference is an important adjunctive proxy for overall metabolic health when combined with BMI [33]. The meta-analysis above did not fully investigate which training style best-reduced waist circumference, because waist circumference was not included as an outcome in studies of high load and high-intensity exercise [31]. However, of the remaining available combinations of aerobic intensity and resistance training load, a combination of *low* load and *low*-intensity training was superior to any individual training style in isolation, like high or low aerobic intensity versus high or low load resistance training. In the context of the other high-intensity/high load benefits noted earlier, combination of high load and high intensity likely would have been the superior exercise plan for reducing waist circumference had outcome data been available. Alternatively, resistance training alone with low-moderate or high load had the lowest impact on waist circumference and cardiorespiratory fitness of the different exercise training types.

Although aerobic/resistance training confers the well-documented benefits described earlier, exercise insufficiently raises daily caloric expenditure to promote meaningful weight loss alone in some individuals for uncertain reasons [34, 35]. Even for these individuals, combinations of aerobic and resistance training are important strategies to prevent weight *regain* in the setting of homeostatic changes that occur after weight loss. These hormonal changes include increased ghrelin, decreased leptin, and decreased conversion of T4 to T3, which result in greater appetite, decreased basal metabolic rate, and subsequent weight gain [36].

Lifestyle Evidence

Preoperative lifestyle modifications like nutritional/supplement optimization paired with exercise can improve candidacy for surgery and increase the likelihood of maximizing postoperative weight loss and improving metabolic disease [37]. With regard to weight loss promoting lifestyle changes, certain medications and nutritional changes can maximize the ratio of fat mass to lean mass loss, allowing the individual to maintain lean mass while in caloric deficit. Nutritional supplements such as high-quality protein like whey protein [38, 39] and creatine [40, 41] promote strength and muscle mass maintenance when paired with resistance training [42, 43]. These supplements have a detailed history of safety and are widely available. As skeletal muscle has pleiotropic effects on promoting insulin sensitivity [44], reducing inflammation [45], increasing BDNF [46], and other short and long-term benefits [47], retaining this muscle mass should be a priority.

Other Nutritional Strategies

Research shows efficacy in programs centered around meal replacement shakes, which often also include regular (typically weekly) shared medical appointments with other patients. In fact, research suggests better weight loss in patients attending these group sessions over individual meetings with their medical team [48, 49].

These programs require specially designed shakes and should not be created with any off-the-shelf protein supplement. These beverages often have higher sodium and potassium, and therefore, clinicians should be mindful in prescribing these for patients with kidney/heart disease. These pre-made meal replacements reduce the cognitive burden of calorie-restricted meal planning, which may at least partially explain the success in nearly half of the participants in the OPTIWIN trial [50]. Using one brand of meal replacement drinks (Optifast), four times the number of participants in the intervention group compared with the food-based diet control successfully lost 15% of their bodyweight in 26 weeks, and overall, the whole Optifast cohort lost 12.4% total bodyweight.

The 26-week timeline of the OPTIWIN trial does not translate directly to the application in bariatric surgery prehabilitation; however, Optifast and other low-calorie meal replacements may be components of a preoperative very low-calorie diet (VLCD) nutritional strategy. VLCD diets are associated with greater total body weight loss preoperatively and shorter postoperative lengths of stay [51, 52]. When paired with resistance training, one study demonstrated significant increases in lean mass with lower fat mass after only 2 weeks [42].

Dietary caloric restriction is the keystone of medical weight loss, and individuals may choose from several strategies to achieve this average weekly deficit. For example, patients can maintain a daily deficit without changing meal frequency or timing by dutifully planning meals with fewer calories. Simple dietary nudges can help achieve this deficit such as removing sugar-sweetened beverages such as fruit juices, and full-sugar soft drinks, and using non-sugar sweeteners in coffee/tea and when cooking. Changing meal sequencing by first eating protein-dense foods before starchy, low-fiber foods prioritize foods with a higher "thermogenic effect" earlier in the meal and increase the likelihood of leaving calorically dense foods uneaten. Others find it easier to restrict the amount of time spent eating during the day (time-restricted feeding, TRF) or during the week (intermittent fasting, IF) to produce an average caloric deficit. Presently, the "ideal" diet for preprocedural weight loss is not well defined, but different dietary compositions are described in greater detail in chapter "Basic Prehabilitation Pillars."

In addition to the myriad benefits above, the psychological impact of sustaining these changes is an important skill for patients prior to bariatric surgery. These nutritional and exercise habits need to become fundamental features of patients' day-to-day lives as they mirror many of the postoperative habits that must become routine including exercise and supplementation.

Sex Hormones

In addition to nutritional supplements, testosterone replacement therapy (TRT) for men with testosterone deficiency or hormone replacement for postmenopausal women may restore lost physiologic "anabolic potential" [53, 54]. Obesity and hypogonadism in men are highly correlated. If a patient continues to have secondary hypogonadism after correcting lifestyle factors like alcohol consumption [55] and repleting hormones to physiologic levels may improve the anabolic potential for building skeletal muscle while increasing a patient's metabolic rate [56]. Further, the patient will likely appreciate the benefits of increased energy and exercise tolerance, allowing for greater activity participation [57]. Data in the pre-bariatric surgery population have not yet been published, but other research shows that supraphysiologic doses of testosterone in men prior to total knee arthroplasty did not significantly decrease the risk of adverse events but did improve functional status at post-op day 3 [58]. Data also propose that obesity-associated hypogonadism in men [59] improves postoperatively in parallel with insulin resistance, which suggests there may only be a temporary need for testosterone replacement therapy in testosterone-deficient men before bariatric surgery.

With regard to hormone replacement therapy in postmenopausal women, patients experiencing the potentially debilitating symptoms of menopause may be able to safely continue HRT. Similar to interpreting TRT safety in men, the surgery-specific data, although limited, suggest hormone replacement therapy for postmenopausal women may *not* increase the risk of venous thromboembolism (VTE) during orthopedic surgery [60]. While not studied in bariatric surgery, VTE is arguably the most likely severe acute complication from HRT in a surgical population among the highest risk (orthopedic surgeries). For some, HRT may be the only hope for tolerating and maximally benefiting from the increased exercise and dietary changes prior to surgery. However, larger scale studies suggest the highest risk for VTE after starting estrogen replacement is within the first year, making HRT initiated exclusively for prehabilitation benefit likely to confer a higher risk.

With considerations like these in mind, the current clinical practice guidelines for bariatric surgery suggest cessation of supplemental estrogen (both as HRT and in use as a contraceptive) prior to surgery [22, 61]. However, for women who have been safely treated with HRT, medical professionals may consider maintaining these regimens for symptomatic benefit, maintenance of bone density, and support of skeletal muscle [62]. Similarly, as for men, sex hormone abnormalities in women improve postoperatively in parallel with insulin resistance [63].

Anti-Obesity Medications

Given the cumulative effects of chronic metabolic disease, the ideal approach to treating obesity is prompt, multifaceted, and often involves the full arsenal of highly effective anti-obesity medications (AOMs).

AOMs are common in medical weight loss programs including, at times, bariatric surgery programs [64]. Some insurance providers and even practitioners require a tiered approach to prescribing these medications; though, this practice is changing. In this approach, patients begin their weight loss with lifestyle changes followed by "first line" AOMs. If the patients are unable to lose weight or have contraindications to the first line, they can trial newer medications like gut peptide analogs. The "step up" approach runs counter to the current literature on medication selection and appropriate treatment of obesity as a chronic disease. This may be borne out of residual stigma attributing obesity to a lack of willpower to control eating habits and activity levels [65]. For this reason, practitioners are shifting from this perspective to strategies targeting specific eating patterns.

Clinicians can enhance weight loss outcomes at a relatively low expense by tailoring anti-obesity medication prescriptions based on eating patterns and substance use history. Researchers at the Mayo Clinic reported substantially higher efficacy of commonly used agents like bupropion/naltrexone, phentermine with increased resistance training (RT), phentermine/topiramate, and a GLP-1 R agonist (liraglutide) relative to their typical outcomes by first categorizing eating behaviors/weight gain etiologies into specific descriptive phenotypes and targeting each phenotype with the medication most likely to reverse the behavior/pathophysiology. These phenotypes and targeted agents are hedonic eating (emotional hunger, bupropion/naltrexone), abnormally low metabolic rate (phentermine and RT), "hungry brain" (delayed satiation-fullness during meals, phentermine/topiramate), and "hungry gut" (reduced satiety-fullness between meals, GLP-1 RA) [66], respectively. Each of these agents targets the suspected pathophysiology of the respective phenotype instead of empirically relying on whichever medication offers the greatest weight loss at any given time.

As part of optimizing weight loss pharmacologically, new gut peptide analogs (i.e., semaglutide, tirzepatide, etc.) offer the largest magnitude of weight loss but come with potential risks including significant gastrointestinal distress, indiscriminate weight loss of both fat and lean mass, and uncertain risks of pancreatitis and medullary thyroid cancer. Further, patients may be required to discontinue AOMs prior to surgery at the discretion of their surgical team due to potential interaction with surgical anesthetics and risk of aspiration [64, 67].

Note, that post-surgically, patients may begin AOM therapy or resume prior therapy, typically initiated as their post-surgical weight loss begins to slow. For these patients, many ask if they are destined to require these medications into perpetuity. Practitioners may reasonably attempt gradually de-escalating medications after achieving sufficient weight loss; although, many patients will require lifelong AOM therapy for maintenance as obesity is a chronic disease even when in remission [68, 69]. As noted previously, strategies that increase the likelihood of successful weight maintenance include combined resistance and aerobic training and nutritional programs with sustained caloric deficit-often built on a high protein diet for muscle support.

Neuropsychiatric Evidence

Targeted interventions within the neuropsychiatric domain (including mood, pain, and sleep) may independently improve health outcomes. However, addressing pathology in these areas will also augment the efficacy of exercise and lifestyle therapies through more consistent participation, reduced fatigue, and improved recovery, amongst other mechanisms.

For example, obstructive sleep apnea (OSA) is one prevalent obesity-related comorbidity, but inadequate sleep quantity and quality from any cause impact health in countless ways. As highlighted in chapter "Basic Prehabilitation Pillars," optimal sleep is necessary for appetite regulation [70] via leptin, ghrelin, and cortisol levels [71], blood glucose and blood pressure homeostasis [72], mood [73], immune system function [74], exercise performance and recovery [75], cognitive health [76], and pain modulation [77, 78]. In the context of patients with obesity and prehabilitation prior to bariatric surgery, screening for sleep disorders is appropriate. BMI has a dose-dependent impact on the risk/severity of OSA, and therefore, the more severe a patient's obesity, the more prudent the assessment of sleep [79]. Instruments such as the STOP-BANG and the Berlin Questionnaire are effective screening tools in this population, whereas the Epworth Sleepiness Scale correlates worse with OSA in patients undergoing bariatric surgery [22, 80].

Patients in the process of qualifying for bariatric surgery will undergo psychologic assessment for behaviors or pathology that may worsen with the stress and the biochemical changes of surgery. Providers should optimize treatment for mood/substance use disorder relative to their impact on weight gain. For example, some antidepressant/neuropathic pain medications like tricyclic and tetracyclic antidepressants [81] are more likely to promote weight gain than others; alternatively, a medication like bupropion may be as effective for mood while promoting weight loss, especially when paired with naltrexone. In the latter case, this provides a highly effective weight loss combination with some added benefits for substance use disorder management.

Nicotine cessation therapy is critical for patients prior to surgery. Nicotine has vasoconstrictive activity, and research has demonstrated various complications associated with smoking across multiple surgery types, including a higher risk of reintubation, prolonged intubation, sepsis, and wound-related complications [82, 83].

Table 2 provides a summary of important risk factors for poor outcomes of metabolic and obesity surgery and available evidence for targeted interventions and outcomes associated with these interventions.

Table 2 Evidence summary table

Domain	Study design	Population	Interventions	Outcomes measured
Lifestyle: nicotine cessation	Møller et al. [82] RCT	108 patients awaiting joint replacement	6–8 week smoking cessation counseling and nicotine replacement therapy	Significant and clinically meaningful reduction in complications-particularly wound-related, cardiovascular, and those requiring a second surgery
Lifestyle: nicotine cessation	Haskins et al. [83] retrospective cohort	41,445 patients who underwent bariatric surgery	Comparing patients who smoked with matched non-smokers	Smoking significantly increased the risk of prolonged intubation/ reintubation, pneumonia, sepsis, LOS, and organ space infection
Multimodal: exercise, nutrition, psychological	Lucini et al. [84] single arm pre-post test design	39 patients awaiting bariatric surgery	Counseled on exercise, rec 30 min/day mod intensity aerobic, recommended 500–1000 calorie reduction in diet, and a 1.5 h psych assessment with counseling to enact behavioral change. Weekly phone call for compliance	Significant decrease in weight (>6 kg average)

(continued)

Table 2 (continued)

Domain	Study design	Population	Interventions	Outcomes measured
Neuropsychiatric: mood	Livhits et al. [48] systematic review; subgroup comparison between presence/ absence of binge eating disorder	Adults awaiting bariatric surgery	Preoperative mandatory weight loss	Preoperative mandatory weight loss predicts postoperative weight loss success and, conversely, "super-obesity" (Class 3 obesity) is associated with less excess body weight loss. Also, personality disorders are negatively associated with postoperative weight loss. Binge eating disorder predicts an increased risk of weight regain at 1 year
Neuropsychiatric: mood	Cassin et al. [49] RCT	47 patients with binge eating disorder before bariatric surgery	Six sessions of preoperative telemedicine-based cognitive behavioral therapy (CBT)	Significant improvements in validated measures of BED (the Binge Eating Scale), Emotional Eating Scale, and Depression (PHQ-9). In the control group, patients had significant *increases* in emotional eating, depression, and anxiety
Multimodal: counseling (exercise, nutrition, goal setting, surgery expectations)	Kalarchian et al. [85] RCT	240 patients preoperatively	60-minute individual/in person therapy sessions weekly ×8, followed by monthly 60-min sessions with additional phone sessions	The intervention group had better weight loss at follow-up and better eating behaviors

(continued)

Table 2 (continued)

Domain	Study design	Population	Interventions	Outcomes measured
Neuropsychiatric: mood	Gandara et al. [86] observational study	110 patients awaiting bariatric surgery	12 once-weekly CBT sessions	Patients had improved depression, anxiety, and disordered eating. When comparing BED/ non-BED groups, patients with BED resolved their preoperative lower ratings of QoL and self-esteem
Exercise	Picó-Sirvent et al. [87] prospective cohort study	20 patients	Including resistance training in the exercise plan	Individuals with obesity awaiting bariatric surgery could avoid the loss of FFM and reduction in BMR seen in aerobic-only exercise plans [88, 89] by adding 1 day of RT per week (second month) and 2 days/week (third month)
Exercise	Picó-Sirvent et al. [28] prospective cohort study	Six patients awaiting bariatric surgery	Combined HIIT + RT for 6 months leading up to surgery. Frequency: 2 days/ week the first month, 3 days/week the second month, and 4 days/week from the third to the last month. 60 minute sessions for the first 2 months and 70 min from the third to the last month. The endurance training days alternated MICT and HIIT. RT followed HIIT sessions	This resulted in significant BMI and EBWL compared with individuals awaiting surgery who did not participate in the supervised exercise program

(continued)

Table 2 (continued)

Domain	Study design	Population	Interventions	Outcomes measured
Exercise	Marc-Hernandez et al. [88] prospective cohort study	23 patients awaiting bariatric surgery	12-week progressively increasing exercise program (4 weeks of 2×/week; 4 weeks of 3×/week; 4 weeks of 4×/week) combining resistance, aerobic, and HIIT	The intervention group had a significantly greater reduction in BMI, and %EWL while FFM remained constant. VO_{2max} and HRQoL (domains in physical functioning, social functioning, and general health perceptions)
Exercise	Gilbertson et al. [89] prospective cohort	14 patients awaiting bariatric surgery	The control group met with dieticians and received a special two-week preoperative diet, had a surgical education session, and received psychologic clearance. In addition to the control group regimen, the exercise group added 30 min/day, 5 days/week of walking at 65–85% peak HR for the 30 days preop	The intervention group had significantly shorter LOS by adding a fast walking program, alone
Multimodal: lifestyle (nutrition) and neuropsychiatric (sleep)	Schiavo et al. [90] RCT	70 patients total	Four weeks preop, the intervention group received a CPAP and low-calorie ketogenic diet (LCKD); the control only received CPAP	Both groups improved AHI, without any significant difference in magnitude of improvement. CPAP + LCKD led to significantly greater improvements in CRP. The intervention group also had significant weight loss, BMI improvement, blood pressure (systolic and diastolic), total and LDL cholesterol, and triglycerides that were not noted in the control group

(continued)

Table 2 (continued)

Domain	Study design	Population	Interventions	Outcomes measured
Neuropsychiatric: sleep	Horvath et al. [80] retrospective cohort study	251 patients before bariatric surgery	Compared polysomnography data and screening questionnaires	STOP-Bang Questionnaire and NoSAS performed the best in terms of sensitivity/ specificity for predicting moderate/ severe OSA
Neuropsychiatric: sleep	Consensus guidelines based on an expert panel of metabolic and bariatric surgeons and a systematic review of the literature [91]			The current position regarding screening tools recommends using the STOP-Bang or, with weaker evidence, the Berlin Questionnaire. Polysomnography (preferably in-lab) is recommended for patients with suspected moderate/ severe OSA and treatment with CPAP if confirmed. Patients may benefit from getting acclimated to CPAP weeks before surgery
Lifestyle: nutrition	Albanese et al. [51] prospective cohort	178 patients awaiting bariatric surgery	The intervention group received a VLCKD with control on VLCD for 3 weeks preoperatively	The intervention group had significantly greater weight loss and significantly fewer required a prolonged (>3 days) hospital stay. Drainage output was lower and postoperative hemoglobin was higher
Lifestyle: nutrition	Leonetti et al. [52] prospective cohort study	80 patients awaiting bariatric surgery	Intervention groups received a progressive diet of VLCKD for 10 days, a VLCD for 10 days, and then an LCD for 10 days; control maintained an LCD for 30 days preoperatively	Intervention group had significant weight loss, BMI reduction, waist and neck circumference decreases by the end of the study compared to baseline; control did not have significant improvements in these parameters

(continued)

Table 2 (continued)

Domain	Study design	Population	Interventions	Outcomes measured
Lifestyle (nutrition) and exercise	Ho et al. [42] prospective cohort study	45 patients awaiting bariatric surgery	The intervention used a VLCD with high protein (1.3 g/kg of adjusted bodyweight) and 7 strength exercises in 3 different aerobic circuits for 2 weeks preoperatively	All patients lost weight while gaining muscle mass and lowered their sarcopenic risk (as measured by the FM/FFM ratio) during the 2-week period; however, patients with BMI <50 gained significantly more muscle but lost less weight than patients with BMI 50+
Lifestyle: endocrine	Saad et al. [57] review article	Men with obesity and hypogonadism	Testosterone repletion to physiologic level	Testosterone supplementation reverses fat accumulation with significant insulin sensitivity and lean body mass improvement. Note, authors also describe how current insights do not support the assumption that testosterone supplementation contributes to prostate malignancy and cardiovascular disease

RCT randomized controlled trial, *LOS* length of stay, *sig* significant, *CBT* cognitive behavioral therapy, *BED* binge eating disorder, *PHQ-9* patient health questionnaire 9, *QoL* quality of life, *FM* fat mass, *FFM* fat-free mass, *BMR* basal metabolic rate, *RT* resistance training, *HIIT* high-intensity interval training, *BMI* body mass index, *EBWL* excess body weight loss, *MICT* medium intensity continuous training, *HRQoL* health-related quality of life, *CPAP* continuous positive airway pressure, *AHI* apnea-hypopnea index, *VLCKD* very low-calorie ketogenic diet with variations (LCKD, VLCD, etc.,), *CRP* C-reactive protein, *OSA* obstructive sleep apnea

5 Preoperative Screening

Serum lab work is a standard preoperative assessment. Patients can also be susceptible to postoperative vitamin deficiencies, and therefore they are assessed preoperatively [92]. Optimization of vitamin levels (especially vitamin C) has been shown to reduce postoperative complications in bariatric patients [93]. Other aspects of this panel include:

- Complete blood count (CBC) and cofactors for red blood cell production such as B12 and methylmalonic acid, folate, and iron level/transferrin/ferritin/TIBC.
- Fat-soluble vitamins/minerals and related values such as 25-hydroxyvitamin D, calcium, parathyroid hormone, vitamin A, zinc, and copper (often as erythrocyte superoxide dismutase).
- HbA1c, lipid profile, renal function panel, given the effect of metabolic syndrome on these; though, the lipid profile is unlikely to have direct implications during the prehabilitation period given the predominantly cumulative negative impact of dyslipidemia.

Patients undergoing surgery participate in these screenings for conditions that may increase their risks of perioperative complications. A truly comprehensive discussion of potentially applicable screenings is beyond the scope of this text; however, these tests comprise some of the most important.

6 Plan Formulation Considerations and Best Practices

Exercise

Best practice considerations for designing an exercise prescription for bariatric surgery prehabilitation must consider unique patient demographic factors identified earlier. With these in mind, recommendations include:

Exercise Type

- Identify the form of physical activity the patient enjoys most or is most likely to enjoy and perform safely. If the patient does not have physical activity preferences, modalities such as aquatic-based exercises have a low impact on joints and minimize heat-discomfort, and pairing individuals with similar capabilities and body habitus in group settings may minimize apprehension about participation.
- Cross-training through different styles may amplify metabolic improvements when compared with any single style alone and may reduce injury risk compared with repeated bouts of one single training style [30].
- For patients who find significant weight bearing to be prohibitively painful, blood flow restriction training (BFRT) can provide an augmented anabolic and metabolic stimulus with a relatively lower joint load [94]. Information on

techniques and precautions for BFRT is provided in greater detail in chapter "Basic Prehabilitation Pillars."

Exercise Initiation and Progression

- For patients without prior exercise participation in whom tolerance is unknown, start with low frequency, intensity, and duration to minimize the risk of injury and overtraining. After assessing a baseline level of tolerance, gradually increase these parameters as able. For example, in a walking program, this may include increasing the frequency of sessions, the number of steps per session, or speed/terrain difficulty.
- Similarly, for land-based resistance training, add body weight exercises such as chair stands, modified push-ups, and/or modified pull-ups to offer muscle-building benefits and mirror important daily functional activities [95, 96].

Unstructured Physical Activity

- Incorporating 5-min walks around an office building every hour can increase an individual's daily step count, brief sets of bodyweight squats punctuating a sedentary workday can meaningfully increase total exercise time, or taking the stairs instead of the elevator can transiently improve insulin resistance [97]. These relative increases in activity use seemingly minor interventions to potentiate the benefits of dedicated exercise [98].

Exercise Goals

- Educate the patient on proper technique, intensity, and frequency of training, to improve his or her aerobic conditioning and to improve body composition. These improvements occur by exploiting the concept of "progressive overload"—gradually increasing variables like the intensity of aerobic training and the weight/volume of resistance training—instead of rigidly adhering to a fixed exercise program.
- Exercise in prehabilitation also serves to establish a lifelong habit of physical activity for patients after bariatric surgery.

Lifestyle

Anti-Obesity Medications (AOMs)

In formulating the most efficacious approach to include AOMs in a prehabilitation program for bariatric surgery, clinicians should choose medications to simultaneously manage comorbidities like diabetes or based on the patient's "obesity phenotype," as described in greater detail previously in chapter "Basic Prehabilitation Pillars" [66].

- Per FDA guidelines [99] as of the time of this writing, for patients with BMI at least 30 or those with BMI at least 27 and conditions such as hypertension, dyslipidemia, or type II diabetes, practitioners may choose AOMs in conjunction with lifestyle changes. If not achieving 3–5% TBWL after 12–16 weeks, consider increasing the dose or adding a complementary medication, particularly if the patient has had *some* success, and these benefits continue to outweigh any side effects.

- If the response is unexpectedly poor, consider the impact that medication administration may be having on absorption. For example, food intake may affect oral medication absorption such as phentermine, which is why prescribers often recommend the patient not eat within 2 h of medication administration [100]. For subcutaneous medications, decreased blood flow to certain body tissues may affect drug absorption.
- As noted previously as well, these medications should be stopped in the immediate preoperative period, typically about a week, as instructed by the anesthesiologist or surgeon in the team.

Testosterone and Hormone Replacement Therapy

With regards to testosterone repletion for men with obesity and hypogonadism, practitioners comfortable managing replacement therapy should discuss the recommended protocol with patients, the full details of which are beyond the scope of this text. Some highlights, however, include:

- Screen for contraindications such as history of prostate cancer, benign prostatic hyperplasia (BPH), erythrocytosis, untreated OSA, and for individuals attempting to conceive. This discussion should include an understanding that exogenous testosterone may suppress the hypothalamic-pituitary-gonadal axis and impair fertility.
- Note, men with hypogonadism and obesity may see improvement in testosterone deficiency after bariatric surgery, and so, testosterone supplementation during prehabilitation may only be a temporary measure [59].

For women who are currently stable on an HRT program, surgical teams should discuss the risks of potential VTE-related events vs the resilience-promoting benefits of continuing therapy [101]. These considerations are highly individualized, and the current literature cannot provide a definitive, comprehensive assessment.

Nutrition and Supplementation

As the data demonstrated previously, patients should follow two core nutritional principles: adherence to a high protein, low-calorie diet.

- These individuals require a caloric deficit to promote weight loss and high protein for exercise recovery and to maintain skeletal muscle [102, 103]. High protein roughly equates to consuming at least 1.2 g/kg of bodyweight daily; although, there is no universally accepted standard cutoff for what constitutes a "high protein diet."
- As these programs are effectively temporizing measures before surgery, the source of protein (i.e., fish, poultry, low-fat dairy, and vegetable sources in lieu

of saturated-fat-containing red meats) is less crucial than it will be in the patient's postoperative diet.
- There are limited data in the specific context of bariatric surgery prehabilitation, but patients may consider supplementing creatine monohydrate for its demonstrated benefit in exercise tolerance, recovery, and adaptation.

Neuropsychiatric Recommendations

Mood and Chronic Pain

While psychiatric illness and chronic pain are traditionally managed by distinct specialists, clinicians who feel comfortable managing both should approach treatment in a targeted, streamlined fashion. Many treatment strategies including medication classes, psychotherapy types, and even exercise prescriptions can have efficacy in managing both pain and mood/anxiety disorders.

- Patients who qualify for surgery and have symptoms of mood disorder should receive treatment as early as possible to increase adherence to other interventions. Acute crises must be appropriately managed with a subsequent timeframe of stability to ensure safety and appropriateness for surgery.
- Similarly, approach pain management in a proactive and aggressive manner with multimodal, opioid-minimizing therapies. Incorporate pain psychologists as able given the bidirectionality of chronic pain and mood disorders.
- Although already the goal in most clinical situations, practitioners should strive to treat multiple conditions with the fewest prescriptions such as targeting both pain and mood with a single serotonin-norepinephrine reuptake inhibitor (SNRI), for example. This will minimize polypharmacy, which is a greater concern in the context of a postoperative nutritional supplementation regimen.
  - Even if multiple providers are comanaging conditions like pain and behavioral health (particularly in remote communities), coordinating care as able can simplify treatment regimens for patients and potentially improve adherence.

Sleep

Published data and the recommendations from the American Society for Metabolic and Bariatric Surgery (ASMBS) simplify the sleep optimization aspect of prehabilitation.

- Screen patients for obstructive sleep apnea using the STOP-BANG or Berlin Questionnaire, two short survey instruments that can be included in intake paperwork. Patients with moderate/high risk for OSA should receive a referral to a sleep specialist, and they will likely undergo subsequent polysomnography, with in-lab testing preferred.
- Prompt referral to a sleep specialist/polysomnography will reduce the lead time in diagnosis/treatment and progressing through the adjustment period patients

often required to habitually utilize nighttime continuous positive airway pressure (CPAP) machines.

Monitoring Program Efficacy

To maximally assess program efficacy, quickly identify complications and stalled progress in real time, and improve patients' overall experience, multidisciplinary care for follow-up is critical. This should include different measurement instruments to objectively track patients' weight loss and body composition.

- Ideally, prehabilitation practitioners monitor clinical improvements with frequent check-ins either virtually or in person, eventually transitioning to less frequent visits. These visits may be with different team members such as registered dieticians [104], weight loss counselors [105], and exercise specialists [106], or as part of shared medical appointments. Even informal messages within a patient portal can maximize the "touchpoints" to ensure accountability, understanding of recommendations, and confidence in proper exercise techniques.
- Tracking body composition is the most direct way to monitor the efficacy of interventions designed to facilitate excess body weight loss (EBWL) and build/maintain lean mass. Typical means of measuring body composition include bioelectric impedance or DEXA here. If using DEXA, patients should utilize the same imaging center to minimize measurement differences between assessments.
- Practices measuring weight/BMI who do not have access to professional-grade bioelectric impedance devices or DEXA scans should at least measure waist circumference to help contextualize simultaneous fat loss and muscle mass gains.

Finally, practitioners can use disease-specific metrics to track the efficacy of discrete interventions.

- Using remote patient monitoring (RPM) devices, patients can track improvements in comorbidities like hypertension that may be falsely worsened in the presence of medical professionals or fasting blood sugar readings without having to delay breakfast until after a morning medical appointment.
- These RPM devices also accurately log activity in real time but will require teaching sessions with patients.

7 Safety Concerns When Designing and Delivering the Intervention

No intervention is without risk, even interventions that ultimately can produce great benefit. Having a few patient-specific potential safety considerations in mind prior to program initiation may minimize the risk of harm as well as provide reassurance to patients who may already be concerned about the acute effects of poor metabolic health.

Atherosclerotic cardiovascular disease (ASCVD) is a primary safety concern when initiating the exercise portion of a prehabilitation program. As outlined in chapter "Basic Prehabilitation Pillars," the American College of Sports Medicine (ACSM) currently [107] recommends pre-participation health screening for individuals with known or suspected (based on signs/symptoms) cardiopulmonary, renal, or vascular disease who are not currently participating in regular exercise. After clearance demonstrates an acceptably low risk of complications, patients should begin with light-moderate-intensity exercise, and if the patient is already exercising regularly, a physician should provide clearance before the patient increases the intensity of exercise.

As introduced previously, novices may also experience modest safety risks once initiating exercise if their technique is poor, they escalate intensity too quickly, or if they are not optimizing recovery after exercise. Mitigate much of this risk with thorough pre-participation counseling, demonstration, and frequent open communication. After initial success, some patients may experience an increase in drive and dedication to their new lifestyle; therefore, a steadying external influence should temper these patients' urge to over-participate by clearly communicating the "long view," explaining that an unexpected injury may risk falling short of his/her goals.

Nutritional safety concerns overlap with recovery, as well. The prescribed caloric deficit for weight loss may also relatively impair recovery from exercise, should the diet lack adequate protein. A high protein diet ensures that, at a physiologic level, mTOR in skeletal muscle is stimulated and promotes anabolism during fat mass loss. In patients with baseline sarcopenic obesity, indiscriminate weight loss including high amounts of fat and muscle mass can worsen sarcopenia, increase the risk of sequelae like frailty, and worsen surgical outcomes.

8 Other Potential Medical Complications

While the previous complications relate to the implementation of the prehabilitation program, patients and their medical teams may lower the risk of surgery-related complications with some consideration during preoperative planning. Overall, bariatric surgical procedures are safe with lower rates of complications than other commonly performed gastrointestinal surgeries like laparoscopic cholecystectomy [108–110].

For example, marginal ulceration around the suture line after bariatric surgery, specifically the Roux-en-Y gastric bypass, is relatively uncommon, and some prehabilitation interventions may further lower the risk. Postoperative smoking is the most significant prehabilitation-related risk factor, bolstering the case for preoperative cessation [111]. Steroid and NSAID use after surgery are other risk factors for marginal ulceration which can be mitigated; though short courses of perioperative NSAIDs may be important parts of pain management [112]. Patients with marginal ulcers may present with epigastric pain, melena, weakness (usually secondary to anemia), and dysphagia.

Similarly, anastomotic complications such as stenoses and leaks are other *relatively* common complications of bypass procedures (and less commonly gastrectomy), should a complication occur. Like marginal ulcers, certain preoperative strategies may reduce the risk of anastomotic complications, as factors like abnormal thiamine levels, diabetes mellitus, thyroid disorders, and postoperative NSAID use for stenoses [113] and elevated BMI, visceral fat mass, nutritional status, and impaired respiratory function [114, 115] may be potentially addressable with preprocedural nutritional and respiratory optimization, weight loss, and education.

Prehabilitation may mitigate select other relevant medical complications with appropriate counseling and/or preventative measures including surgical site infections (SSIs), addiction (as noted earlier), dumping syndrome, weight regain, and vitamin deficiencies with secondary neurologic injury.

Like other complications, modifiable risk factors for SSIs include obstructive sleep apnea [116] and diabetes [117]. Appropriate screening and management of OSA and DM during the prehabilitation period may reduce the risk of postoperative infection.

Dumping syndrome comprises two phenomena—early dumping syndrome occurs approximately 30 min after eating, whereas late dumping occurs 1–3 h afterward. This may occur in any bariatric surgical procedure but is significantly more common following bypass procedures than in gastrectomy procedures [118]. Preoperative education on reducing processed carbohydrate and fat intake, increasing protein and fiber consumption, adhering to portion control, and reducing fluid intake during meals (particularly milk/dairy) may reduce the incidence/severity of these phenomena [119].

9 Post-surgery Rehabilitation Planning

In rare cases, surgeons may refer patients for inpatient rehabilitation after a complex postoperative course, as may similarly occur following any complicated hospitalization. More typically, however, patients will be discharged home following surgery and may instead participate in home-based therapies, outpatient rehabilitation, or exercise programs under the guidance of a certified trainer. These may focus on reconditioning or managing musculoskeletal pain issues in anticipation of advancing their activity and exercise as they recover. Data on admission/referral rates in these populations are not readily available, likely due to their infrequent nature.

10 Recommendations and Action Points

- Substance use: At least 8 weeks prior to surgery, patients should have begun nicotine replacement therapy and stopped smoking [82]. Patients with substance use disorder should undergo therapy and medication-assisted treatment, as needed. Cannabis users should abstain for at least 4–6 weeks preoperatively to minimize interaction with anesthesia and medications.

- Exercise: Patients should participate in 30 min/day of moderate-intensity aerobic exercise (as able) and at least 3 days/week of resistance training (RT) with a day of rest between each RT session. Introduce resistance training gradually (1 day/week) and increase the frequency as tolerated. Motivated patients may substitute high-intensity interval training in lieu of moderate-intensity continuous aerobic training some days for variety and added benefit in reduced time.
- Psychiatric: Patients with binge eating disorder should participate in cognitive or dialectical behavioral therapy. Those with other mood and personality disorders should receive targeted treatment including preferred weight neutral or weight negative medications, as able.
- Sleep: Patients should complete a screening questionnaire like the STOP-BANG or the Berlin Questionnaire early in preoperative evaluation to allow those with moderate/high likelihood of obstructive sleep apnea to receive a thorough evaluation and learn to comfortably tolerate CPAP/BiPAP therapy.
- Nutrition: Preoperative diets should include caloric deficit with high protein. Some studies have shown improved outcomes with a low carbohydrate or ketogenic diet during the preoperative period [51, 120]. Patients should meet with a nutritionist for ongoing nutritional guidance and to improve diet adherence. Patients intending to maintain the ketogenic diet long term should ensure they do not have adverse changes in their lipid profiles, though these changes are unlikely to impact the prehabilitation period [121, 122].
- Other lifestyle: Men with persistent hypogonadism despite lifestyle optimization may benefit from exogenous testosterone. Practitioners should discuss the risks/benefits of continuing hormonal contraception or perimenopausal hormone replacement in women already established on therapy.

References

1. Rey-Lopez J, De Rezende L, Pastor-Valero M, Tess BH. The prevalence of metabolically healthy obesity: a systematic review and critical evaluation of the definitions used. Obes Rev. 2014;15(10):781–90.
2. Blüher M. Metabolically healthy obesity. Endocr Rev. 2020;41:3.
3. Fitch AK, Bays HE. Obesity definition, diagnosis, bias, standard operating procedures (SOPs), and telehealth: an Obesity Medicine Association (OMA) Clinical Practice Statement (CPS) 2022. Obes Pillars. 2022;1:100004.
4. Kawarazaki W, Fujita T. The role of aldosterone in obesity-related hypertension. Am J Hypertens. 2016;29(4):415–23.
5. Kang YM, Jung CH, Cho YK, Lee SE, Lee MJ, Hwang JY, et al. Fatty liver disease determines the progression of coronary artery calcification in a metabolically healthy obese population. PLoS One. 2017;12(4):e0175762.
6. Saponaro C, Sabatini S, Gaggini M, Carli F, Rosso C, Positano V, et al. Adipose tissue dysfunction and visceral fat are associated with hepatic insulin resistance and severity of NASH even in lean individuals. Liver Int. 2022;42(11):2418–27.

7. Brunner KT, Henneberg CJ, Wilechansky RM, Long MT. Nonalcoholic fatty liver disease and obesity treatment. Curr Obes Rep. 2019;8:220–8.
8. Tutunchi H, Naeini F, Ebrahimi-Mameghani M, Najafipour F, Mobasseri M, Ostadrahimi A. Metabolically healthy and unhealthy obesity and the progression of liver fibrosis: a cross-sectional study. Clin Res Hepatol Gastroenterol. 2021;45(6):101754.
9. Gaillard M, Tranchart H, Maitre S, Perlemuter G, Lainas P, Dagher I. Preoperative detection of sarcopenic obesity helps to predict the occurrence of gastric leak after sleeve gastrectomy. Obes Surg. 2018;28(8):2379–85.
10. Pinotti E, Montuori M, Borrelli V, Giuffrè M, Angrisani L. Sarcopenia: what a surgeon should know. Obes Surg. 2020;30(5):2015–20.
11. Chung F, Elsaid H. Screening for obstructive sleep apnea before surgery: why is it important? Curr Opin Anesthesiol. 2009;22(3):405–11.
12. Susmallian S, Nikiforova I, Azoulai S, Barnea R. Outcomes of bariatric surgery in patients with depression disorders. PLoS One. 2019;14(8):e0221576.
13. Jumbe S, Hamlet C, Meyrick J. Psychological aspects of bariatric surgery as a treatment for obesity. Curr Obes Rep. 2017;6(1):71–8.
14. Castaneda D, Popov VB, Wander P, Thompson CC. Risk of suicide and self-harm is increased after bariatric surgery—a systematic review and meta-analysis. Obes Surg. 2019;29(1):322–33.
15. Meany G, Conceição E, Mitchell JE. Binge eating, binge eating disorder and loss of control eating: effects on weight outcomes after bariatric surgery. Eur Eat Disord Rev. 2014;22(2):87–91.
16. Steffen KJ, Engel SG, Wonderlich JA, Pollert GA, Sondag C. Alcohol and other addictive disorders following bariatric surgery: prevalence, risk factors and possible etiologies. Eur Eat Disord Rev. 2015;23(6):442–50.
17. Berkovic MC, Bilic-Curcic I, Mrzljak A, Varzic SC, Cigrovski V. Prehabilitation of overweight and obese patients with dysglycemia awaiting bariatric surgery: predicting the success of obesity treatment. World J Diabetes. 2022;13(12):1096.
18. Avci BS, Saler T, Avci A, Bankir M, Tuzun Z, Nazik H, et al. Relationship between morbidity and mortality and HbA1c levels in diabetic patients undergoing major surgery. J Coll Physicians Surg Pak. 2019;29:1043.
19. Kanji S, Wong E, Akioyamen L, Melamed O, Taylor VH. Exploring pre-surgery and post-surgery substance use disorder and alcohol use disorder in bariatric surgery: a qualitative scoping review. Int J Obes. 2019;43(9):1659–74.
20. Ibrahim N, Alameddine M, Brennan J, Sessine M, Holliday C, Ghaferi AA. New onset alcohol use disorder following bariatric surgery. Surg Endosc. 2019;33(8):2521–30.
21. Stenberg E, dos Reis Falcao LF, O'Kane M, Liem R, Pournaras DJ, Salminen P, et al. Guidelines for perioperative care in bariatric surgery: Enhanced Recovery After Surgery (ERAS) Society recommendations: a 2021 update. World J Surg. 2022;46:729–51.
22. Carter J, Chang J, Birriel TJ, Moustarah F, Sogg S, Goodpaster K, et al. ASMBS position statement on preoperative patient optimization before metabolic and bariatric surgery. Surg Obes Relat Dis. 2021;17(12):1956–76.
23. Cassie S, Menezes C, Birch DW, Shi X, Karmali S. Effect of preoperative weight loss in bariatric surgical patients: a systematic review. Surg Obes Relat Dis. 2011;7(6):760–7.
24. Benotti PN, Still CD, Wood GC, Akmal Y, King H, El Arousy H, et al. Preoperative weight loss before bariatric surgery. Arch Surg. 2009;144(12):1150–5.
25. Kushner BS, Eagon JC. Systematic review and meta-analysis of the effectiveness of insurance requirements for supervised weight loss prior to bariatric surgery. Obes Surg. 2021;31:5396.
26. Campanha-Versiani L, Pereira DAG, Ribeiro-Samora GA, Ramos AV, de Sander Diniz MFH, De Marco LA, et al. The effect of a muscle weight-bearing and aerobic exercise program on the body composition, muscular strength, biochemical markers, and bone mass of obese patients who have undergone gastric bypass surgery. Obes Surg. 2017;27(8):2129–37.

27. Morales-Marroquin E, Kohl HW, Knell G, de la Cruz-Muñoz N, Messiah SE. Resistance training in post-metabolic and bariatric surgery patients: a systematic review. Obes Surg. 2020;30(10):4071–80.
28. Picó-Sirvent I, Aracil-Marco A, Pastor D, Moya-Ramón M. Effects of a combined high-intensity interval training and resistance training program in patients awaiting bariatric surgery: a pilot study. Sports. 2019;7(3):72.
29. Schroeder EC, Franke WD, Sharp RL, Lee D-C. Comparative effectiveness of aerobic, resistance, and combined training on cardiovascular disease risk factors: a randomized controlled trial. PLoS One. 2019;14(1):e0210292.
30. Shaw I, Shaw B, Brown G, Shariat A. Review of the role of resistance training and musculoskeletal injury prevention and rehabilitation. Int J Clin Exp Med. 2016;2016:1–5.
31. O'Donoghue G, Blake C, Cunningham C, Lennon O, Perrotta C. What exercise prescription is optimal to improve body composition and cardiorespiratory fitness in adults living with obesity? A network meta-analysis. Obes Rev. 2021;22(2):e13137.
32. Jawade SS. Prediction of the one repetition maximum to design strength training protocol. J Clin Diagn Res. 2021;15(3) https://doi.org/10.7860/JCDR/2021/46131.14648.
33. Ross R, Neeland IJ, Yamashita S, Shai I, Seidell J, Magni P, et al. Waist circumference as a vital sign in clinical practice: a Consensus Statement from the IAS and ICCR Working Group on Visceral Obesity. Nat Rev Endocrinol. 2020;16(3):177–89.
34. Miller WC, Koceja DM, Hamilton EJ. A meta-analysis of the past 25 years of weight loss research using diet, exercise or diet plus exercise intervention. Int J Obes. 1997;21(10):941–7.
35. Cadieux S, McNeil J, Lapierre MP, Riou M-È, Doucet É. Resistance and aerobic exercises do not affect post-exercise energy compensation in normal weight men and women. Physiol Behav. 2014;130:113–9.
36. Fothergill E, Guo J, Howard L, Kerns JC, Knuth ND, Brychta R, et al. Persistent metabolic adaptation 6 years after "The Biggest Loser" competition. Obesity. 2016;24(8):1612–9.
37. Cigrovski Berkovic M, Bilic-Curcic I, Mrzljak A, Canecki Varzic S, Cigrovski V. Prehabilitation of overweight and obese patients with dysglycemia awaiting bariatric surgery: predicting the success of obesity treatment. World J Diabetes. 2022;13(12):1096–105.
38. Verreijen AM, Verlaan S, Engberink MF, Swinkels S, de Vogel-van den Bosch J, Weijs PJ. A high whey protein–, leucine-, and vitamin D–enriched supplement preserves muscle mass during intentional weight loss in obese older adults: a double-blind randomized controlled trial. Am J Clin Nutr. 2014;101(2):279–86.
39. Meckling KA, Sherfey R. A randomized trial of a hypocaloric high-protein diet, with and without exercise, on weight loss, fitness, and markers of the metabolic syndrome in overweight and obese women. Appl Physiol Nutr Metab. 2007;32(4):743–52.
40. Harmon KK, Stout JR, Fukuda DH, Pabian PS, Rawson ES, Stock MS. The application of creatine supplementation in medical rehabilitation. Nutrients. 2021;13(6):1825.
41. Bernat P, Candow DG, Gryzb K, Butchart S, Schoenfeld BJ, Bruno P. Effects of high-velocity resistance training and creatine supplementation in untrained healthy aging males. Appl Physiol Nutr Metab. 2019;44(11):1246–53.
42. Ho C, Samwil SNM, Kahairudin Z, Jamhuri N, Abd AA. Pre-habilitation with high whey-protein-based meal replacement therapy and exercise promote weight loss and preserve muscle mass before bariatric surgery. Asian J Surg. 2023;46:3716.
43. Henriques HKF, Kattah FM, Piccolo MS, Rosa COB, de Araújo Ventura LH, Cerqueira FR, et al. Effect of whey protein supplementation on body composition of patients undergoing bariatric surgery. Arch Health. 2023;4(1):44–55.
44. Eckardt K, Görgens SW, Raschke S, Eckel J. Myokines in insulin resistance and type 2 diabetes. Diabetologia. 2014;57:1087–99.
45. Benatti FB, Pedersen BK. Exercise as an anti-inflammatory therapy for rheumatic diseases—myokine regulation. Nat Rev Rheumatol. 2015;11(2):86–97.
46. Lee JH, Jun H-S. Role of myokines in regulating skeletal muscle mass and function. Front Physiol. 2019;10:42.

47. Severinsen MCK, Pedersen BK. Muscle–organ crosstalk: the emerging roles of myokines. Endocr Rev. 2020;41(4):594–609.
48. Livhits M, Mercado C, Yermilov I, Parikh JA, Dutson E, Mehran A, et al. Preoperative predictors of weight loss following bariatric surgery: systematic review. Obes Surg. 2012;22(1):70–89.
49. Cassin SE, Sockalingam S, Du C, Wnuk S, Hawa R, Parikh SV. A pilot randomized controlled trial of telephone-based cognitive behavioural therapy for preoperative bariatric surgery patients. Behav Res Ther. 2016;80:17–22.
50. Ard JD, Lewis KH, Rothberg A, Auriemma A, Coburn SL, Cohen SS, et al. Effectiveness of a total meal replacement program (OPTIFAST program) on weight loss: results from the OPTIWIN study. Obesity. 2019;27(1):22–9.
51. Albanese A, Prevedello L, Markovich M, Busetto L, Vettor R, Foletto M. Pre-operative very low calorie ketogenic diet (VLCKD) vs. very low calorie diet (VLCD): surgical impact. Obes Surg. 2019;29:292–6.
52. Leonetti F, Campanile FC, Coccia F, Capoccia D, Alessandroni L, Puzziello A, et al. Very low-carbohydrate ketogenic diet before bariatric surgery: prospective evaluation of a sequential diet. Obes Surg. 2015;25(1):64–71.
53. Kelly DM, Jones TH. Testosterone and obesity. Obes Rev. 2015;16(7):581–606.
54. Sørensen MB, Rosenfalck AM, Højgaard L, Ottesen B. Obesity and sarcopenia after menopause are reversed by sex hormone replacement therapy. Obes Res. 2001;9(10):622–6.
55. Smith SJ, Lopresti AL, Fairchild TJ. The effects of alcohol on testosterone synthesis in men: a review. Expert Rev Endocrinol Metab. 2023;18(2):155–66.
56. Mangolim AS, de Andrade Rodrigues Brito L, dos Santos Nunes-Nogueira V. Effectiveness of testosterone replacement in men with obesity: a systematic review and meta-analysis. Eur J Endocrinol. 2022;186(1):123–35.
57. Saad F, Aversa A, Isidori AM, Gooren LJ. Testosterone as potential effective therapy in treatment of obesity in men with testosterone deficiency: a review. Curr Diabetes Rev. 2012;8(2):131–43.
58. Amory JK, Chansky HA, Chansky KL, Camuso MR, Hoey CT, Anawalt BD, et al. Preoperative supraphysiological testosterone in older men undergoing knee replacement surgery. J Am Geriatr Soc. 2002;50(10):1698–701.
59. Botella-Carretero JI, Balsa JA, Gómez-Martin JM, Peromingo R, Huerta L, Carrasco M, et al. Circulating free testosterone in obese men after bariatric surgery increases in parallel with insulin sensitivity. J Endocrinol Investig. 2013;36(4):227–32.
60. Hurbanek JG, Jaffer AK, Morra N, Karafa M, Brotman DJ. Postmenopausal hormone replacement and venous thromboembolism following hip and knee arthroplasty. Thromb Haemost. 2004;92(08):337–43.
61. Mechanick JI, Apovian C, Brethauer S, Garvey WT, Joffe AM, Kim J, et al. Clinical practice guidelines for the perioperative nutrition, metabolic, and nonsurgical support of patients undergoing bariatric procedures—2019 update: cosponsored by American Association of Clinical Endocrinologists/American College of Endocrinology, The Obesity Society, American Society for Metabolic & Bariatric Surgery, Obesity Medicine Association, and American Society of Anesthesiologists. Surg Obes Relat Dis. 2020;16(2):175–247.
62. Tiidus PM, Lowe DA, Brown M. Estrogen replacement and skeletal muscle: mechanisms and population health. J Appl Physiol. 2013;115(5):569–78.
63. Lv B, Xing C, He B. Effects of bariatric surgery on the menstruation-and reproductive-related hormones of women with obesity without polycystic ovary syndrome: a systematic review and meta-analysis. Surg Obes Relat Dis. 2022;18(1):148–60.
64. Vosburg RW, El Chaar M, El Djouzi S, Docimo S, Choi D, LaMasters T, et al. Literature review on antiobesity medication use for metabolic and bariatric surgery patients from the American Society for Metabolic and Bariatric Surgery Clinical Issues Committee. Surg Obes Relat Dis. 2022;18(9):1109–19.
65. Puhl RM, Heuer CA. Obesity stigma: important considerations for public health. Am J Public Health. 2010;100(6):1019–28.

66. Acosta A, Camilleri M, Abu Dayyeh B, Calderon G, Gonzalez D, McRae A, et al. Selection of antiobesity medications based on phenotypes enhances weight loss: a pragmatic trial in an obesity clinic. Obesity. 2021;29(4):662–71.
67. Curatolo C, Trinh M. Challenges in the perioperative management of the patient receiving extended-release naltrexone. A A Case Rep. 2014;3(11):142–4.
68. Rippe JM, Crossley S, Ringer R. Obesity as a chronic disease: modern medical and lifestyle management. J Am Diet Assoc. 1998;98(10 Suppl):S9–S15.
69. Fujioka K. Management of obesity as a chronic disease: nonpharmacologic, pharmacologic, and surgical options. Obes Res. 2002;10(S12):116S–23S.
70. Tasali E, Wroblewski K, Kahn E, Kilkus J, Schoeller DA. Effect of sleep extension on objectively assessed energy intake among adults with overweight in real-life settings: a randomized clinical trial. JAMA Intern Med. 2022;182(4):365–74.
71. Knutson KL. Impact of sleep and sleep loss on glucose homeostasis and appetite regulation. Sleep Med Clin. 2007;2(2):187–97.
72. Makarem N, Alcántara C, Williams N, Bello NA, Abdalla M. Effect of sleep disturbances on blood pressure. Hypertension. 2021;77(4):1036–46.
73. Ford DE, Cooper-Patrick L. Sleep disturbances and mood disorders: an epidemiologic perspective. Depress Anxiety. 2001;14(1):3–6.
74. Prather AA. Chapter 24: Sleep, stress, and immunity. In: Grandner MA, editor. Sleep and health. Academic Press; 2019. p. 319–30.
75. Samuels C. Sleep, recovery, and performance: the new frontier in high-performance athletics. Neurol Clin. 2008;26(1):169–80.
76. Yaffe K, Falvey CM, Hoang T. Connections between sleep and cognition in older adults. Lancet Neurol. 2014;13(10):1017–28.
77. Bowen ME, Ji X, Griffioen MA. Poor sleep predicts increased pain perception among adults with mild cognitive impairment. Nurs Res. 2021;70(4):310–6.
78. Lautenbacher S, Kundermann B, Krieg J-C. Sleep deprivation and pain perception. Sleep Med Rev. 2006;10(5):357–69.
79. Romero-Corral A, Caples SM, Lopez-Jimenez F, Somers VK. Interactions between obesity and obstructive sleep apnea: implications for treatment. Chest. 2010;137(3):711–9.
80. Horvath CM, Jossen J, Kröll D, Nett PC, Baty F, Brill A-K, et al. Prevalence and prediction of obstructive sleep apnea prior to bariatric surgery—gender-specific performance of four sleep questionnaires. Obes Surg. 2018;28:2720–6.
81. Fava M. Weight gain and antidepressants. J Clin Psychiatry. 2000;61(11):37–41.
82. Møller AM, Villebro N, Pedersen T, Tønnesen H. Effect of preoperative smoking intervention on postoperative complications: a randomised clinical trial. Lancet. 2002;359(9301):114–7.
83. Haskins IN, Amdur R, Vaziri K. The effect of smoking on bariatric surgical outcomes. Surg Endosc. 2014;28:3074–80.
84. Lucini D, Malacarne M, Pagani M, Morizzo C, Kozakova M, Nannipieri M, et al. A four-week prehabilitation program in candidates for bariatric surgery improves hemodynamic load, metabolism and cardiac autonomic regulation. Acta Diabetol. 2021;58(4):517–20.
85. Kalarchian M, Marcus M, Courcoulas A, Cheng Y, Levine M. Preoperative lifestyle intervention in bariatric surgery: initial results from a randomized, controlled trial. Obesity. 2013;21(2):254–60.
86. Gandara N, Abilés V, Abilés J, Rodríguez-Ruiz S, Luna V, Obispo A, et al. Effectiveness of cognitive-behavioral therapy in morbidity obese candidates for bariatric surgery with and without binge eating disorder. Nutr Hosp. 2013;28(5):1523–9.
87. Picó-Sirvent I, Manresa-Rocamora A, Aracil-Marco A, Moya-Ramón M. A combination of aerobic exercise at Fatmax and low resistance training increases fat oxidation and maintains muscle mass, in women waiting for bariatric surgery. Obes Surg. 2022;32(4):1130–40.
88. Marc-Hernandez A, Ruiz-Tovar J, Aracil A, Guillen S, Moya-Ramon M. Impact of exercise on body composition and cardiometabolic risk factors in patients awaiting bariatric surgery. Obes Surg. 2019;29:3891.

89. Gilbertson NM, Gaitán JM, Osinski V, Rexrode EA, Garmey JC, Mehaffey JH, et al. Preoperative aerobic exercise on metabolic health and surgical outcomes in patients receiving bariatric surgery: a pilot trial. PLoS One. 2020;15(10):e0239130.
90. Schiavo L, Pierro R, Asteria C, Calabrese P, Di Biasio A, Coluzzi I, et al. Low-calorie ketogenic diet with continuous positive airway pressure to alleviate severe obstructive sleep apnea syndrome in patients with obesity scheduled for bariatric/metabolic surgery: a pilot, prospective, randomized multicenter comparative study. Obes Surg. 2022;32(3):634–42.
91. De Raaff CA, Gorter-Stam MA, De Vries N, Sinha AC, Bonjer HJ, Chung F, et al. Perioperative management of obstructive sleep apnea in bariatric surgery: a consensus guideline. Surg Obes Relat Dis. 2017;13(7):1095–109.
92. Parrott J, Frank L, Rabena R, Craggs-Dino L, Isom KA, Greiman L. American Society for Metabolic and Bariatric Surgery integrated health nutritional guidelines for the surgical weight loss patient 2016 update: micronutrients. Surg Obes Relat Dis. 2017;13(5):727–41.
93. O'Kane M, Parretti HM, Pinkney J, Welbourn R, Hughes CA, Mok J, et al. British Obesity and Metabolic Surgery Society Guidelines on perioperative and postoperative biochemical monitoring and micronutrient replacement for patients undergoing bariatric surgery—2020 update. Obes Rev. 2020;21(11):e13087.
94. Karabulut M, Garcia SD. Hemodynamic responses and energy expenditure during blood flow restriction exercise in obese population. Clin Physiol Funct Imaging. 2017;37(1):1–7.
95. Dobek JC, White KN, Gunter KB. The effect of a novel ADL-based training program on performance of activities of daily living and physical fitness. J Aging Phys Act. 2007;15(1):13–25.
96. Paterson DH, Jones GR, Rice CL. Ageing and physical activity: evidence to develop exercise recommendations for older adults. Appl Physiol Nutr Metab. 2007;32(S2E):S69–S108.
97. Li X, Zhou T, Ma H, Liang Z, Fonseca VA, Qi L. Replacement of sedentary behavior by various daily-life physical activities and structured exercises: genetic risk and incident type 2 diabetes. Diabetes Care. 2021;44(10):2403–10.
98. Villablanca PA, Alegria JR, Mookadam F, Holmes DR, Wright RS, Levine JA. Nonexercise activity thermogenesis in obesity management. Mayo Clin Proc. 2015;90(4):509–19.
99. Bays HE, Fitch A, Christensen S, Burridge K, Tondt J. Anti-obesity medications and investigational agents: an Obesity Medicine Association (OMA) Clinical Practice Statement (CPS) 2022. Obes Pillars. 2022;2:100018.
100. Bray GA. A concise review on the therapeutics of obesity. Nutrition (Burbank, Los Angeles County, Calif). 2000;16(10):953–60.
101. Nedergaard A, Henriksen K, Karsdal MA, Christiansen C. Menopause, estrogens and frailty. Gynecol Endocrinol. 2013;29(5):418–23.
102. Moon J, Koh G. Clinical evidence and mechanisms of high-protein diet-induced weight loss. J Obes Metab Syndr. 2020;29(3):166.
103. Campos-Nonato I, Hernandez L, Barquera S. Effect of a high-protein diet versus standard-protein diet on weight loss and biomarkers of metabolic syndrome: a randomized clinical trial. Obes Facts. 2017;10(3):238–51.
104. Kirk S, Woo JG, Jones MN, Siegel RM. Increased frequency of dietitian visits is associated with improved body mass index outcomes in obese youth participating in a comprehensive pediatric weight management program. Child Obes. 2015;11(2):202–8.
105. Tsai AG, Wadden TA, Rogers MA, Day SC, Moore RH, Islam BJ. A primary care intervention for weight loss: results of a randomized controlled pilot study. Obesity. 2010;18(8):1614–8.
106. Graffagnino CL, Falko JM, La Londe M, Schaumburg J, Hyek MF, Shaffer LE, et al. Effect of a community-based weight management program on weight loss and cardiovascular disease risk factors. Obesity. 2006;14(2):280–8.
107. Riebe D, Franklin BA, Thompson PD, Garber CE, Whitfield GP, Magal M, et al. Updating ACSM's recommendations for exercise preparticipation health screening. Med Sci Sports Exerc. 2015;47:2473.
108. Gulinac M, Miteva DG, Peshevska-Sekulovska M, Novakov IP, Antovic S, Peruhova M, et al. Long-term effectiveness, outcomes and complications of bariatric surgery. World J Clin Cases. 2023;11(19):4504.

109. Goel R, Nasta AM, Goel M, Prasad A, Jammu G, Fobi M, et al. Complications after bariatric surgery: a multicentric study of 11,568 patients from Indian bariatric surgery outcomes reporting group. J Minim Access Surg. 2021;17(2):213–20.
110. Agarwal S, Joshi AD. Perioperative complications of laparoscopic cholecystectomy: a cross-sectional observational study. Int Surg J. 2020;7(5):1490–5.
111. Dittrich L, Schwenninger M-V, Dittrich K, Pratschke J, Aigner F, Raakow J. Marginal ulcers after laparoscopic Roux-en-Y gastric bypass: analysis of the amount of daily and lifetime smoking on postoperative risk. Surg Obes Relat Dis. 2020;16(3):389–96.
112. Hariri K, Hechenbleikner E, Dong M, Kini SU, Fernandez-Ranvier G, Herron DM. Ketorolac use shortens hospital length of stay after bariatric surgery: a single-center 5-year experience. Obes Surg. 2019;29(8):2360–6.
113. Nath A, Yewale S, Tran T, Brebbia JS, Shope TR, Koch TR. Dysphagia after vertical sleeve gastrectomy: evaluation of risk factors and assessment of endoscopic intervention. World J Gastroenterol. 2016;22(47):10371.
114. Bracale U, Peltrini R, De Luca M, Ilardi M, Di Nuzzo MM, Sartori A, et al. Predictive factors for anastomotic leakage after laparoscopic and open total gastrectomy: a systematic review. J Clin Med. 2022;11(17):5022.
115. Mocanu V, Dang JT, Birch DW, Karmali S, Switzer NJ. Factors implicated in discharge disposition following elective bariatric surgery. Surg Obes Relat Dis. 2021;17(1):104–11.
116. Chopra T, Marchaim D, Lynch Y, Kosmidis C, Zhao JJ, Dhar S, et al. Epidemiology and outcomes associated with surgical site infection following bariatric surgery. Am J Infect Control. 2012;40(9):815–9.
117. Martin ET, Kaye KS, Knott C, Nguyen H, Santarossa M, Evans R, et al. Diabetes and risk of surgical site infection: a systematic review and meta-analysis. Infect Control Hosp Epidemiol. 2016;37(1):88–99.
118. Poljo A, Pentsch A, Raab S, Klugsberger B, Shamiyeh A. Incidence of dumping syndrome after sleeve gastrectomy, Roux-en-Y gastric bypass and one-anastomosis gastric bypass. J Metab Bariatr Surg. 2021;10(1):23.
119. Scarpellini E, Arts J, Karamanolis G, Laurenius A, Siquini W, Suzuki H, et al. International consensus on the diagnosis and management of dumping syndrome. Nat Rev Endocrinol. 2020;16(8):448–66.
120. Barrea L, Verde L, Schiavo L, Sarno G, Camajani E, Iannelli A, et al. Very low-calorie ketogenic diet (VLCKD) as pre-operative first-line dietary therapy in patients with obesity who are candidates for bariatric surgery. Nutrients. 2023;15(8):1907.
121. Goldberg IJ, Ibrahim N, Bredefeld C, Foo S, Lim V, Gutman D, et al. Ketogenic diets, not for everyone. J Clin Lipidol. 2021;15(1):61–7.
122. Nizamuddin J, Turner Z, Rubenstein JE, Pyzik PL, Kossoff EH. Management and risk factors for dyslipidemia with the ketogenic diet. J Child Neurol. 2008;23(7):758–61.

Amputation Prehabilitation

Robin T. Tipps and Jeffrey T. Heckman

1 Overview: Prehabilitation Considerations for Individuals Undergoing Lower Limb Amputation

This is a general recommendation for the sequence of the steps a patient will transition through from the initial discussion for potential amputation surgery through the postoperative recovery period.

- Patient education on the medical necessity of the surgery with easily understood verbal and written descriptions.
- Gathering a detailed history of activities of daily living, ambulation level, and community/recreational involvement to understand the potential for a return to functional independence with appropriate assistive devices and adaptive equipment.
- Screening for exercise tolerance, malnutrition, frailty, and depression/anxiety.
- Family involvement addressing anticipated practical limitations as well as unspoken concerns.
- Interprofessional consultations to understand functional potential at different limb levels of amputation surgery.
- Ongoing medical therapy to optimize blood pressure, cholesterol, and glycemic control.
- Interprofessional surgical discussions for peripheral nerve management.
- Dietician consultation for nutritional education and increased protein intake with oral protein supplementation as needed.

R. T. Tipps (✉)
University of Pittsburgh Medical Center, Pittsburgh, PA, USA
e-mail: tippsrt@upmc.edu

J. T. Heckman
University of South Florida, Tampa, FL, USA
e-mail: jeffrey.t.heckman@va.gov

A. Watson, K. Barr (eds.), *A Prehabilitation Guide for All Providers*,
https://doi.org/10.1007/978-3-031-72862-4_8

- Therapy services consultations include physical, occupational, recreational, and vocational rehabilitation to develop rapport with the patient and assess their preoperative functional status, postoperative ambulation potential, and adaptive equipment or assistive device needs.
- Rehabilitation psychology services including opportunities for individual certified peer visitors and peer-matched support group programs.
- Immediate preoperative period: ERAS perioperative protocol.
- Immediate postoperative care with dietary progression and consideration for rehabilitation environment for the preprosthesis training phase.

2 Specialized Treatment Team

- Surgical team: Members of the surgical team vary from hospital to hospital but generally include vascular surgeons, orthopedic surgeons, and podiatrists. Trauma surgeons may also be involved depending on the events leading to amputation. Preoperative care from the vascular surgery team is especially important to evaluate blood flow and assess for wound healing potential. Ideally, the surgical team will educate patients on the pathology, and the reasons necessitating the amputation procedure, and provide education on what to expect during the perioperative course.
- Physiatrist leading the rehabilitation team: Physiatrists are experts in caring for individuals who have undergone limb amputations. They optimize pain control and overall health overseeing therapies designed to improve the functional and ambulatory status of the patient. Physiatrists are also well-versed in evaluating patients for assistive devices and prostheses based on their predicted level of ambulation.
- Medical management team: Optimize the patient's health status prior to surgery. For example, endocrinologists create antihyperglycemic medication regimens that provide tight control of blood glucose levels in patients with diabetes mellitus to support wound healing and minimize postoperative complications. Members of the vascular team assess the degree of peripheral artery disease and offer interventions to maximize the ankle-brachial index, potentially delaying amputation procedures, preserving residual limb length, and improving postoperative wound healing.
- Rehabilitation nurses: They work closely with patients to manage pain, provide wound care, encourage mobility and participation in therapies, support patients and their families during a psychologically demanding time, monitor for preoperative health complications, set realistic daily goals, and coordinate care with other healthcare professionals. Rehab nurses are familiar with disabling conditions and chronic illnesses that impact daily function and mobility. They specialize in helping patients optimize function, adapt to an altered lifestyle, and progress toward independence.
- Rehabilitation psychologist: Ideally, a rehab psychologist should meet with the patient and their family/significant others to identify the emotions and unspoken

fears involved with undergoing an amputation surgery, assess social supports, attend to caregiver concerns, emphasize healthy coping responses, and address any underlying mood disorders that may arise from or be exacerbated by limb loss.

- Registered dietician: Optimize nutrition prior to the procedure to maximize wound healing, particularly regarding protein intake, broadly, and carbohydrate control in patients with diabetes mellitus.
- Certified prosthetist/orthotist: Work with the patient to determine the best prosthesis type for his or her mobility needs after an amputation surgery. Identify orthotic solutions that contribute to preventive care for secondary conditions. Develop a timeline for early fitting and prosthetic training.
- Physical therapist: Assess the patient's functionality and expectations for postoperative mobility. Develop exercise and education programs to maintain mobility, activity, and range of motion in the affected and unaffected limbs. Also, focus on strength and function preservation. Anticipate any practical challenges that may arise as a result of the amputation surgery, such as ambulation and workplace modification requirements, or adaptive activities of daily living. Begin educating the patient on exercises that will take place during the rehabilitation period.
- Occupational therapist: Work with the patient to develop a customized treatment plan to maximize the patient's level of functional independence prior to and after amputation surgery. Educate patients on the use of assistive devices, environmental modifications, bed and wheelchair transfer training, and residual limb care. Practice adaptive techniques to help patients with activities of daily living, dressing, grooming, bathing, writing, electronic communications, medication management, money management, cooking, and cleaning. In some cases, the occupational therapist may be the primary professional involved in helping the patient cope with losing their locus of control, especially if he or she functioned as the head of the household prior to the amputation procedure.
- Recreational therapy: Design therapeutic activities and interventions to assist in maintaining the health status, functional capabilities, recovery, and quality of life for individuals who undergo limb amputations. This non-pharmacological approach assists in reintegrating individuals into the community, maintaining engagement with other therapies, and promoting functional independence through mental health strategies, art therapy, music therapy, dance and movement therapy, pet therapy, and physical activity. Recreational therapists also help interested patients find opportunities for participation in adaptive sports, which might include but are not limited to, sled hockey, skiing, surfing, billiards, rock climbing, bowling, wheelchair basketball, fishing, sailing, mountain biking, horseback riding, wheelchair rugby, dragon boat racing, curling, and golf.
- Vocational rehabilitation counselor: They counsel and guide patients on work opportunities available that match their individual skills, abilities, and interests. They assist with training opportunities, job placement resources, and workplace environment accessibility.
- Case manager or social worker: They screen patients for any unanticipated needs or barriers to discharge. They connect patients with social services and resources

that can assist with the increased costs of healthcare that patients undergoing amputation surgery may face as well as services that provide environmental modifications to their home and/or workplace.
- Pain management specialists: Utilize the biopsychosocial model and create multimodal pain control plans prior to and after surgery to optimize physical functioning and ability to participate in therapy services.

3 Defining the Problem in Prehabilitation Phase for Patients Undergoing Lower Limb Amputation

Preoperative preparation for patients undergoing limb amputation procedures is a complex and under-researched area of prehabilitation, largely due to the circumstances necessitating limb amputations and the comorbidities of the populations most likely to undergo these procedures. However, coordinated, multidisciplinary prehabilitation for individuals undergoing limb amputations can be crucial in optimizing functional independence and mobility for a population at significant risk of social isolation and continued health status deterioration.

Limb amputation surgery is a life-altering procedure that changes the ways in which patients function and adapt to perform the basic activities of daily living. The most common reasons for amputation are peripheral vascular disease, diabetes mellitus with underlying foot ulcer, severe trauma, neoplasia, infection, and congenital defects [1]. The acute nature of limb amputations resulting from trauma, sepsis, gas gangrene, or osteomyelitis generally precludes organized prehabilitation efforts. However, over 80% of all amputations in the United States are due to dysvascular causes, which may allow for a longer prehabilitation period. Ninety-seven percent of these amputations involve the lower extremity, including transmetatarsal, transtibial, and transfemoral amputations [2]. For the populations who make up the majority of limb amputation patients, pre-and postoperative conditioning tends to be limited due to increased age, comorbidities that prevent physical activity, and reduced motivation to maintain physical fitness [3].

Limb amputation procedures are life-changing events that require substantial energy and psychosocial engagement to regain ambulatory status. Goals of prehabilitation include improving respiratory and cardiac capacities as well as muscular strength prior to surgery. These are vital for obtaining successful surgical outcomes, quickly progressing to postoperative rehabilitation, adapting to a new prosthesis, and maintaining independence with activities of daily living. This strategy is often challenged by non-weight-bearing recommendations requiring prolonged wheelchair use due to chronic healing from diabetic foot ulcers that ultimately lead to the requirement for lower extremity amputation surgery. Additionally, preventing disease progression of diabetes mellitus and peripheral vascular disease through physical activity might allow for a more distal amputation, which is generally associated with improved post-rehabilitation outcomes [4].

Patients undergoing limb amputation procedures present a special prehabilitation challenge in that the circumstances leading to their amputation make it difficult to create preoperative interventions that patients readily adhere to in the weeks leading up to surgery. Prehabilitation typically involves a 4–6-week program of physical and occupational therapy to maximize physical function, nutritional education with trained dieticians, psychosocial counseling to prepare patients for psychological changes following surgery, and mixed endurance and resistance training to improve the patient's cardiorespiratory reserves and muscle strength in anticipation of postoperative rehabilitation [5]. Patients with significant comorbidities might have difficulty participating in the physical aspects of these programs or have developed long-standing health habits that impair program compliance. This, in turn, can delay participation in rehabilitation, increase hospital length of stay, and increase surgical complications, all of which make it more difficult for patients to return to a premorbid ambulatory status. Comorbidities such as advanced coronary artery disease, end-stage renal disease, and uncontrolled diabetes mellitus also lead to increased intraoperative complications [6].

Risk Factors for Poor Outcomes and Prehabilitation Challenges

Age

The prevalence of dysvascular diseases and diabetes mellitus increases with age. As such, the number of amputation surgeries for the geriatric population in the United States is predicted to increase as the general population ages. Individuals over 60 years old are already the most common patients undergoing lower limb amputation [7]. Studies suggest that each year increase in patient age increases the mortality rate following amputation surgery by 4.6% [8]. Patients over the age of seventy are one-third as likely to wear their prosthesis and four times as likely to lose functional independence within 1 year of the procedure [9].

Heart Disease

Risk factors for amputation, such as diabetes and vascular disease also place patients at higher risk of cardiac comorbidities prior to their procedure. Patients with a medical history of myocardial infarction, atrial fibrillation, or congestive heart failure face a mortality risk equivalent to that of a 26-year increase in age when undergoing a lower limb amputation [10].

Frailty and Other Confounding Medical Issues

The majority of dysvascular patients are over age 65 and present with multiple comorbidities including cardiomyopathy, renal failure, and pulmonary conditions. These individuals are less likely to be functionally ambulatory prior to amputation and more likely to acutely decondition following the procedure [11]. They may experience chronic pain that precludes participation in exercise programs without extensive modifications.

Difficulty Adhering to Medical Recommendations and Lifestyle Changes

Critical limb ischemia and non-healing ulcers leading to limb amputation are typically end-stage complications in patients with peripheral vascular disease and diabetes mellitus. These are most often the result of inadequate control of risk factors and baseline reduced physical activity levels. Proper preoperative assessments should consider the patient's current level of physical fitness, independence, and health habits when designing a prehabilitation program and determining the potential for prosthesis use. An individual with critical limb ischemia has often received recommendations to improve their health through smoking cessation, regular exercise, dietary changes, or other modifications for years leading up to their procedure, and yet have not made changes. For these patients, adherence to prehabilitation recommendations may be a continuation of this long-term difficulty. In contrast, other patients are already physically active, have stopped smoking, and adopted healthy eating habits, and are generally likely to continue them in the weeks leading up to their procedure. Sorting out a patient's past experience with lifestyle modification adoption is essential to determine the best way to support them during the prehabilitation phase. An already active individual is a good candidate to enroll in physical and occupational therapy programs that rehearse the exercises and activity modifications they will perform after surgery, and these individuals would benefit from working with an interdisciplinary amputation specialty clinic including a physiatrist and prosthetist to ensure early prescription, fitting and delivery of a prosthesis. A patient with less success in making these changes in the past may need more intensive support such as psychological counseling from an expert in behavioral change.

Additionally, the constraints resulting from living with chronic disease may reduce the ability of individuals to participate in exercise programs regardless of motivation levels [2]. This is why an individual approach that takes into account comorbidities, past experiences, resources and support, and personal preference is essential (Table 1).

Contralateral Limb Comorbidity

Preoperative assessment should also consider the unaffected or contralateral limb. Individuals with peripheral vascular disease or diabetes mellitus are at high risk of secondary amputation, and the development of new or worsening ulcers negatively impacts the patient's ability to ambulate successfully after amputation [13]. A complete assessment of the limb will include Semmes-Weinstein monofilament

Table 1 Ankle-brachial index normative values [12]

ABI measurement	Interpretation
>1.4	Poorly compressible vessels due to calcification
1.0–1.4	Normal
0.9–1.0	Borderline peripheral arterial disease
0.8–0.9	Mild peripheral arterial disease
0.4–0.8	Moderate peripheral arterial disease
<0.4	Severe peripheral arterial disease

examination and noninvasive vascular studies to measure the ankle-brachial index (ABI), which allows for classifying the severity of peripheral arterial disease. This, in turn, provides the operative team with a better sense of the patient's wound healing potential and assists with predicting the risk of additional amputation procedures.

Therapists emphasize strengthening the unaffected limb during the prehabilitation process in order to optimize post-operative transfers and maximize standing tolerance. The unaffected limb will also experience greater mechanical forces during rehabilitation and prosthesis use. Therefore, a complete monofilament examination of the unaffected limb should be done to ensure the patient has proper protective sensation in this area, particularly as the patient increases reliance on this limb. Individuals lacking protective sensation require prescription footwear and accommodative custom-molded foot orthoses for the prevention of secondary amputation. Single-legged standing times on the unaffected limb should be assessed to determine the level of exercise and ambulation tolerance the patient and rehabilitation team can expect before and after surgery. The vascular team should also collect ABIs of the unaffected limb. Throughout the prehabilitation process, appropriate footwear and orthoses should be provided for the intact limb in order to compensate for the greater mechanical forces and accommodate for foot deformity (Fig. 1; Table 2).

Nonexistent, Truncated, or Interrupted Time for Prehabilitation

With regard to prehabilitation in patients undergoing amputation procedures, two limitations emerge. First, unlike other procedures wherein prehabilitation has shown to be beneficial, the time window for amputation is often uncertain. For amputations resulting from trauma, embolic or thrombotic events, or overwhelming infection, the acute nature of the event precludes the development of or participation in prehabilitation. However, such individuals may have a higher pre-procedure functional

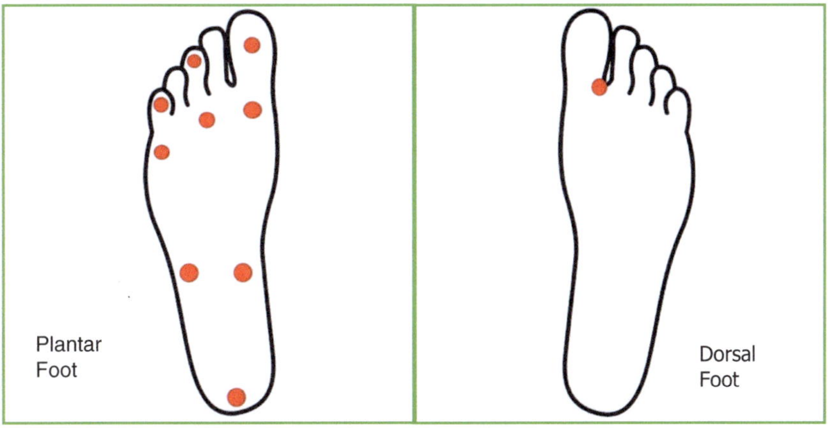

Fig. 1 Diagram of monofilament testing locations [14]

Table 2 Risk factors and associated complications

Risk factor	How risk factor has been measured	Known negative effects of risk factor
Age	>60 years old	Each year increase in age resulted in a 4.6% mortality rate increase [8]
Cardiac co-morbidities	Medical history of myocardial infarction, atrial fibrillation, or congestive heart failure	Adjusted hazard ratio of 3.3, which is equivalent to a 26-year increase in age [10]
Malnutrition	BMI, Patient-Generated Subjective Global Assessment Short Form (PG-SGA SF), Malnutrition Universal Screening Tool (MUST)	Patients with a medium risk factor for malnutrition had a 1.39× higher comprehensive complication index; prolonged stay, higher mortality due to dampened immune response, and impaired wound healing [15]
Current smoking	Pack-year history	Increases cardiopulmonary complications, impairs wound healing, increases the likelihood of wound infections, and increases the risk of prolonged hospitalization [16]
Preoperative anemia	Hemoglobin level <13 g/dL	Impairs functional capacity and increases the risk of perioperative blood transfusion as well as post-operative morbidity and mortality [17]
Low pre-operative physical activity level	Preoperative functional assessment, Activity Measure for Post-Acute Care (AM-PAC)	Difficulties participating in group exercise programs need for specifically-tailored aerobic activities, poor habitual lifestyle tendencies [18]

capacity, increasing their chances of ambulation after the procedure or being able to utilize a prosthesis.

Even for patients with peripheral vascular disease or diabetes mellitus, the timing of amputation can be unpredictable. Focus groups of specialists regarding the feasibility of prehabilitation in lower limb amputations noted that patients frequently delay seeking medical care until critical ischemia develops and progresses to include severe pain, ulcers, sores, or gangrene [19]. Most prehabilitation plans for other conditions outlined in this textbook broadly recommend 6–12 weeks of exercise therapy and 4–8 weeks of lifestyle interventions prior to their various procedures [20]. However, clinicians note that the timeframe between hospital presentation and surgery is often a number of days rather than weeks or months because patients do not present to the doctor until they are unable to ambulate entirely. For patients undergoing lower extremity amputation procedures, the evolving nature of their unique disease process makes close physiatry-led coordination between the multidisciplinary team especially critical. Even procedures that are planned months in advance may require a number of minor procedures prior to the major amputation surgery, thereby necessitating modifications to the original prehabilitation plan and timeline.

Despite these challenges, several successful prehabilitation programs are described in the literature and summarized in Table 3.

Table 3 Evidence summary table

Domain	Study design	Population	Interventions	Outcome measured
Availability of prehabilitation services and assessments	Bates et al. [21]	VAMC patients who underwent transtibial or transfemoral amputations	Evidence of a preoperative rehabilitation assessment after the index surgical stay but before the surgical date	Only 8.2% of VA patients overall received prehab services, but preoperative services varied by location with those treated in the South Central and Mountain Pacific regions being more likely to receive preoperative consultation
Co-morbidities prior to surgery	Taylor et al. [22]	553 lower limb amputation patients	Preoperative functional assessment	Younger patients (<60 years) without coronary or renal disease with below-knee amputations achieve functional outcomes similar to lower extremity revascularization and amputation can be seen as extending functionality
Preoperative functionality assessment to determine prosthesis suitability and optimize postoperative functional independence	Pinzur et al. [23]	Patients treated by lower extremity amputations for peripheral vascular insufficiency	95 patients were preoperatively evaluated by physical therapists, psychologists, social workers, and physiatrists and underwent cardiopulmonary stress testing. This information was used to determine the patient's physical capacity to undergo intensive rehabilitation, identify psychosocial barriers, predict rehab potential, and evaluate metabolic reserve. Surgeons then used this data to determine amputation level selection and guide early prosthetic limb fitting	Two years following their amputation, 84% of patients ambulated within one functional level of their preamputation status. Prosthetic use increased and the use of walking aids decreased for patients who underwent intensive preoperative functionality assessments

(continued)

Table 3 (continued)

Domain	Study design	Population	Interventions	Outcome measured
Multimodal preoperative training and education	O'Banion et al. [24]	141 vascular patients undergoing lower extremity amputation	LEAP protocol with social team making pre-op functional and quality of life survey, social work providing discharge options and discussing expectations for discharge, PT/OT assessing functionality and discussing rehab exercises and mobility expectations, prosthetics discussing timeline, and anesthesiology discussing pain control options	LEAP patients were more likely to be discharged to acute rehab, receive a prosthesis, ambulate with a prosthesis, receive PT/OT 2 days sooner, and have a shorter post-op LOS (3 days versus 6 days)
Prehabilitation-plus programming prior to amputation	Fulton et al. [25]	Seven patients receiving prehabilitation-plus were retrospectively matched with seven control patients undergoing planned major lower limb amputation	One- to four-week multidisciplinary program involving strength and endurance exercises, home assessment and modifications, assistive device assessment and training, peer support group referrals, psychological counseling, PT/OT, and diet education	Patients who received prehabilitation-plus had shorter acute hospital and total hospital length of stay, but no significant difference was seen for in patient rehabilitation length of stay

4 Preoperative Screening

Similar to any surgical procedure, individuals undergoing limb amputation in a non-acute setting should be screened for anemia and undergo a dietary assessment to assess for malnutrition [26]. A registered dietician should optimize caloric intake and protein consumption prior to surgery to promote wound healing. Cigarette smokers should undergo smoking cessation in the weeks leading up to their procedure. Obtain serum labs to assess the patient's risk for surgical complications resulting from malnutrition, anemia, or uncontrolled diabetes mellitus.

Such labs include:

- Complete blood count, B12, folate, ferritin/TIBC.
- HbA1c, lipid profile, and basic metabolic panel to assess renal function and electrolyte status.

The patient should undergo a thorough preoperative physical examination of all extremities, including Semmes-Weinstein monofilament testing of the feet as illustrated in Fig. 1 to determine his or her protective sensation. Perform vibratory sensation testing using a tuning fork and pinprick sensation testing using a safety pin to test the patient for peripheral neuropathy. The physical exam should also test functional mobility, including testing balance, timed single-leg stance tolerance, bed mobility, transfers, and an assessment of the patient's gait using assistive devices. All existing wounds need assessment with an accompanying broader assessment of the presence, color, and skin temperature of both limbs. Test the joint integrity and spasticity of the hip and knees, as well as the strength and range of motion of all limbs. Strength and fine motor skills of the hands are critical for determining the patient's capacity to use a manual wheelchair or don and doff a prosthesis independently. Noninvasive vascular studies should be done to calculate the ABI of the affected and unaffected limbs.

A comprehensive interdisciplinary baseline assessment of the patient's functional status, psychosocial profile, social barriers to care, and rehabilitation goals should be made prior to surgery. If pre-operative time allows, assessing walking distance, gait velocity, and level of independence will inform the design of individualized prehabilitation and rehabilitation plans that align with the patient's abilities and post-operative goals. Using a risk calculator such as AMPREDICT may provide the medical and surgical teams with a better understanding of the patient's risk of mortality, re-amputation, and mobility potential after surgery [27].

5 Plan Formulation Considerations and Best Practices

Exercise

Regular physical activity increases aerobic capacity, lean body mass to fat mass ratios, insulin sensitivity, and cardiorespiratory reserves. Conversely, poor preoperative fitness scores and levels of functional ambulation increase surgical mortality, increase the likelihood of post-operative deconditioning, and lengthen the time before the patient can participate in rehabilitation [11]. Patients undergoing limb amputations may need exercise programs specially tailored to their levels of ability and ambulation; individuals with comorbidities or functional limitations due to pain, balance, or existing limb deformity may have difficulty participating in standard group exercise therapy. Although similar studies have not been completed involving individuals undergoing amputations, individuals participating in regular exercise and cardiopulmonary therapy prior to orthopedic, abdominal, and cardiac surgeries experienced fewer surgical complications, shortened lengths of stay, and less of a decline in functional ability [5] as noted in earlier chapters of this text.

Patients should engage in at least 30 min of moderate-intensity exercise a day [28]. Individuals who are hampered by pain or limited mobility may participate in activities that reduce stress on affected limbs or joints, including water aerobics, arm bikes, or zero-gravity treadmills. Blood flow restriction training, detailed in other chapters, is likely not appropriate for individuals with dysvascular complications though research supporting/refuting this is currently unavailable given that their comorbidities tend to place them in a higher risk category that is not frequently included in studies [29]. As able, patients may benefit from a prescribed walking program by their PCP, physiatrist, or other qualified professional with adaptive equipment as needed. Patients should first be assessed for baseline ambulatory status and activity tolerance before starting at a lower level of intensity and working their way up as safely tolerated.

In addition to aerobic activity, patients should participate in three 30–60 min sessions of resistance training at least 2–3 days/week with a day of rest between each session [30]. Ideally, this would start up to 12 weeks before the procedure, but other programs have demonstrated success in as short as a 4–6-week timeframe [25, 31, 32]. These strength training sessions would incorporate resistance bands and free weights to maintain strength and functionality in the unaffected limbs as well as to prepare the muscle groups in the affected limb for increased load bearing should the patient be suitable for prosthesis use. On days without strength training, patients should participate in other exercise routines with repeated contractions of proximal muscles and a motor imagery program that might include watching themselves or others perform tasks [33]. Sessions could also include the techniques that the patients will perform during rehabilitation sessions in preparation for the postoperative recovery period. In addition, it would be helpful to begin practicing transfers and wheelchair mobility to prepare for the initial post-operative phase. A physical therapist or exercise specialist should oversee any exercise intervention, given the inherently elevated risk in this population for injury. At the same time, patients and their families should be educated on the extent and rigors of rehabilitation required to achieve the patient's optimal function [34].

Maintaining good physical fitness prior to surgery decreases the patient's recovery time, expedites participation in rehabilitation, and reduces the incidence of intraoperative complications [35]. This, in turn, increases the patient's chance for ambulatory recovery and recovering/maintaining independence after the procedure. With regards to individuals undergoing amputations, ambulation using a prosthesis requires increased energy expenditure after the amputation [36]. Increasing or maintaining physical activity prior to the procedure helps individuals accommodate this higher energy demand. As a result, if the timeline and patient factors allow, it is crucial to design a program tailored to the individual in the weeks leading to surgery.

Psychosocial Interventions

Limb amputation is a life-changing event that can result in reduced mobility and independence, decreased postoperative psychological conditioning, and new or worsened depression [37]. As such, psychosocial interventions are oftentimes as important as exercise interventions to facilitate overall wellness and adherence to other recommendations. Great care should be taken to ensure all patients undergo a psychosocial assessment and receive adequate support via therapists, certified peer visitors or support groups.

If able, patients should receive a baseline cognitive assessment to ensure cognitive ability for safely donning and doffing a prosthesis and for properly evaluating the intact limb for sores or ulcerations [38]. Family members should provide collateral historical information since factors like delirium, infection, pain medications, and depression postoperatively may impact cognition. Speech pathology consultants can also help with the evaluation, and geriatricians may administer a Montreal Cognitive Assessment (MoCA) or other executive functioning assessment to determine the need for further comprehensive neurocognitive evaluation.

Undergoing an amputation is associated with increased rates of depression even in individuals with no prior history of mood disorder [39]. Preexisting mood disorders and substance use disorders may also contribute to difficulty with prosthesis fitting and decreased post-operative quality of life. A psychiatrist consultant would be helpful to optimize treatments for individuals and provide resources for therapy or medications as needed.

The patient's primary medical team should provide an early acknowledgment of the possibility of an amputation procedure, so the patient is adequately prepared in the event this becomes necessary. If the condition progresses, the care team should provide a firm, clear indication of the necessity of the amputation and review previous attempts to prevent loss, including their outcomes. These discussions should also include a clear verbal description of the procedure and what the patient can expect during the perioperative recovery stage, with written supplementation as needed. Finally, the primary team should assure the patient that no procedure will be done without the patient's informed consent [40].

All patients, regardless of prior psychiatric history, should be offered counseling or therapy from a rehabilitation psychologist. Some have also found benefits in peer support groups to learn from others about their experiences with amputations and prosthesis use [41]. For individuals unable to participate in or unsure about attending in-person meetings, organizations such as the Amputee Coalition host weekly virtual interactive sessions led by experienced peer support team members and trained support group leaders from their National Support Group Network via Zoom [42]. The Amputee Coalition also offers caregivers support meetings and specialized meetings for members of the Black, Indigenous, and other People of Color (BIPOC) community. It is likely that the patient's family and loved ones will also be impacted by the amputation, so they should remain involved in psychological support conversations, as well. Undergoing an amputation is likely to elicit many emotions, including anger, grief, and depression. It is important that the patient be given space to recognize and identify these emotions. Heroic cheerfulness should also be challenged in these settings as it often masks the true emotions an individual is feeling prior to undergoing such a significant procedure. At the same time emphasize the continuity of personal characteristics that the patient will maintain after the procedure and highlight the ways in which the patient has responded in the past to distressing events.

Therapy sessions are also an important time to elicit unspoken fears that the patient might have about the procedure and life after the amputation. Sessions should be a safe space for patients to speak about their fear of death, mutilation, social rejection, loss of independence, employment and housing issues, and a change in sexual function. It is also important to attend to caregiver concerns, such as what assistance the patient might need, how the procedure will impact their living situation or ability to provide an income and determining a care schedule. Interventions such as relaxation techniques, breathing exercises, meditation, mindfulness, and cognitive behavioral therapies could be introduced at this stage so the patient can use them in the time leading up to and following the procedure.

Including a social worker or case worker in some conversations could also assist with anticipating practical concerns that could arise as a result of the procedure, including occupational limitations, housing modifications, complying with the Americans with Disabilities Act, modifying or finding someone to assist with activities of daily living, and adaptive recreational activities that the patient can pursue.

Lifestyle Interventions

Nutritional care is key when undergoing any major procedure to provide the energy needed for rehabilitation therapy, to promote muscle repair, and to support post-operative wound healing. Individuals who are malnourished face worse surgical outcomes and post-operative quality of life as a result of their lacking the protein and glycogen reserves necessary to endure the metabolic stress of surgery [43]. Those who are able should be placed on a high-protein diet designed to promote exercise recovery and build skeletal muscle. A registered dietician should be involved early in the process to ensure the patient is receiving 1.5 g/kg/day of protein. The dietician can also help with special dietary needs the patient has, such as carbohydrate-controlled meals for individuals with diabetes mellitus or cardiac healthy diets for those with cardiac comorbidities. Should the patient not be getting sufficient protein through their regular diet, oral supplementation should be added with high-protein drinks. While there are no specific pre-operative guidelines for individuals undergoing amputation procedures, nutritional support would theoretically support a faster recovery from the metabolic stress of surgery and increase the benefits of physical activity before and after surgery.

6 Rehabilitation Planning

In general, the immediate health concerns necessitating surgical intervention are the most important aspect of an amputation procedure, be it due to trauma, infection, vascular disease, cancer, or diabetes mellitus. However, whenever possible, it is important to discuss long-term outcomes and rehabilitation goals with the patient prior to a procedure. Evidence suggests that earlier involvement in structured physical therapy leads to improved functional scores for individuals undergoing lower limb amputations [44]. As previously described in the preoperative assessment section, a comprehensive interdisciplinary baseline assessment should be done to determine the patient's functional status, psychosocial profile, social barriers to care, and rehabilitation goals. Tools like the AMPREDICT risk calculator take into account the patient's age, socioeconomic factors, co-morbidities, renal and hematologic function, and pre-operative functional status to predict the 1 year mortality rate, the likelihood of re-amputation, and the chance of achieving independent mobility within 1 year of the operation [27]. This, in turn, assists in designing an individualized prehabilitation plan for each patient based on their likelihood of ambulation and suitability for the use of a prosthesis.

The level of amputation should also be taken into account as studies suggest the preservation of longer residual limbs improves walking distance, speed, and quality of life [45]. However, longer residual limbs might also increase the likelihood of needing revision surgery, which is why the risks and benefits of the procedure should be discussed with the patient [46]. For individuals undergoing a planned amputation, such as those with prolonged traumatic injuries or chronic diabetic foot ulcers, a tool similar to AMPREDICT exists to aid in the decision-making process. AMPDECIDE [47] allows patients to better understand the risks and benefits of each level of amputation being considered within the context of their own priorities and values. Patients using the AMPDECIDE tool first select whether they are deciding between a transmetatarsal versus transtibial amputation or a transtibial versus transfemoral amputation. Educational videos clearly explain each option and illustrate the risks and benefits of each procedure including the likelihood of healing problems and re-amputation, the chance of independent ambulation, the average life expectancy, and rehabilitation and prosthetic needs after surgery. Patients then see the tradeoffs associated with their chosen level of amputation.

Performing a baseline assessment of the patient's functional status allows for the design of a rehabilitation program that matches the physical capabilities of the individual with their postprocedure mobility goals. Assessments should take into account the patient's strength, range of motion, balance, and training in adaptive activities of daily living. The patient should also be educated on skin care routines for the residual limb as well as the unaffected limb. For individuals, whose functional status allows prosthetic options could be discussed prior to surgery, the rehabilitation plan can be designed with the patient's specific prosthesis in mind [48]. Assessment tools such as AMPREDICT can assist with developing plans that align with the patient's likelihood for and level of ambulatory status following surgery, which, in turn, allows for a more selective choice of adaptive device. The cause of amputation also plays a factor as individuals undergoing surgery due to trauma or planned surgeries following prolonged limb trauma like severe fractures with subsequent non-union despite surgical fixation may be more apt to need and use prosthetic devices.

Postamputation mobility exercises are introduced in an "as-tolerated" fashion. Evidence supporting out-of-bed activities and mobility training early in the postoperative period is limited, but patients should begin mobility and strength training as early as feasible [34, 49]. This includes therapeutic exercise progression, range of motion, balance, and transfer training without a prosthesis. The medical stability of the patient, hemodynamic status, limb healing, and mental status among other patient-specific factors may impact the timing, frequency, and intensity of training. A timely and comprehensive pain management plan will allow for meaningful therapy participation and minimize the risk of mental health deterioration and delirium in the post-operative phase.

If the operation is planned, home visits help determine whether the patient's home is accessible by a wheelchair or other adaptive devices. If necessary, modifications should be made prior to the operation to ensure a safe discharge to the community without delay. The baseline preoperative assessment should also consider whether an immediate postoperative prosthesis (IPOP) will be used in postoperative rehabilitation. Early use of a postoperative prosthesis is associated with early mobilization, gait reeducation, accelerated residual limb healing, fewer postsurgical complications, and faster definitive prosthesis fitting [50]. However, early use of a prosthesis might also increase the risk of skin breakdown, complicate pain management, and result in more post-operative falls [51]. Multiple options exist for immediate postoperative prostheses, including simple pylon and foot structures with adjustable sockets or sockets with pneumatic bladders that can be initiated within the first week following an amputation if the patient's overall recovery picture allows.

Accepted postoperative care of patients undergoing amputation procedures includes multidisciplinary rehabilitation using open and closed-chain exercises and progressive resistance programs to improve gait, mobility, strength, cardiopulmonary reserve, and adaptive activities of daily living. Physical rehabilitation involves physical therapists, occupational therapists, recreational therapists, certified prosthetists, and wound care specialists. Rehabilitation providers should use training that mimics real-world situations in anticipation of community integration, such as stair training and vehicle transfers. There is some evidence suggesting that more intensive exercise therapy results in better cognitive outcomes and improved ambulatory function, such as better performance on the 2-minute walk test [52]. Additionally, higher-intensity exercise during the rehabilitation process may help maintain basal metabolic rate, which could improve exercise participation and prevent weight fluctuations that complicate the artificial limb fitting process. Ideally, the patient should be familiar with many of these exercises from the prehabilitation phase, particularly those aimed at maintaining strength and range of motion in the unaffected limb.

Work with occupational therapy should include functional ADLs, such as bed-to-chair, sit-to-stand, chair-to-toilet, chair-to-tub, and vehicle transfers done with and without a prosthesis. Therapy sessions should also include training in adaptive dressing, feeding, grooming, bathing, and toileting both with and without the prosthesis in place. Patients should have access to neuropsychological therapy and peer-to-peer sessions to help address the psychosocial barriers patients face when reintegrating into the larger community postamputation. Such sessions may help address unexpressed or unanticipated concerns such as mood disorders, adaptive workplace issues, navigating crowded spaces that might not be simulated in therapy, and intimacy with significant others.

Working with a prosthetist is a key component of rehabilitation as these professionals are well-positioned to educate the patient on the type of prostheses available, managing skin breakdown, fabricating and fitting the socket, delivering and repairing the device, and assessing gait. Utilizing microprocessor knee units has been shown to improve one's ability to walk faster on level ground and uneven surfaces, which, in turn, decreases the risk of falling and increases the patient's confidence in utilizing a prosthesis [53]. If the patient is prescribed a prosthesis, he or she should continue working with physical and occupational therapy throughout the prosthesis training phase. Outcome measures such as the Comprehensive High-Level Activity Mobility Predictor, Amputee Mobility Predictor, 10-minute walk test, and 6-minute walk test can assess the patient's progression through therapy [54].

7 Summary of Recommendations

- Smoking cessation: Patients should stop smoking as early as possible prior to their procedure. If the amputation is planned and non-emergent, the patient should ideally start nicotine replacement therapy 1–2 months prior to surgery.
- Exercise: Patients should undergo moderate-intensity aerobic exercise for at least 30 min/day for at least 4–6 weeks prior to surgery. Additionally, patients should undergo at least 3 days/week of high-intensity resistance training using bands or free weights, as able. This can be done in a group setting, but many patients will need regimens tailored to their individual physical capabilities. Ideally, exercises will focus on improving strength and maintaining mobility in the unaffected limbs. If possible, patients should work with PT to begin practicing the adaptive exercises they will be performing in postoperative rehabilitation.
- Psychiatric: Patients should undergo neurocognitive testing to assess for the possibility of postoperative delirium. Patients with mood and personality disorders should undergo targeted treatment for their conditions, such as cognitive behavioral therapy. All patients should undergo counseling sessions with rehabilitation psychiatrists to identify the emotions undergoing the procedure, including anger, grief, and depression. Sessions should also elicit unspoken fears that patients might not verbalize with their medical team, including fear of death, mutilation, social rejection and isolation, and sexual function. Family and caretakers should be involved in anticipating practical concerns, such as occupational limitations, adaptive recreation, and lifestyle changes to maximize independence.
- Education: Patients should receive a firm, clear indication of the necessity of the procedure from the medical team, including a verbal description of the procedure and perioperative recovery process with written supplementation. If needed, the care team can review previous attempts at measures to prevent limb loss.
- Nutrition: Patients should undergo malnutrition screening with the Malnutrition Universal Screening Tool and meet with a dietician to ensure a protein intake of at least 1.5–2 g/kg/day. Oral nutrition can be supplemented with high-protein drinks. Carbohydrate intake should be monitored to ensure the patient is receiving the proper calories to promote healing while also maintaining glycemic control.
- Prosthesis preparation: Patients should meet with a certified prosthetist to become familiar with the adaptive devices they might use after the procedure and how these devices can be used to maximize postoperative ambulation. The

prosthetist can prepare the patient for anticipated difficulties or complications that might deter prosthetic compliance, which is associated with worse outcomes. Appointments can be made in advance for prosthesis fitting and training to help ensure the patient is not lost to follow-up.

- Pain management: Patients should work with a specialist in Anesthesia or Pain Medicine to create a medication regimen that will optimize their ability to participate in pre-and postoperative rehabilitation therapies. Steps should be taken to prepare the patient for the levels of pain they might face after the amputation, including phantom limb pain, and options for addressing these stressors.

Action Points for Patients

Action Points for Patients:

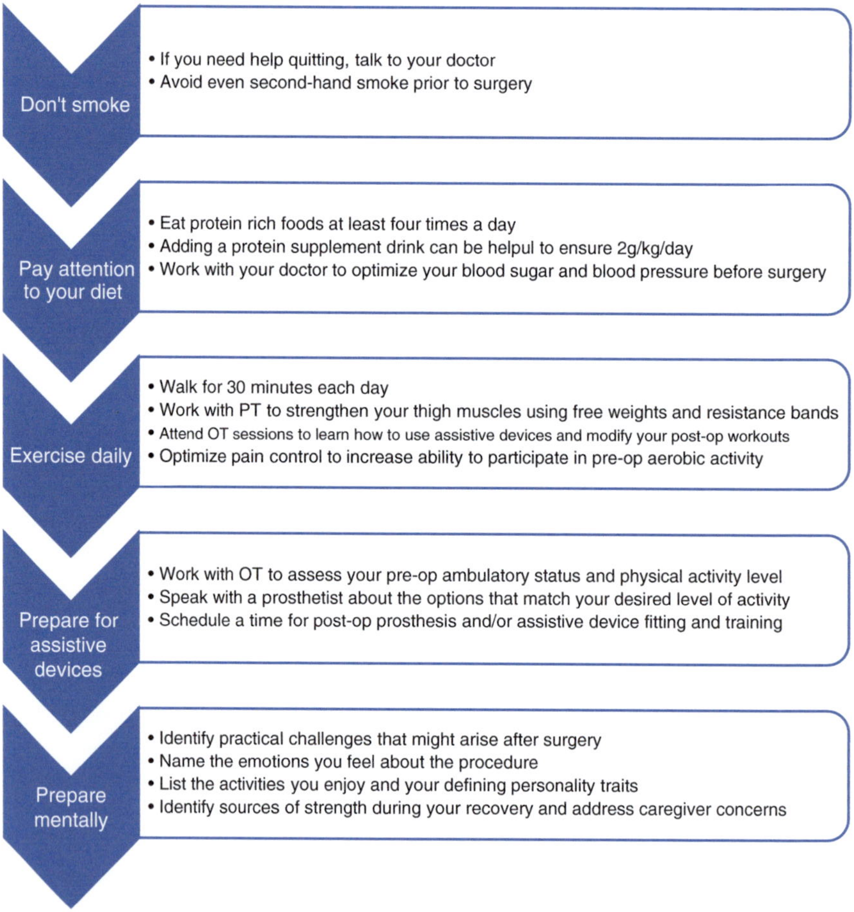

References

1. Dillingham TR, Pezzin LE, MacKenzie EJ. Limb amputation and limb deficiency: epidemiology and recent trends in the United States. South Med J. 2002;95(8):875–83.
2. Hakimi KN. Pre-operative rehabilitation evaluation of the dysvascular patient prior to amputation. Phys Med Rehabil Clin N Am. 2009;20(4):677–88.
3. Bragaru M, Dekker R, Geertzen JH, Dijkstra PU. Amputees and sports: a systematic review. Sports Med. 2011;41(9):721–40.
4. Dillon MP, Quigley M, Fatone S. Outcomes of dysvascular partial foot amputation and how these compare to transtibial amputation: a systematic review for the development of shared decision-making resources. Syst Rev. 2017;6(1):54.
5. Ditmyer MM, Topp R, Pifer M. Prehabilitation in preparation for orthopaedic surgery. Orthop Nurs. 2002;21(5):43–54.
6. Hasanadka R, McLafferty RB, Moore CJ, Hood DB, Ramsey DE, Hodgson KJ. Predictors of wound complications following major amputation for critical limb ischemia. J Vasc Surg. 2011;54(5):1374–82.
7. Ziegler-Graham K, MacKenzie EJ, Ephraim PL, Travison TG, Brookmeyer R. Estimating the prevalence of limb loss in the United States: 2005–2050. Arch Phys Med Rehabil. 2008;89(3):422–9.
8. Thorud JC, Plemmons B, Buckley CJ, Shibuya N, Jupiter DC. Mortality after nontraumatic major amputation among patients with diabetes and peripheral vascular disease: a systematic review. J Foot Ankle Surg. 2016;55(3):591–9.
9. Pomeranz B, Adler U, Shenoy N, Macaluso C, Parikh S. Prosthetics and orthotics for the older adult with a physical disability. Clin Geriatr Med. 2006;22(2):377–94, ix.
10. Stern JR, Wong CK, Yerovinkina M, et al. A meta-analysis of long-term mortality and associated risk factors following lower extremity amputation. Ann Vasc Surg. 2017;42:322–7.
11. Suckow BD, Goodney PP, Cambria RA, et al. Predicting functional status following amputation after lower extremity bypass. Ann Vasc Surg. 2012;26(1):67–78.
12. Rac-Albu M, Iliuta L, Guberna SM, Sinescu C. The role of ankle-brachial index for predicting peripheral arterial disease. Maedica (Bucur). 2014;9(3):295–302.
13. Kwasniewski M, Mitchel D. Post amputation skin and wound care. Phys Med Rehabil Clin N Am. 2022;33(4):857–70.
14. Nather A, Neo SH, Chionh SB, Liew SC, Sim EY, Chew JL. Assessment of sensory neuropathy in diabetic patients without diabetic foot problems. J Diabetes Complications. 2008;22(2):126–31. https://doi.org/10.3402/dfa.v2i0.6367.
15. Banning LBD, Ter Beek L, El Moumni M, et al. Vascular surgery patients at risk for malnutrition are at an increased risk of developing postoperative complications. Ann Vasc Surg. 2020;64:213–20.
16. Lind J, Kramhøft M, Bødtker S. The influence of smoking on complications after primary amputations of the lower extremity. Clin Orthop Relat Res. 1991;267:211–7.
17. Rammell J, Perre D, Boylan L, et al. The adverse impact of pre-operative anaemia on survival following major lower limb amputation. Vascular. 2023;31(2):379–86.
18. Pernot HF, de Witte LP, Lindeman E, Cluitmans J. Daily functioning of the lower extremity amputee: an overview of the literature. Clin Rehabil. 1997;11(2):93–106.
19. Dekker R, Hristova YV, Hijmans JM, Geertzen JHB. Pre-operative rehabilitation for dysvascular lower-limb amputee patients: a focus group study involving medical professionals. PLoS One. 2018;13(10):e0204726.
20. Durrand J, Singh SJ, Danjoux G. Prehabilitation. Clin Med J. 2019;19(6):458–64.
21. Bates BE, Hallenbeck R, Ferrario T, et al. Patient-, treatment-, and facility-level structural characteristics associated with the receipt of preoperative lower extremity amputation rehabilitation. PM R. 2013;5(1):16–23.
22. Taylor SM, Kalbaugh CA, Blackhurst DW, et al. Preoperative clinical factors predict postoperative functional outcomes after major lower limb amputation: an analysis of 553 consecutive patients. J Vasc Surg. 2005;42(2):227–35.

23. Pinzur MS, Littooy F, Daniels J, et al. Multidisciplinary preoperative assessment and late function in dysvascular amputees. Clin Orthop Relat Res. 1992;281:239–43.
24. O'Banion LA, Qumsiyeh Y, Matheny H, et al. Lower extremity amputation protocol: a pilot enhanced recovery pathway for vascular amputees. J Vasc Surg Cases Innov Techn. 2022;8(4):740–7.
25. Fulton S, Baird T, Naik S, Stiller K. Prehabiliation-plus for patients undergoing major lower limb amputation may reduce acute hosptial and total hospital length of stay: a retrospective, matched, case-controlled pilot service evaluation. Int J Ther Rehabil. 2022;29(3):1.
26. Shovel L, Morkane C. Prehabilitation for vascular surgery patients: challenges and opportunities. Can J Cardiol. 2022;38(5):645–53.
27. Center for Limb Loss and Mobility. AMPREDICT decision support tool. Department of Veterans Affairs. 2023. ampdecide.org/ampredict.
28. Piercy KL, Troiano RP, Ballard RM, Carlson SA, Fulton JE, Galuska DA, George SM, Olson RD. The physical activity guidelines for Americans. JAMA. 2018;320(19):2020–8.
29. Nascimento DDC, Rolnick N, Neto IVS, Severin R, Beal FLR. A useful blood flow restriction training risk stratification for exercise and rehabilitation. Front Physiol. 2022;13:808622.
30. Corr AM, Liu W, Bishop M, et al. Feasibility and functional outcomes of children and adolescents undergoing preoperative chemotherapy prior to a limb-sparing procedure or amputation. Rehabil Oncol. 2017;35(1):38–45.
31. Tew GA, Ayyash R, Durrand J, Danjoux GR. Clinical guideline and recommendations on pre-operative exercise training in patients awaiting major non-cardiac surgery. Anaesthesia. 2018;73(6):750–68.
32. Santa Mina D, Clarke H, Ritvo P, et al. Effect of total-body prehabilitation on postoperative outcomes: a systematic review and meta-analysis. Physiotherapy. 2014;100(3):196–207.
33. Saruco E, Guillot A, Saimpont A, et al. Motor imagery ability of patients with lower-limb amputation: exploring the course of rehabilitation effects. Eur J Phys Rehabil Med. 2019;55(5):634–45.
34. Webster JB, Crunkhorn A, Sall J, Highsmith MJ, Pruziner A, Randolph BJ. Clinical practice guidelines for the rehabilitation of lower limb amputation: an update from the Department of Veterans Affairs and Department of Defense. Am J Phys Med Rehabil. 2019;98(9):820–9.
35. Valkenet K, van de Port IG, Dronkers JJ, de Vries WR, Lindeman E, Backx FJ. The effects of preoperative exercise therapy on postoperative outcome: a systematic review. Clin Rehabil. 2011;25(2):99–111.
36. Chin T, Sawamura S, Fujita H, et al. Physical fitness of lower limb amputees. Am J Phys Med Rehabil. 2002;81(5):321–5.
37. Webster JB, Hakimi KN, Williams RM, Turner AP, Norvell DC, Czerniecki JM. Prosthetic fitting, use, and satisfaction following lower-limb amputation: a prospective study. J Rehabil Res Dev. 2012;49(10):1493–504.
38. Lee DJ, Costello MC. The effect of cognitive impairment on prosthesis use in older adults who underwent amputation due to vascular-related etiology: a systematic review of the literature. Prosthet Orthot Int. 2018;42(2):144–52.
39. Jo SH, Kang SH, Seo WS, Koo BH, Kim HG, Yun SH. Psychiatric understanding and treatment of patients with amputations. Yeungnam Univ J Med. 2021;38(3):194–201.
40. Sobti N, Park A, Crandell D, et al. Interdisciplinary care for amputees network: a novel approach to the management of amputee patient populations. Plast Reconstr Surg Glob Open. 2021;9(2):e3384.
41. Richardson LJ, Molyneaux V, Murray CD. Being a peer support mentor for individuals who have had a lower limb amputation: an interpretative phenomenological analysis. Disabil Rehabil. 2020;42(26):3850–7.
42. The Amputee Coalition. Amputee coalition virtual support group meetings. support groups & peer support. 2023. https://www.amputee-coalition.org/support-groups-peer-support/virtual-support-group-meetings.
43. Mignini EV, Scarpellini E, Rinninella E, et al. Impact of patients nutritional status on major surgery outcome. Eur Rev Med Pharmacol Sci. 2018;22(11):3524–33.

44. Rau B, Bonvin F, de Bie R. Short-term effect of physiotherapy rehabilitation on functional performance of lower limb amputees. Prosthet Orthot Int. 2007;31(3):258–70.
45. Ihmels WD, Miller RH, Esposito ER. Residual limb strength and functional performance measures in individuals with unilateral transtibial amputation. Gait Posture. 2022;97:159–64.
46. Dillingham TR, Pezzin LE, Shore AD. Reamputation, mortality, and health care costs among persons with dysvascular lower-limb amputations. Arch Phys Med Rehabil. 2005;86(3):480–6.
47. Center for Limb Loss and Mobility. AMPDECIDE patient decision aids. Department of Veterans Affairs. 2023. ampdecide.org/decision-making.
48. O'Keeffe B, Rout S. Prosthetic rehabilitation in the lower limb. Indian J Plast Surg. 2019;52(1):134–43.
49. Esquenazi A, Meier RH 3rd. Rehabilitation in limb deficiency. 4. Limb amputation. Arch Phys Med Rehabil. 1996;77(3):S18–28.
50. Stineman MG, Kwong PL, Kurichi JE, Prvu-Bettger JA, Vogel WB, Maislin G, Bates BE, Reker DM. The effectiveness of inpatient rehabilitation in the acute postoperative phase of care after transtibial or transfemoral amputation: study of an integrated health care delivery system. Arch Phys Med Rehabil. 2008;89(10):1863–72.
51. Christiansen CL, Fields T, Lev G, Stephenson RO, Stevens-Lapsley JE. Functional outcomes after the prosthetic training phase of rehabilitation after dysvascular lower extremity amputation. PM R. 2015;7(11):1118–26.
52. Bouzas S, Molina AJ, Fernández-Villa T, Miller K, Sanchez-Lastra MA, Ayán C. Effects of exercise on the physical fitness and functionality of people with amputations: systematic review and meta-analysis. Disabil Health J. 2021;14(1):100976.
53. Kaufman KR, Levine JA, Brey RH, McCrady SK, Padgett DJ, Joyner MJ. Energy expenditure and activity of transfemoral amputees using mechanical and microprocessor-controlled prosthetic knees. Arch Phys Med Rehabil. 2008;89(7):1380–5.
54. Sansam K, Neumann V, O'Connor R, Bhakta B. Predicting walking ability following lower limb amputation: a systematic review of the literature. J Rehabil Med. 2009;41(8):593–603.

Solid Organ Transplant Prehabilitation

Haylie C. Kromer and Karen Barr

1 Overview: The Continuum of Care in Solid Organ Transplantation

- Screening and identification of chronic end-organ disease involving the primary care physician and medical subspecialists and risk factor mitigation
- Prehabilitation begins: maximization of lifestyle and medical interventions including exercise, nutrition, substance use, and psychosocial counseling; guideline-directed medical therapies
- Assistance with frailty assessment and prehabilitation program refinement as patients attempt to qualify for transplant and maintain function during listing
- Surgery
- Immediate postoperative care: early mobilization in the context of management of the consequences of major surgery and screening for any emerging complications. Transplantation-related issues vary at this stage such as restrictions on forces through the upper body after chest surgery
- Post-transplantation rehabilitation
- Long-term lifestyle and medical management

Prehabilitation to improve patients' readiness for transplant has become an essential phase of care for patients with end-stage organ disease. Common comorbidities such as the high incidence of frailty and the conditions that lead to frailty such as deconditioning, sarcopenia, and nutritional deficiencies transcend diagnoses for patients with end-stage organ disease. The mechanisms behind these deficits vary, as do the research insights on how best to address them. This chapter outlines organ-specific issues in prehabilitation, and then concludes with a summary of best practices for prehabilitation in organ transplantation.

H. C. Kromer · K. Barr (✉)
University of Pittsburgh, Pittsburgh, PA, USA
e-mail: kromerhc2@upmc.edu; barrkp@upmc.edu

A. Watson, K. Barr (eds.), *A Prehabilitation Guide for All Providers*,
https://doi.org/10.1007/978-3-031-72862-4_9

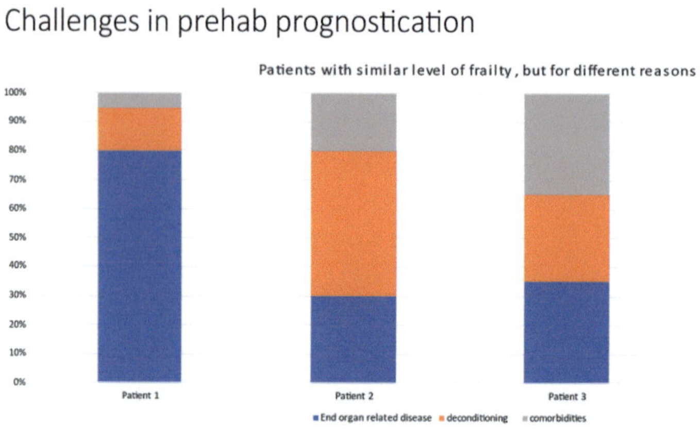

Fig. 1 Challenges in prehabilitation prognostication

Successful prehabilitation interventions for this group need to be multifaceted, multidisciplinary, and individualized so that they are feasible and effective. The challenging goal in the prehabilitation phase of organ transplantation is to identify modifiable risk factors for poor outcomes and to address issues that contribute to poor quality of life during the patient's attempt to qualify for transplantation. As outlined in each organ section, end-stage organ disease profoundly impacts the entire body's function. Understanding the fascinating interdependence of these body systems can help us tactfully proceed in determining the aspects of a patient's condition that only responds to transplantation, which responds to interventions such as exercise and improved nutrition and are attributable to another addressable comorbidity. These considerations are demonstrated in Fig. 1. Determining this makes up the art and science of prehabilitation of the patient in need of organ transplantation.

2 Renal Transplantation

The Need for Prehabilitation in Candidates for Kidney Transplant

Patients with end-stage renal disease (ESRD) have a high need for prehabilitation because of the consequences of the disease process as well as risk factors that are contributory to renal failure such as a sedentary lifestyle, obesity/metabolic disease, and smoking. Research has shown prehabilitation prior to kidney transplant improves physical function, mitigates frailty, and likely improves patient outcomes [1].

Frailty and Kidney Transplantation

One common theme in risk stratification of patients pursuing solid organ transplants is the concept of frailty. Frailty is a risk factor for poor outcomes including delayed recovery and death following kidney transplantation [2]. In ESRD, rates of frailty increase with disease severity, quantified by glomerular filtration rate, with 73% of patients with ESRD considered to have frailty [3]. Although currently there is no gold standard assessment of frailty, the most recognized tool in chronic kidney disease is the fried frailty phenotype (FFP), also known as the physical frailty phenotype (PFP) [2, 4]. Based on the FFP, frailty is the presence of three out of five of the following: shrinking (unintentional weight loss), weakness, poor endurance, slowness (gait speed), and low physical activity [4]. In the context of chronic kidney disease and end-stage renal disease, these elements are closely linked to disease-specific risk factors such as sarcopenia, protein-energy wasting, bone mineral disorders, metabolic derangements, and chronic inflammation. Poor nutrition and low activity levels compound these factors leading to accelerated deconditioning. Studies have revealed an increased risk of hospitalization, delayed graft function, and graft rejection in patients with frailty; therefore, identifying modifiable factors related to frailty is essential for implementing effective prehabilitation strategies [2, 5].

One metric that serves as a simple, efficient method to assess frailty is lower extremity physical function through the Short Physical Performance Battery (SPPB). This test is composed of three elements, balance, sit-to-stand, and four-meter walk tests. Hartmann et al. compared the SPPB scores of patients with renal failure to patients with COPD, heart failure, and cardiovascular risk factors and found that patients with renal failure had significantly lower SPPB scores, especially in gait speed and balance [6]. Physical performance appears to be an important indicator of mortality even prior to end-stage disease. In a study of physical performance and all-cause mortality in stage II-IV CKD, reduced gait speed and increased time in a timed up-and-go test were both associated with a higher risk for death [7]. Combining these functional tests with serum biomarkers better predicted 3-year mortality than serum biomarker testing alone [7]. Generally, in elderly patients, gait speeds <1.0 m/s correlate with patient-reported persistent difficulty walking, hospitalization within 1 year, and all-cause mortality [8]. Furthermore, a pretransplant balance score less than four on the SPPB was associated with more than a three-fold higher rate of prolonged post-transplant hospital length of stay (>4 days) and a five-fold increased risk of rehospitalization after transplant [9]. In another study evaluating the relationship between pre- and post-transplant SPPB scores and post-transplant mortality, impaired patients were those achieving less than or equal to 10 on the SPPB. Impaired patients had a 2.3-fold increased risk of mortality after transplant and a 5-year risk of mortality of 21%, compared with a 5% risk in unimpaired patients [10].

Although not explicitly included as an aspect of the physical frailty phenotype, falls occur more frequently in patients with end-stage renal disease and frailty. Falls prior to transplant are associated with an increased risk for wait list mortality and poor outcomes in the first year post-transplant including increased risk of graft rejection, three-fold longer hospital length of stay, and twofold increased likelihood of skilled nursing facility placement or death [11, 12]. Factors associated with increased fall risk include vitamin D deficiency, orthostatic and autonomic hypotension, diabetic neuropathy, and sarcopenia [13].

Identification of Other Modifiable Risk Factors for Poor Outcomes Besides Global Frailty Assessment

Sarcopenia and Osteoporosis Are Consequences of ESRD That May Be Modifiable

Inflammation, endocrine dysfunction, and uremia contribute to a multitude of cellular changes. These include damage to muscles that cause both muscle loss and decreased functional capacity of the muscle that remains [3].

Both bone synthesis and resorption are critical to maintain proper bone density. Uremic toxins and secondary hyperparathyroidism lead to decreased activity of both osteoblasts and osteoclasts leading to *adynamic bone disease*, a state of absent or reduced bone turnover. Thus, patients with advanced CKD are at heightened risk for fracture, and this risk directly correlates with the duration of hemodialysis therapy [14]. These patients are four times more likely to sustain a hip fracture, which itself independently carries mortality risk [14].

Central Obesity and Visceral Adiposity Are Modifiable Risk Factors

Obesity is an independent disease-modifying factor in the development and progression of chronic kidney disease. Traditionally, obesity has been defined using the body mass index (BMI >30 kg/m^2). With increases in BMI, there is an associated increase in glomerular filtration rate leading to direct injury to nephrons [15]. Studies are conflicting, however, regarding higher BMI and transplant outcomes in ESRD. The *obesity paradox*, in which elevated BMI confers survival benefits, has been observed across numerous end-stage organ diseases, including ESRD [16]. This paradox may be due to the high variability of body composition when utilizing BMI to identify obesity. When comparing BMI and the waist-to-hip ratio (WHR), a measure of central obesity as a proxy for visceral fat, elevated BMI is associated with a decreased risk of mortality in CKD, while elevated WHR is associated with increased risk [17, 18]. Body composition, therefore, is a more accurate metric for assessing risk. In addition to WHR, dual-energy X-ray absorptiometry (DEXA) and bioelectrical impedance analysis (BIA) are commonly used tools to further characterize body composition [19]. Central adiposity directly induces inflammation through adipokine release, which in turn promotes insulin resistance and muscle catabolism. In patients with metabolic syndrome, adiposity suppresses the release of insulin-like growth factor and testosterone, limiting anabolic capacity [16]. These pathways promote the development of a phenotype of increased visceral adiposity and low muscle mass known as *sarcopenic obesity*. This is potentially why transplant recipients with obesity have demonstrated an increased incidence of delayed graft function, acute rejection, surgical site infections, and mortality [15, 20–22].

A patient's body composition is bidirectionally associated with the etiology of ESRD as well, with the metabolic syndrome predisposing to visceral adiposity, and visceral adiposity promoting/worsening metabolic syndrome. Alternatively, other etiologies of renal failure such as chronic viral infections or autoimmune disorders trend toward a phenotype of cachexia with fat and muscle loss. Although low muscle mass and visceral adiposity are associated with poorer outcomes, increasing muscle mass has not been shown to improve outcomes [23–25]; however, improved muscle strength demonstrated with functional metrics imparts survival and outcome benefits.

Nutrition: A Major Concern in ESRD

Protein-energy wasting (PEW) is a significant driver of the frailty phenotype in ESRD, especially in patients undergoing maintenance dialysis. The Interventional Society of Renal Nutrition and Metabolism (ISRNM) has defined protein-energy wasting as a state of "low serum albumin, transthyretin, or cholesterol, reduced body mass, and reduced muscle mass" [26]. The physiologic basis for this phenomenon is a complex and synergistic disruption of nutrition, metabolism, hormones, electrolytes, and inflammation along with other comorbidities that drive a chronic catabolic state [27]. A distinctive characteristic of PEW is the degree of preferential muscle breakdown compared to individuals without CKD due to decreased muscle insulin-sensitivity and insulin-growth factor-1 signaling in the setting of increased oxidative stress from chronic inflammation and metabolic acidosis [27]. Additionally, in patients undergoing dialysis, resting energy expenditure increases due to chronic inflammation as opposed to declining as traditionally seen in states of starvation without PEW [27]. Comorbidities can exacerbate the state of PEW due to compounded states of inflammation, elevated resting energy expenditure, and insulin resistance as in congestive heart failure, chronic obstructive lung disease, and diabetes, respectively [27]. Therefore, PEW is not solely due to low energy intake but is rather a complex, multifactorial process. The PEW-Score 2014 is a reliable and efficient metric to both identify protein-energy wasting and stratify the severity of malnutrition in patients who are on dialysis. The score is derived from serum creatinine divided by body surface area (sCr/BSA) [28].

As renal function declines, there is an associated decline in caloric intake in patients with chronic kidney disease. Estimates suggest up to 50% of patients with end-stage renal disease experience anorexia [27]. Uremia decreases appetite via several mechanisms. Animal models of renal failure suggest that uremia drives a decline in the appetite-stimulating hormone ghrelin and contributes to gastric dysmotility [29, 30].

Furthermore, the diets of patients with end-stage renal disease on hemodialysis may require dietary restrictions due to the impairment of electrolyte homeostasis and the risk for systemic toxicity [31, 32]. Unfortunately, foods containing electrolytes like phosphorus and potassium include fruits and vegetables which are otherwise recommended for a healthy diet. This has been shown to generate confusion and frustration in patients on such diets [33]. Protein-energy wasting along with poor appetite and food restrictions all contribute more broadly to malnutrition in ESRD [34].

Other Lifestyle Considerations

Smoking remains prevalent among individuals with chronic and end-stage renal disease with approximately 14% of hemodialysis patients actively smoking [35]. Smoking contributes heavily to cardiovascular diseases which remains the most common cause of death in patients on hemodialysis [35, 36].

Table 1 Summary of risk factors amenable to prehabilitation in ESRD

Risk factor	How risk factor has been measured	Known negative effect of risk factor
Protein-energy wasting and malnutrition	Serum creatinine/body surface area 5% weight loss in 3 months or 10% in 6 months	Increased all-cause mortality Delayed graft function Graft rejection
Weakness	Short physical performance battery Gait speed Hand grip strength Lean whole body mass	Increased all-cause mortality Increased hospital length of stay
Low physical activity	Self-reported	Increased all-cause mortality
Falls	Self-reported Hospital admission diagnosis	Increased all-cause mortality Increased hospital length of stay
Obesity	BMI	Delayed graft function

Table 1 provides a summary of modifiable risk factors to address for patients with ESRD prior to renal transplantation.

Prehabilitation Interventions that Reduce Risk Factors and Improve Outcomes

Exercise Interventions

Based on the National Institute of Health's physical activity guidelines, Kidney Disease: Improving Global Outcomes (KDIGO) has adopted the recommendation for patients with chronic kidney disease to perform a total of 150 min of moderate-intensity physical activity each week, or 30-min of activity 5 days a week. Patients on hemodialysis show improved rates of morbidity and mortality when physically active between 2 and 5 days/week [37]; although, some studies show that higher doses of exercise of 50 min/day are necessary to preserve walking ability [38]. Despite this, levels of physical activity remain low in this population with a majority of patients exercising less than once per week [37].

Numerous studies have assessed physical activity interventions in patients with advanced CKD and patients receiving dialysis therapy. One proposed method of increasing physical activity participation in patients with end-stage renal disease is intradialytic exercise. Patients, on average, attend dialysis for 4 h, three times per week. Time spent at dialysis is traditionally sedentary but may provide an opportunity to implement regular, supervised exercise. Several studies have investigated intradialytic stationary cycling for its effects on cardiovascular capacity via measuring outcomes including self-reported activity tolerance (Yale Physical Activity Survey), the six-minute walking distance test (6MWD), spiroergometry, and VO_2 max. Chung et al. conducted a systematic review and meta-analysis including 17 studies of intradialytic exercise involving 651 participants on hemodialysis therapy.

The typical dose of stationary cycling in these studies was 30–60 min three times per week during hemodialysis. Overall, compared with no-exercise control groups, intradialytic cycling improved peak oxygen consumption, the physical component of quality of life assessments, and depression scores; participants did not demonstrate significantly improved 6MWD [39]. However, a 4-month intradialytic program combining aerobic and strength training revealed statistically significant improvements in 6MWD, handgrip strength, and body composition.

Compared to home-based programs, intradialytic therapy increases weekly physical activity as measured by metabolic equivalents multiplied by min/week [40]. Conversely, one study comparing intradialytic cycling with a home-based pedometer program revealed no significant difference in aerobic capacity between the two groups, suggesting that patients who prefer to exercise at home can effectively do this, provided they are able to match the same intensity/frequency [40]. Considering the length of dialysis sessions, intradialytic therapy is a reasonable solution to increasing the overall activity level for patients struggling to find the necessary time or motivation to exercise on their own.

Given the concern for muscle wasting in ESRD and other end-stage organ diseases, there is growing attention on resistance training to mitigate these effects. Even in the setting of ESRD, resistance exercise has been shown to improve muscle protein synthesis and improve inflammatory markers [41, 42]. Over a course of 12–24 weeks, supervised, progressive intradialytic resistance training can increase muscle mass, strength, and exercise capacity (assessed via 6MWD) when participants trained at an exertion of 15–17 ("hard" to "very hard") on the Borg Scale [43, 44].

Due to concerns for fatigue in end-stage renal disease as a barrier to physical activity tolerance, Dobsak et al. explored the utilization of electric myostimulation applied to the lower extremities during dialysis sessions as a method of passive muscle activation and mobilization [45, 46]. This study revealed improvement in the 6MWD and maximal muscle power (F_{max}) of leg extensors [46].

In addition to benefitting preoperative quality of life and physical functioning, exercise also likely improves surgical outcomes. Relevant to both renal and liver transplant, Barberan et al. conducted a randomized-controlled trial investigating post-surgical outcomes after the implementation of a personalized, supervised high intensity endurance training prehabilitation program in 144 high-risk patients undergoing elective abdominal surgery. High risk patients were defined as age greater than 70 years and/or American Society of Anesthesiologists score III/IV. The intervention group performed one to three 50-min sessions of supervised endurance training on a stationary bicycle per week. Progression through the study, such as increased intensity was personalized to the patient's peak work rate. After the above intervention (total duration was not defined in the study), there was a decrease in hospital length of stay from 13 to 8 days and decrease in intensive care unit days from four to one. Postoperative complications declined from 62% in the control to 31% in the intervention group with significant reductions in cardiovascular and infectious complications. Furthermore, there was a statistically significant increase in patient endurance time and the Yale physical activity scale index [47].

Dietary Interventions

Optimized nutrition is essential to counter the catabolic state of ESRD. The National Kidney Foundation's Kidney Disease Outcomes Quality Initiative (KDOQI) has outlined dietary recommendations for patients with ESRD on hemodialysis or peritoneal dialysis. The goal protein intake is 1.0–1.2 g/kg/day [31]. Recommended daily electrolyte intake, including phosphorus and potassium, is determined on a case-by-case basis which emphasizes the role of registered dietician nutritionists [31]. Like intradialytic exercise, researchers have investigated intradialytic nutrition interventions in their implications for mitigating PEW, both in the form of oral and parenteral nutrition. Increased energy and protein intake, improved biochemical measures including albumin and prealbumin, and improved quality of life are some of the potential benefits of intradialytic nutrition supplementation [48].

With the goal of simplifying the complexity of a renal diet, one meta-analysis explored the concept of "dietary patterns" versus specific dietary component elimination or inclusion. Patients with end-stage renal disease self-reported their intake via a variety of recall questionnaires and food records. The analysis revealed that those with a dietary pattern including a higher intake of fruit, vegetables, legumes, whole grains, fiber, and fish, and a lower intake of red meat, salt, and refined sugar had lower 5-year all-cause mortality [49]. In Japan, a study of dietary patterns compared individuals consuming a well-balanced diet that contained levels of protein and potassium within physician-prescribed ranges, and those with unbalanced diets who consumed exceedingly higher levels of sodium, potassium, phosphorus, and protein. Unbalanced diets were associated with higher rates of cardiovascular-related hospitalizations and death due to any cause [47].

Pharmacologic Interventions

Growth hormone supplementation of nandrolone decanoate in patients on hemodialysis increased lean body mass; however, no studies have shown outcome improvements. Supplementation of whey protein, creatine, and beta-hydroxy-beta-methylbutyrate has failed to result in gait speed and the timed up-and-go test [50].

3 Liver Transplant

The Need for Prehabilitation in Liver Transplant Candidates

End-stage liver disease (ESLD) is a major cause of morbidity and mortality across the world. Its etiologies stem from causes of acute and chronic liver diseases including cholestatic liver disorders, viral liver disease, alcoholic liver disease, vascular liver disease, metabolic-associated fatty liver disease, and primary liver malignancies [51]. The development of liver cirrhosis is an indication for consideration of transplantation due to its high risk of mortality compared to the general population [51]. With improved awareness, diagnostics, and overall success with liver transplantation, the number of patients on liver transplant wait lists has dramatically increased while the supply of donor organs remains limited, leading to longer transplant wait times and risk of death while on the waitlist. This waitlist time window provides a critical opportunity to address modifiable risk factors that influence the success and longevity of liver transplantation.

Frailty and Liver Transplantation

Frailty enhances the risk of waitlist mortality, hospitalization, and post-transplant hospital length of stay independent of liver disease severity [52, 53]. The liver frailty index is an objective, performance-based metric consisting of grip strength, chair stands, and balance. Adding this functional assessment to the model for end-stage liver disease score (MELD), improves the identification of patients at the greatest risk of mortality [54].

Similar to patients with ESRD, there are inherent factors in the disease process of end-stage liver disease that contribute to the frailty phenotype which are discussed below. In addition, some behaviors that contribute to the development of ESLD also contribute to poor outcomes if not addressed.

Identification of Modifiable Risk Factors for Poor Outcomes Besides Global Frailty Assessment

Sarcopenia and Osteoporosis Are Potentially Modifiable Consequences of ESLD

Like end-stage renal disease, sarcopenia plays a significant role in the frailty phenotype of end-stage liver disease (ESLD) [55–58]. Sarcopenia is present in approximately 25–70% of patients with ESLD) [56]. Numerous factors impact the loss of skeletal muscle including chronic inflammation, a hypermetabolic state, hormone dysregulation, anorexia, dietary restrictions, and low physical activity. Identifying sarcopenia is important due to its influence on transplant waitlist mortality. Waitlist patients with sarcopenia experience nearly twice the risk of mortality as their non-sarcopenic counterparts [57]. Pretransplant sarcopenia also impacts post-transplant outcomes including overall survival, 1-year mortality, 5-year mortality, and 1-year complications. Across all outcomes, there were fewer events in patients with larger dorsal muscle group size on CT imaging [58].

The most widely utilized measure of sarcopenia in studies investigating prevalence and mortality associated with sarcopenia in ESLD is computed tomography (CT) derived skeletal muscle index (SMI) which is obtained from the skeletal muscle area at the third lumbar vertebrae [59]. Dual-energy X-ray absorptiometry (DEXA) is another tool to identify lean body mass but DEXA accuracy is affected by volume status which tends to fluctuate in the setting of decompensated cirrhosis, making it an unreliable measure in ESLD [60]. Handgrip strength (HGS) functions as a surrogate to identify sarcopenia. Although a less sensitive test, HGS combined with MELD score is a stronger predictor for mortality of men with ESLD on a liver transplant waitlist [61].

Unique to end-stage liver disease are the myotoxic effects of hyperammonemia, which directly impacts skeletal muscle nitrogen balance leading to a net loss of muscle mass [62, 63]. High levels of ammonia in skeletal muscle not only induce transcription of myostatin, which downregulates muscle synthesis but also stimulate autophagy [64]. Myostatin-mediated muscle loss in ESLD is also triggered by low testosterone levels and insulin resistance as testosterone is an anabolic hormone that stimulates myocyte proliferation and muscle hypertrophy [65]. Ammonia-lowering therapy shows promise in reducing myostatin expression, improving skeletal mass, and increasing muscle strength [66]. Increased physical activity and proper nutrition may downregulate the effects of myostatin, as well [63].

Bone mineral disease is also a concern in this population. Patients with cirrhosis have significantly lower vitamin D2 and D3 levels than the general population due to fat-soluble vitamin deficiency, and 43% have osteoporosis based on DEXA screening [67]. As the disease state progresses in severity, bone mineral density worsens [67]. Roughly 15% of patients undergoing organ transplants will suffer a new fracture within 1 year post-transplant [68, 69]. Falls, smoking and alcohol use, sedentary lifestyle, and nutritional status are several important modifiable risk factors for osteoporosis post-transplant to consider during prehabilitation [68, 70].

Obesity/Adiposity

Obesity may confound visual identification of sarcopenia by obscuring reduced muscle mass, but sarcopenic obesity especially in nonalcoholic steatohepatitis is important to identify [55, 71]. In 2021, nearly half of the patients on the liver transplant waitlist had a BMI >30, and there were higher rates of waitlist mortality in patients with nonalcoholic steatohepatitis [71]. Patients with a BMI >30 also experience higher rates of transplant complications including increased operative time, blood product usage, ICU length of stay, infectious complications, and biliary complications. The risk of these complications does not continue to rise with higher BMI [72]. Rather, fat distribution is important to consider when assessing the risk associated with obesity. Visceral adiposity predicts increased mortality 1 year post-transplant, considering the metabolic syndrome comorbidities such as diabetes and heart disease also associated with this phenotype. Whereas, low levels of subcutaneous fat, indicating energy wasting, increase the risk of cirrhosis-related complications and death prior to transplant [73].

Physical Activity

Many of the behaviors that contribute to the development of end-stage liver disease also elevate the risk of poor waitlist and post-transplant outcomes. One component is low physical activity level and the resulting deconditioning, often with chronic fatigue in ESLD as a major contributing factor. Patients with ESLD tend to be sedentary with very low step counts per day and very low percentages of time in physical activity [74]. Physical activity is necessary to achieve improved cardiovascular conditioning and muscle strength, two areas associated with better transplant outcomes.

Cardiopulmonary Function

Poor aerobic capacity is prominent in patients with ESLD and is associated with poor post-transplant outcomes. Peak oxygen uptake (VO_2 peak) during cardiopulmonary exercise testing (CPET) and the six-minute walk test (6MWT) are commonly used tools to assess cardiopulmonary endurance in patients with ESLD. In a study of 149 patients referred for a liver transplant, the VO_2 peak was only normal in 12% of patients but was severely impaired in over half of patients [75]. Poor aerobic capacity, VO_2 peak <60% of predicted is associated with longer post-liver transplant hospital length of stay, longer need for oxygen, and increased mortality independent of MELD score [75]. Similarly, patients on a transplant waitlist achieved a significantly reduced distance on the 6MWT. A pretransplant 6MWD <250 m increases the risk of death while on the waitlist, whereas, increases of 100 m were associated with increased survival [76].

Endocrine Dysfunction

Hypogonadism is present in a large percentage of patients with cirrhosis. Low testosterone in male patients with ESLD is a marker of increased risk of mortality [77]. Although hormone replacement therapy in hypogonadal men with cirrhosis can increase muscle mass, its widespread use is controversial [65]. Roughly 50% of patients with cirrhosis have preexisting type 2 diabetes [78]. In patients with NASH, diabetes doubles the risk of hepatic decompensation and quadruples the risk of death or transplant compared to patients with NASH without diabetes [78, 79]. A high percentage of these patients also have obesity and dyslipidemia consistent with metabolic syndrome [78, 79].

Nutrition

Malnutrition affects 50–90% of patients with liver cirrhosis and independently predicts a higher risk of post-transplant graft dysfunction, infection, prolonged hospitalization, and mortality [80]. Prior to transplant, malnutrition increases the incidence of decompensation manifesting as ascites, hepatorenal syndrome, prolonged hospitalization, and mortality [81]. Malnutrition is multifactorial, stemming from physiologic changes directly related to loss of liver function as well as indirectly from symptoms of nausea, vomiting, and overall anorexia [80]. The liver is a quintessential center for metabolism, and therefore, with ESLD, numerous metabolic derangements result. At the cellular level, there is impaired glycogen production to provide energy reserves [80]. Decreased fat absorption due to reduced bile production leads to fat-soluble vitamin deficiencies including vitamins A, D, E, and K [80]. Nutrients that are absorbed from the GI tract may also bypass the liver for processing due to portosystemic shunting induced by portal hypertension [80]. Additionally, as in ESRD, chronic inflammation induces numerous metabolic changes such as worsening insulin resistance, increased catabolism, and elevated resting energy expenditure. These mechanisms lead to an accelerated and persistent state of relative starvation with increased lipolysis, proteolysis, and ultimately decreased BMI and lean muscle mass [82, 83]. The Liver Disease Undernutrition

Screening Tool for ambulatory patients with cirrhosis has a sensitivity and specificity of 72% and 75%, respectively with a positive predictive value of 93% [84].

The European Society for Clinical Nutrition and Metabolism (previously the European Society for Parenteral and Enteral Nutrition) (ESPEN) has recommended a target protein intake of 1.2–1.5 g/kg/day in patients with cirrhosis to mitigate skeletal muscle losses [85]. Despite this, there is still a high prevalence of inadequate protein intake in patients with cirrhosis on a transplant waitlist. Patients with protein intake <0.8 g/kg/day had a higher risk of waitlist mortality and were more likely to have malnutrition [82]. Despite efforts to improve nutrition, the presence of hepatic encephalopathy may limit a patient's ability to tolerate oral intake requiring alternative enteral routes of nutrition and the assistance of dietician evaluation.

Cognitive Dysfunction

While not directly factored into the Liver Frailty Index (LFI), cognitive function certainly influences performance in the various physical domains of the LFI and, therefore, is associated with frailty in liver cirrhosis [86, 87]. Individuals with frailty across disease states demonstrate deficits in processing speed, verbal fluency, and recognition tasks [88].

Hepatic encephalopathy (HE) is a unique phenomenon in end-stage liver disease defined as "brain dysfunction caused by liver insufficiency and/or porto-systemic shunting manifesting as a wide spectrum of neurological or psychiatric abnormalities ranging from subclinical alterations to coma" [89]. Subclinical hepatic encephalopathy is defined as "a condition in which patients with cirrhosis, regardless of its etiology, demonstrate a number of quantifiable neuro-psychiatric defects, yet have a normal mental and neurologic status to clinical examination" [90]. The high variability of hepatic encephalopathy makes the diagnosis of more subtle presentations challenging. Several classification methods attempt to assist in identifying and grading the severity of HE. A per the West Haven criteria, which is a largely subjective grading scale, Grade I HE (the least severe phenotype) may present with a trivial lack of awareness, inattention, and anxiety, all subtle signs of cognitive impairment. Grade IV is defined as coma, a very well-defined clinical state. Many patients with low grade or subclinical HE may remain undiagnosed and untreated, which is a significant concern as HE is the most likely reason for hospitalization prior to transplant [91]. Some estimates suggest subclinical HE is present in greater than 60% of patients with liver cirrhosis [90]. Even in its mildest forms, HE is associated with impaired quality of life and a heightened risk for mortality [92]. There is a 50% risk of mortality within 1 year after the development of HE.

Neuropsychometric assessments can aid in detecting low grades of HE. Combining the Montreal Cognitive Assessment (MoCA) and clinical frailty score (CFS) helps to predict 6-month hospitalization risk. Poor scores on both scales (MoCA <24 and CSF >4) are associated with increased rates of all-cause mortality and hospital admission within 6 months for any reason [91]. Specific areas of the MoCA associated with admission included naming, recall, and attention [91], all of which are subtle findings consistent with Grade I HE, emphasizing its utility in predicting outcomes. In considering the Liver Frailty Index (LFI), which is commonly used in the prehabilitation phase, executive function and reaction time significantly contribute to frailty [87]. These cognitive impairments also influence the ability of the patient to learn and adapt to therapeutic interventions during the prehabilitation phase, making them essential elements to identify and address.

Ammonia-lowering therapies have been the mainstay of HE treatment and secondary prevention. Intrinsically, muscle plays a critical role in ammonia detoxification, and, thus, sarcopenia inherently increases a patient's risk for HE. There is a higher prevalence of HE during hospitalizations in patients with muscle depletion and decreased muscle strength [93].

Chronic alcohol use seen in patients with alcoholic steatohepatitis places patients at heightened risk for cognitive decline independent of the development of HE. The brain demonstrates global atrophy especially in the cerebral cortex, hippocampus, hypothalamus, mammillary bodies, and the cerebellum when exposed to chronic alcohol use [94]. The most extreme state is Korsakoff syndrome which is a state of inattention, confabulation, and anterograde amnesia [95].

Risk factors for obesity like inactivity and metabolic syndrome also contribute to cognitive impairment as demonstrated in animal and human models. Obesity influences learning, memory, and executive functioning in the setting of preferential brain atrophy within the temporal and frontal lobes, lower levels of brain-derived neurotrophic factor, and reduced synaptic plasticity [96–98]. Changes in microglial morphology also suggest active, chronic neuroinflammation. These structural changes are appreciated in even early stages of obesity and the development of the metabolic syndrome [96]. These underlying structural changes and inflammation common in both alcohol use disorder and obesity enhance a patient's risk for the development of HE. More recent theories suggest hyperammonemia alone is unlikely to induce HE, but rather is a component in a two-hit model of inflammation and hyperammonemia provoking clinical HE [92].

Mood Dysregulation

The above disorders may mask underlying psychiatric disorders [99]. Depression is present in about 30% of patients with chronic liver disease across disease etiologies [100]. Even higher rates of depression are present in patients with liver disease secondary to Hepatitis C infection and alcohol-related liver disease [100, 101]. Depression in cirrhosis is associated with poor quality of life, decreased functional status, and increased risk of mortality while on a transplant waitlist [101]. There is no known association between the severity of cirrhosis and the incidence of depression [101]. In alcoholic steatohepatitis, a history of depression and alcohol consumption within a year of liver transplant is linked to alcohol recidivism, and depression in this population is an independent risk factor for decreased survival after liver transplantation [102]. In a prospective assessment of outcomes in patients on a liver and kidney transplant waitlist, patients with depression during screening were more likely to live alone, be actively smoking, and not be working [103]. Even prior to the progression to ESLD, the risk factors for cirrhosis like substance use disorders and metabolic syndrome have higher associations with mood disorders; progression to ESLD likely only worsens this. Table 2 provides a summary of modifiable risk factors to address for patients with ESLD prior to liver transplantation.

Table 2 Summary of risk factors amenable to prehabilitation in ESLD

Risk factor	How risk factor has been measured	Known negative effects of risk factor
Sarcopenia	Skeletal muscle index DEXA Handgrip strength	Increased all-cause waitlist mortality Increased post-surgical all-cause mortality Increased post-surgical complications Increased graft rejection
Malnutrition	BMI	Post-transplant graft dysfunction, infection, prolonged hospitalization, and mortality
Weakness	Gait speed Hand grip strength Thigh circumference Quadriceps strength	Increased all-cause mortality Increased hospital length of stay
Low physical activity	Self-reported Daily step count	Increased all-cause mortality
Low aerobic capacity	VO_2 peak, 6MWT	Increased mortality Increased readmission risk Increased length of hospitalization
Obesity/metabolic disease	BMI, A1C/OGTT	Increased operative time Increased blood product usage Increased ICU length of stay Increased infectious complications
Low bone mineral density	DEXA	Increased risk of fractures and mortality

Prehabilitation Interventions to Mitigate Risk Factors and Improve Outcomes

Exercise Interventions

Per data from the Organ Procurement and Transplantation Network (OPTN), the average wait time for liver transplantation in the United States is between 3 months to 3 years. Within that time frame, the implementation of exercise-based interventions may improve fatigue, aerobic capacity, muscle strength, frailty metrics, self-perceived health status, and quality of life in patients with ESLD [104–111]. Exercise is safe, feasible, and generally well-tolerated during the prehabilitation phase of care in pre-transplantation ESLD. Concerns regarding the safety of exercise in cirrhosis stemmed from a small 1996 study in which Garcia-Pagan et al. demonstrated that moderate-intensity exercise induces a rise of portal pressures in patients with cirrhosis and therefore may increase the risk of variceal bleeding and, consequently, risk of variceal bleeding [112]. However, more recent literature has established the safety of exercise in patients with cirrhosis [107, 108, 110].

Despite low levels of baseline physical activity in many patients with end-stage liver disease, feasibility studies reveal patients have overall good compliance with a standardized exercise program [105]. Participants in a supervised intensive aerobic exercise program completed 94% of sessions over a period of 6 weeks, and there was no significant dropout from the study due to exercise intolerance [105]. Compliance in a prehabilitation program is associated with improved survival and performance in frailty metrics [109]. In a systematic review of exercise interventions prior to liver transplantation, there were no reported adverse events, further supporting the safety of exercise interventions [111].

Both aerobic and strength training offer benefits to patients with cirrhosis. Walking and stationary cycling improve VO_2 peak values and 6MWD. Patients are more likely to demonstrate significant changes in VO_2 peak when participating in structured and supervised programs as demonstrated by a 6-week aerobic exercise program incorporating intensity interval training with specific intensity targets [105]. Home-based exercise programs, typically involving walking as the primary aerobic activity, led to improvements in 6MWT but were inconsistent in improving VO_2 peak [106]. Control groups not involved in any form of physical activity program experienced a decline in VO_2 peak and 6MWT from their baseline indicating the importance of continuing some "maintenance" level of physical activity to preserve aerobic capacity [105, 106]. Those participating in an exercise also often experience improvement in fatigue [110].

Due to the heterogeneity of baseline physical and cognitive function in patients anticipating liver transplantation like age, comorbidities, severity of liver disease, and the sequelae of liver disease such as bone mineral disease, malnutrition, fatigue, and hepatic encephalopathy, patients may require a personalized physical activity program to improve transplant outcomes including mortality [108]. The implementation of an adapted physical activity program, modeled after recommendations for patients with COPD, incorporated both aerobic (via cycling) and strengthening (via weight bench) training. Participants' programs were tailored to patients' baseline performance on cardiopulmonary exercise testing and strength testing. Progressive load was added to both elements of the program based on these same measures. Key measures linked to mortality including VO_2 peak, 6MWT, and muscle strength were significantly improved [108].

In another study with a personalized approach, physical therapists assigned an activity program including cardiovascular and strength training to participants based on the presence of frailty, baseline functional deficits, and available resources for exercise. This study showed significant improvement in the LFI in participants, and reductions in LFI score >3 provided a survival benefit, suggesting that this degree of change in LFI may provide an objective goal in designing and monitoring prehabilitation progress [109].

Along with improved measures of frailty conferring a survival benefit, exercise training reduces time to transplant, post-transplant hospital length of stay [105], and post-transplant readmission rate [104]. Follow-up and counseling throughout exercise interventions are especially important for adherence to programs both in the ESLD and general population. In one study, participants with activity trackers and biweekly counseling in addition to a home-based exercise program demonstrated significant increases in steps and improved 6MWT [106]. Further, smartphone applications and activity trackers present an emerging opportunity to encourage adherence to exercise programs. Overall, patients report positive interactions with mobile apps not only due to accountability measures but also because they allow for the structuring of activity planning and networking opportunities with other users [113].

Dietary Interventions

A 6-month dietician-supported home-based intensive nutrition therapy significantly improved the liver frailty index, skeletal muscle index, and liver disease severity scores, decreased hospitalizations, and improved survival. The intervention group consumed a high-calorie, protein-rich, and low-sodium diet with a target caloric intake of 34–40 kcal/kg/day and protein intake of 1.4–1.7 g/kg/day, and sodium of 2 g/day divided across three meals and three snacks. Also, 64% of the intervention group were adherent to the diet regimen and experienced a significant improvement in their MELD score. However, this study excluded patients with BMI >25 kg/m^2, and therefore few participants with nonalcoholic steatohepatitis were included [114]. There is also increasing attention toward branched-chain amino acid (BCAA) supplementation in addressing protein-energy malnutrition, hepatic encephalopathy, and immune function [115]. BCAA supplementation of 12 g/day improved MELD and CP scores and decreased mortality by 35% [115]. At the molecular level, BCAA supplementation stimulated mTOR1 signaling promoting anabolism and decreased autophagy on muscle biopsy [116].

Psychosocial Interventions

PHQ-9 or BDI (Beck depression inventory) are the traditional instruments for identifying depression/anxiety. If positive, patients typically start psychotherapy, a selective serotonin reuptake inhibitor, or both. Likewise, screening for anxiety utilizes the generalized anxiety disorder (GAD)-7 instrument with initial treatment also involving psychotherapy and/or SSRI implementation [99]. Due to decreased rates of first-pass metabolism due to direct liver damage, patients will typically require lower doses of serotonergic agents; however, these drugs are still safe and effective in chronic liver disease [99, 100].

Pharmacologic Interventions

Metformin use in patients with nonalcoholic steatohepatitis reduces the risk of death or liver transplantation, hepatic decompensation, and HCC. Of note, patients with MELD >15 were excluded from the study [79].

4 Lung Transplantation

The Need for Prehabilitation in Lung Transplant Candidates

Prehabilitation is a key phase in determining candidacy for a lung transplant. Over time, with refinement in pre- and post-transplant care, older patients are now able to qualify for transplants when they previously would have been deemed ineligible. With increased age and a longer time period living with chronic lung disease, individuals have an increased risk of frailty and subsequent poor outcomes. This shift has forced transplant centers to determine whether individuals have the physical and psychological reserve to survive the procedure and succeed in regaining function and quality of life in the postoperative period. When issues are anticipated, prehabilitation is a way that patients can bolster their candidacy.

Beyond its role in candidate selection, prehabilitation is important, because it improves long-term outcomes. After the transplant, patients have large improvements in pulmonary function but typically have physical limitations in exercise capacity (about half of the predicted levels) [117] and skeletal muscle weakness. Although this would be expected in the early post-transplant period after an extensive surgery and hospital course, these limitations may persist for years after transplantation. Research suggests that a year after the transplant, patients' daily sedentary time is increased and walking time is decreased compared to healthy patients [117]. Pretransplant frailty predicts lower posttransplant function, so addressing this with prehabilitation may likely improve outcomes [118].

Frailty and Lung Transplantation

Depending on how it is measured, about 30% of patients with advanced lung disease are deemed frail at assessment for lung transplantation, about three-fold greater incidence than community-dwelling older adults. Although frailty was initially conceptualized as an aging-associated syndrome, it is thought that this occurs in younger patients with end-stage organ disease because of accelerated biological aging. Features of accelerated aging found in patients with lung disease include mitochondrial dysfunction, increased cellular senescence, and telomere shortening. Frailty is also related to inflammation. Lung transplant candidates with frailty have higher levels of inflammatory biomarkers such as of IL-6 and TNF-1 compared to nonfrail patients, but it is unclear whether this association is causal or related in another way [119]. Despite multiple promising areas of investigation, there are currently no well-established panels of markers or cutoff values that are applied in clinical practice to diagnose frailty. This is likely because multiple external factors such as deconditioning and poor nutrition create a physiologic vulnerability that leads to poor health outcomes.

Frailty status correlates with the severity of lung disease but not the diagnostic cause—for example, patients with chronic obstructive lung disease (COPD) and interstitial lung disease (ILD), the two most common diseases that lead to lung transplantation, equally increased risk of frailty [120]. However, there is a distinct contribution of frailty to poor outcomes that is not linked to lung disease. For patients with both COPD and ILD severe enough to consider transplantation, frailty predicts mortality, extent of dyspnea, and quality of life impairment better than lung disease severity. This is why functional assessments are so essential in this population.

The challenge in lung transplant prehabilitation is not only in identifying frailty indicative of poor reserve and likely inability to tolerate the physiologic stress of transplantation but also in defining the modifiable components of frailty. To improve the transplantation process, the prehabilitation evaluation needs to differentiate risk factors that can improve outcomes, versus limitations that can only improve with transplantation. Lung disease is a large contributor to frailty, and therefore some patients with significant pre-transplantation frailty will gain meaningful function and quality of life benefits with transplantation [119]. However, rehabilitation techniques may better address other contributors to frailty. These include sarcopenia, nutritional deficits, comorbidities such as musculoskeletal pain, and cognitive issues including depression [121]—see Fig. 1 for related considerations.

Identification of Frailty Causes Outside of Lung Disease Severity

The short physical performance battery (SPPB) is a useful frailty measure because it appears to measure frailty that is distinct from lung function. SPPB predicts wait-list and post-transplant mortality in lung transplantation independent of the severity of lung disease, and it is responsive to improvement with exercise. A study by Singer et al. defined frailty by SPPB as equal to or less than seven. In this study, frail patients had a tenfold increased risk of death during the first year after transplant, and an increased risk of death persisted years after transplantation. For each one-point worsening in SPPB, there is a 20% increased risk of death. Other functional measures supply additional information. The standard 6-minute walk distance (6MWD) may not adequately differentiate global frailty from limitations related to dyspnea and hypoxemia as a standalone test, but it does supply complementary information. 6MWD is a good predictor of mortality while awaiting transplantation independent of lung disease severity. Interestingly, pretransplant 6MWD also predicts survival after transplant, and this association occurs as a continuous variable from 30 days after transplant to 3 years later [122]. The 6MWD only partially correlates with SPPB, making them good complementary tests [123].

Although not well studied in lung transplant candidates, patient-reported outcomes add another important dimension to frailty assessments. In one study of patients seen in an academic vascular surgery clinic, the patient-reported physical function was better at predicting 1-year mortality than the validated clinical frailty scale completed by healthcare professionals [124]. A study in patients with IPF found that patient-reported outcomes that assessed symptoms and physical activity predicted mortality independent of disease severity [125].

A formalized protocol that employs multiple measures for a composite estimate of frailty appears to be the best current approach-frailty is multifaceted and cannot be captured by any single measure.

Identification of Modifiable Risk Factors for Poor Outcomes Besides Global Frailty Assessment

Sarcopenia

Sarcopenia is a hallmark of frailty in patients with severe lung disease. Sarcopenia is defined as both low muscle mass and decreased muscle strength and function [126]. The biological factors that link sarcopenia and lung disease are still being investigated. Poor nutrition and activity levels contribute as well [120]. It is extremely common and found in upwards of 70% of patients listed for transplantation [127].

The ways sarcopenia has been measured in this population are varied. Muscle mass measurements used include whole body dual X-ray absorptiometry (DXA), bioelectrical impedance (BIA), and focal MRI and CT measurements such as quadricep or iliopsoas cross-sectional area; though a wide variety of muscle groups and locations have been analyzed. The use of thoracic CT to diagnose sarcopenia is particularly appealing as it is already routinely performed for clinical care of chronic lung disease [128].

Whatever the technique used to define it, low muscle mass independent from BMI is associated with adverse lung transplant outcomes, such as longer length of stay, increased readmissions, and decreased survival [129]. However, this is not universally true. One likely reason for this variable association between muscle mass and outcomes is the absence of standard measurements or normative values of muscle mass, non-standardized timing of obtaining these measurements pretransplant, and differences in muscle measurement techniques and statistical analysis [130]. For example, clinicians may measure muscle function via isokinetic and isometric methods including grip strength, lower extremity strength, and endurance measures. Patients may demonstrate particular strengths and weaknesses in each domain by virtue of normal variance in muscle physiology and premorbid activity preferences.

Adiposity/Obesity

In patients with severe lung disease, the contributions to frailty or sarcopenic obesity appear to be linked through common mechanisms with sarcopenia: systemic inflammation, oxidative stress, nutrition, and sedentary lifestyle. However, systemic effects of obesity like chronic inflammation are heavily influenced by the distribution of visceral versus subcutaneous fat, and shared causes of obesity and other chronic diseases such as activity level and nutritional status have an unequal impact on overall health status. For example, an individual with obesity and chronic lung disease due to occupational exposure (i.e., pneumoconiosis) who had maintained an active lifestyle until the recent progression of pulmonary disease past a "tipping point" will likely have a substantially lower risk of incident frailty than an individual with end-stage pulmonary sarcoidosis who has relied on chronic steroids throughout his or her disease progression.

BMI is often used to assess candidacy, although it has significant drawbacks as it does not always correlate well with adiposity. Elevated BMI is common in lung transplant candidates. For example, a cohort study of patients who received lung transplants found that 50% were overweight and 13% had clinical obesity [131]. Obesity levels greater than BMI of 35 (i.e., class II or class III) are associated with a twofold increase in mortality and are often a contraindication to transplant [132]. High amounts of abdominal visceral adiposity as measured by cross-sectional CT and central adiposity measured by waist circumference are associated with frailty [120]. Truncal adiposity is associated with an increased risk of postoperative complications and decreased survival as well as an increased risk of primary graft dysfunction thought to be from inflammation associated with fat [130].

Table 3 Summary of risk factors amenable to Prehabilitation in lung disease

Sarcopenia	CT and MRI muscle mass measurements, DXA, BIA	Weakness, decreased survival, longer length of stay in the hospital and ICU
Poor physical function	Short physical performance battery Gait speed Hand grip strength	Increased all-cause mortality Increased hospital length of stay
Obesity	BMI	Poor surgical outcomes
Malnutrition	BMI, nutritional risk index	Increased all-cause mortality Increased hospital length of stay

Nutritional Risk

Researchers have attempted to identify biological markers of poor nutrition, and some of these correlate with lung transplant outcomes. For example, the nutritional risk index and the prognostic nutritional index both utilize low albumin as a marker of nutritional risk and are associated with worse lung transplant outcomes [133, 134]. Low BMI, typically associated with malnutrition, is a risk factor for poor outcomes, and thus low BMI can be a barrier to transplantation [135].

Psychological Risk Factors

The prehabilitation phase can be an opportunity to optimize psychological as well as physical health. Those awaiting lung transplantation have high levels of stress, anxiety, and depression-related symptoms, with studies finding more than 40% of patients have anxiety and depressive symptoms, and many of those with symptoms do not have a prior diagnosis of depression or anxiety [136]. The longer patients are on the waitlist, the more psychological symptoms they develop [137]. The association between mood and outcomes is still being established. Research has found high negative affect has been associated with mortality while on the wait list [138]. However, limited data suggest that pretransplant anxiety and depression may not be associated with worse post-transplant outcomes [139].

Table 3 provides a summary of modifiable risk factors to address for patients with advanced pulmonary disease prior to lung transplantation.

Prehabilitation Interventions That Improve Risk Factors and Improve Outcomes

Exercise Interventions

Physical inactivity is a big driver of frailty, and good evidence suggests exercise may reverse aspects of frailty in lung transplant candidates. A large study of lung transplant candidates who participated in 90-min exercise sessions that included stretching, resistance training, and aerobic exercise three times per week increased short physical performance battery (SPPB) scores. After 6 weeks of this program, most patients became "nonfrail" as defined by SPPB of 10–12. They noted that improvement in the chair stand component drove overall SPPB score increases

[118]. Other studies stimulated increases in 6MWD with combinations of strength and aerobic exercise training in lung transplant candidates [117]. Both inpatient and outpatient-based exercise programs and interval and continuous training were effective strategies to increase 6MWD. Available research shows participating in pulmonary rehabilitation improves survival and other outcome measures after transplant [140]. Given the functional improvements facilitated by these exercise strategies, quality of life measures typically demonstrate improvement even before transplant [141].

A recent review of exercise training in lung transplant candidates noted that, despite these individuals' significant illnesses, exercise training did not provoke any adverse events in the included studies [117]. However, inspiring frail patients to participate in strenuous exercise may be challenging, and patients with frailty are at high risk of not completing pulmonary rehabilitation. For example, one study of an 8-week pulmonary rehabilitation found that patients with frailty were twice as likely to not finish the program, but in those who did, 61% did not meet frailty criteria at program completion [142]. Interval training may cause less dyspnea symptoms and therefore be better tolerated [117]. Single limb, low load/high repetition training results in less dyspnea during training compared to two limbs, yet with equal or greater increase in 6MWD [143].

An initial individual assessment should inform the exercise prescription. Exercise will likely need to begin at a low intensity but should gradually progress to the highest tolerated intensity while maintaining adequate oxygenation, typically not falling below 88%. Exercise should include both aerobic training and upper and lower-extremity resistance training. Some patients will require continuous monitoring to ensure safety. Participation in formal pulmonary rehabilitation is typically the best means of accomplishing this, and additional physical therapy is often beneficial, as well. In addition to the supervision for safety during exercise, therapists can educate patients in real time about managing dyspnea, provide encouragement, and coach them on establishing a home program for suitable patients. Therapists should also be vigilant about investigating acute functional decline to find the etiology [144].

Overall, studies show that exercise pre-transplant can improve quality of life and exercise capacity, particularly the 6-minute walk distance. These gains occur with various exercise types, including continuous and interval training, aerobic exercise, and progressive resistive exercises, and improvements can occur no matter what the primary pulmonary diagnosis.

Nutritional Interventions and Attainment of Normal BMI

Even in the presence of end-stage lung disease, patients are able to improve BMI during the listing process and experience potentially significant benefits. Greater pretransplant weight loss in patients with concomitant obesity was associated with a dose-response improvement in survival, independent of initial weight [131]. A large cohort of patients at one center found that two-thirds of patients were able to achieve a BMI of less than 30 between listing and transplantation. The remaining one-third of patients had worse outcomes such as increased mortality and increased medical and surgical complications. In this same cohort, only about half of those with a low BMI were able to attain a BMI greater than 18.5, but there were no outcome differences between those who gained weight and those who did not. This suggests that adequate nutritional treatment likely contributed to improved outcomes, even in the absence of lean mass gain, which might not be possible for subgroups of patients in whom catabolism and inflammation limit the response to anabolic stimuli [145].

Current insights limit the ability to provide generalizable recommendations about the best nutrition for lung transplant candidates. The wide age range, number of diseases that lead to end-stage lung damage, comorbidities, and lifestyles are too varied. The best course appears to be for each patient to undergo an individualized nutritional assessment and to focus on both normalizing BMI and obtaining optimal nutrition. Typical recommendations include ensuring adequate protein intake, eating smaller and more frequent meals (often better tolerated in those with severe shortness of breath), reducing processed foods that contribute to inflammation and have low nutrition, and determining whether supplementation with shakes or other methods is indicated.

Psychological Support

The effect of increasing psychological support during the prehabilitation phase has not been studied. Mitigating the high levels of psychological comorbidities that patients have may improve the motivation for participating fully in prehabilitation, such as by adhering to a healthy diet and exercise routine. Seeking counseling, optimizing medications, drawing on family support, employing meditation and other relaxation practices, and purposefully seeking out enjoyable activities are some plausibly helpful strategies.

5 Cardiac Transplant

The Need for Prehabilitation in the Heart Transplant Candidate

Cardiovascular disease and heart failure are very common, and just as in other organ failure disorders, the number of patients who would benefit from transplantation far exceeds available donors. Over time, guidelines have liberalized age restrictions which, combined with medical advances in heart failure management including better medications and ventricular assist devices have led to greater focus on frailty assessment for the heart transplant candidate.

Frailty in Cardiac Disease

Physiology maladaptation due to structural changes in the heart plays a significant role in reduced quality of life, increased disability, and worsened mortality in heart failure. Inflammation, oxidative stress, low levels of endogenous anabolic steroids, and micronutrient deficiency are likely underlying mechanisms that improve with transplant. As with end-stage kidney, liver, and lung diseases, comorbidities and deconditioning also drive many of these maladaptations [146].

As seen in other conditions, there is only a fair correlation between clinician estimates of frailty and formal validated frailty assessments in patients with heart failure [147]. Therefore, systematic evaluation of frailty is recommended for all heart transplant candidates. A 2019 consensus statement from the American Society of Transplant Surgeons and the American Society of Transplantation Heart Group recommends the use of the Fried Frailty Phenotype as having the best evidence to measure frailty in this population while suggesting employing modifications to make this more appropriate for heart transplant [148] (see table). Patients with frailty defined as three or greater on this scale have an increased risk of mortality and prolonged hospitalization after transplant independent of other medical factors [148, 149]. Physical measures such as reduced gait speed and reduced grip strength are associated with poor outcomes and can be followed over time.

Recommendations for modified Fried criteria frailty assessment for use in patients with heart failure

Fried criteria: points indicate worse frailty	Applicable to heart failure population?	Modification recommendation
Self-reported weight loss of 10 lbs; documented >5% of total body weight	No: edema confounds	Decreased appetite for 3 months
Slow gait speed (15 ft distance)	Sometimes	1 pt if nonambulatory
Grip strength (based on gender, BMI simplified normative value)	Yes, but better normative data available	3 attempts, 2 SD below sex and age-adjusted normative data
Physical exhaustion "I felt like everything I did was an effort in the last week". Positive if answer moderate, most, or all of the time	Yes, but symptoms are dynamic, subjective, and susceptible to confounders	Yes to "in the last week, did you feel at least 3 days everything you did was an effort"
Low energy per Minnesota leisure time	No: some questions are too high level (such as question related to "jogging")	Duke Activity Status Index (DASI)
No cognition component	No: cognition assessment is important domain in this population	MOCA less than 26/30

Scores of three or greater considered frail

Identification of Modifiable Risk Factors for Poor Outcomes Besides Global Frailty Assessment

Sarcopenia

One clearly established risk for poor outcomes while on a heart transplant waitlist and post-transplant is *cardiac cachexia*. This refers to the phenomenon of skeletal muscle restructuring and atrophy that occurs in chronic heart failure [150–153].

Cachexia is an independent risk factor for mortality across classes and stages of heart failure [154]. There is no unifying definition for cachexia; however, it is frequently defined as unintentional edema-free weight loss of 5% over 12 months [153]. Sarcopenia, a component of cachexia, is also independently associated with poor outcomes in heart failure [152]. Low muscle mass is also associated with an increased risk of post-transplant infection and late graft failure [155, 156]. Muscle weakness contributes to physical disability and lower ADL performance in patients with chronic heart failure [157]. A handgrip strength <25% of body weight portends an increased risk of mortality, increased postoperative complications, and lower survival after ventricular-assist device implantation [158].

A chronic adrenergic state, as seen in end-stage renal, liver, and lung diseases induces a physiologic shift to unimpeded catabolism, leading to skeletal muscle atrophy and sarcopenia. Although not fully understood, molecular and cellular changes of skeletal muscle contribute to physical activity intolerance, which is a hallmark symptom of heart failure and a source of poor health-related quality of life. Muscles in patients with heart failure have fewer mitochondria and transition from slow-twitch type 1 muscle fibers to fast-twitch type II fibers [159–161]. Ultimately, this results in reduced oxidative capacity, translating into poor cardiorespiratory endurance [160, 161]. Furthermore, due to the sympathetic stress to maintain adequate perfusion to tissues in a low-flow state, there is a cycle of neuromuscular and neurohormonal signaling which further contributes to dyspnea on exertion and poor activity tolerance [152, 162].

Aerobic Capacity

Heart failure, by definition, "is the inability of the heart to maintain or increase cardiac output at a rate commensurate with systemic aerobic requirement" [163]. Heart rate and stroke volume are the components of cardiac output, and aberrant heart rates, decreases in diastolic and systolic cardiac function, and increased peripheral vascular resistance contribute to declines in cardiac output in heart failure. Due to deleterious changes in the primary oxidative metabolizer of the body, skeletal muscle, there is also a decline in arteriovenous oxygen difference, as muscle become inefficient in the extraction and utilization of oxygen. VO_2 max (or VO_2 peak) is a well-established predictor of survival preceding and after LVAD placement or cardiac transplant [164–167]. Improvements in VO_2 peak are not guaranteed after LVAD placement or heart transplantation [168, 169], partially due to disruptions of sympathetic chronotropic signaling secondary to cardiac allograft denervation, which limits heart rate responses to increased activity [170]. Additionally, pretransplant deconditioning and low muscle mass limit post-transplant function; therefore, many patients continue to demonstrate low exercise capacity, secondary reduced quality of life and a decline in ADL performance [169, 170].

Evidence of Effects of Prehabilitation and Comparative Effectiveness of Various Interventions

Exercise Interventions

Despite good evidence that physical activity can mitigate negative physiologic adaptions in heart failure, cardiopulmonary rehabilitation remains underutilized, likely due in part to early concerns regarding the safety of exercise as well as the result of poor activity tolerance, as previously discussed. Mounting evidence from exercise interventions in heart failure shows that exercise is safe in all severities of heart failure, even in patients with bridging therapies such as mechanical circulatory support devices [171–173]. Initial concern regarding the safety of resistance training was due to recognizing the inherent increases in afterload during Valsalva maneuvers, which theoretically decrease cardiac output. Contrary to this, studies of resistance training in heart failure have failed to demonstrate adverse cardiac effects and, in fact, identified improved cardiac structure and function [174]. As such, there is an enhanced benefit to combined aerobic-resistance training [175]. At the cellular level, aerobic exercise promotes antioxidant production and is cardioprotective against ischemia-reperfusion injury [176]. Resistance training induces reversal of aberrant myofibril cross-bridging which may improve muscle strength, performance of ADLs, and activity tolerance [177]. Further, resistance training provides greater anabolic stimulus for lean muscle accrual.

These physiologic changes drive increased functional capacity, exercise capacity, quality of life, and survival seen with exercise interventions. Exercise training prior to heart transplantation helps prevent a wait list-associated decline in functional capacity and quality of life, and training decreases the incidence of hospitalization, hospital length of stay, and pharmaceutical costs while on a transplant waitlist, even with bridge mechanical circulatory support devices (MCSD) therapies [172]. Not only can further decline be halted, but functional capacity, measured via the 6-minute walk distance test and/or VO_2 peak, increases with participation in aerobic training and combined aerobic-resistance training programs [157, 172, 174, 175, 178–180]. Quality of life significantly improves with aerobic training and the addition of resistance training augments these improvements [172, 174, 175, 178, 180].

Pharmacotherapies

SGLT2 inhibitors have become a standard addition to guideline-directed medical therapy in heart failure with reduced ejection fraction. Growing evidence suggests that these agents improve aerobic metabolism in skeletal muscle which can, in turn, improve aerobic exercise capacity [181]. Studies are ongoing regarding the efficacy of supplementing inorganic nitrates (found in beetroot), which may play a role in augmenting vasodilation and supporting cardiac output via afterload reduction [182].

Nutrition

One of the most studied diets for cardiovascular risk reduction is the dietary approaches to stop hypertension (DASH) diet. This diet focuses on the reduced consumption of processed foods containing saturated fat, sodium, and added sugar and increasing consumption of whole foods including whole grains, vegetables, fruits, nonfat and low-fat dairy, potassium, fiber, calcium, and vitamin D [183]. The DASH diet in combination with a sodium restriction of 2300 mg daily also significantly reduces blood pressure, ultimately reducing the risk of heart failure [184–186]. The OmniHeart trial showed that there is a benefit to a whole-food, DASH diet of any macronutrient composition (higher in carbohydrates, lean protein, or unsaturated fats) [186].

6 Summary of Recommendations for Prehabilitation in Organ Transplantation

- **Structured assessment of frailty** is beneficial for candidate selection and timing of transplantation, yet no gold standard for this exists. Because frailty is a multidimensional construct, assessing from complementary perspectives appears superior to overreliance on any one test or scale.
- **Objective measures of physical function** such as grip strength, the short physical performance battery (SPPB), and gait speed should be used to set prehabilitation goals and track program response, as they are more accurate than the provider or patient assessment of functional gains alone.
- **Exercise**: This is a safe and effective treatment for patients attempting to receive organ transplantation, but provider expertise and plan personalization are necessary for safety, efficacy, and facilitating consistent participation despite feeling poorly.
- **Nutrition**: Although the cause is varied, all patients with end-organ disease have significant nutritional impairments best addressed by a team-comprehensive approach. Addressing these is essential to make functional gains and improve surgical outcomes.
- **Psychological health**: Living with chronic disease, facing mortality, and the prospect of undergoing transplantation are major stressors that should be addressed in the prehabilitation phase. Just as in physical comorbidities, psychological comorbidities such as anxiety and depression can be aggravated by end-stage organ disease and should be treated.

References

1. McAdams-DeMarco MA, Ying H, Van Pilsum Rasmussen S, Schrack J, Haugen CE, Chu NM, et al. Prehabilitation prior to kidney transplantation: results from a pilot study. Clin Transpl. 2019;33(1):e13450.

2. Alfieri C, Malvica S, Cesari M, Vettoretti S, Benedetti M, Cicero E, et al. Frailty in kidney transplantation: a review on its evaluation, variation and long-term impact. Clin Kidney J. 2022;15(11):2020–6.
3. Chao CT, Lin SH. Uremic toxins and frailty in patients with chronic kidney disease: a molecular insight. Int J Mol Sci. 2021;22(12):6270.
4. Fried LP, Tangen CM, Walston J, Newman AB, Hirsch C, Gottdiener J, et al. Frailty in older adults: evidence for a phenotype. J Gerontol A Biol Sci Med Sci. 2001;56(3):M146–56.
5. McAdams-DeMarco MA, Isaacs K, Darko L, Salter ML, Gupta N, King EA, et al. Changes in frailty after kidney transplantation. J Am Geriatr Soc. 2015;63(10):2152–7.
6. Hartmann EL, Kitzman D, Rocco M, Leng X, Klepin H, Gordon M, et al. Physical function in older candidates for renal transplantation: an impaired population. Clin J Am Soc Nephrol. 2009;4(3):588–94.
7. Roshanravan B, Robinson-Cohen C, Patel KV, Ayers E, Littman AJ, de Boer IH, et al. Association between physical performance and all-cause mortality in CKD. J Am Soc Nephrol. 2013;24(5):822–30.
8. Cesari M, Kritchevsky SB, Penninx BW, Nicklas BJ, Simonsick EM, Newman AB, et al. Prognostic value of usual gait speed in well-functioning older people—results from the Health, Aging and Body Composition Study. J Am Geriatr Soc. 2005;53(10):1675–80.
9. Lorenz EC, Cheville AL, Amer H, Kotajarvi BR, Stegall MD, Petterson TM, et al. Relationship between pre-transplant physical function and outcomes after kidney transplant. Clin Transpl. 2017;31(5) https://doi.org/10.1111/ctr.12952.
10. Nastasi AJ, McAdams-DeMarco MA, Schrack J, Ying H, Olorundare I, Warsame F, et al. Pre-kidney transplant lower extremity impairment and post-kidney transplant mortality. Am J Transplant. 2018;18(1):189–96.
11. Lynch RJ, Patzer RE, Pastan SO, Bowling CB, Plantinga LC. Recent history of serious fall injuries and posttransplant outcomes among US kidney transplant recipients. Transplantation. 2019;103(5):1043–50.
12. Chu NM, Shi Z, Berkowitz R, Haugen CE, Garonzik-Wang J, Norman SP, et al. Poor outcomes in kidney transplant candidates and recipients with history of falls. Transplantation. 2020;104(8):1738–45.
13. Papakonstantinopoulou K, Sofianos I. Risk of falls in chronic kidney disease. J Frailty Sarcopenia Falls. 2017;2(2):33–8.
14. Maalouf NM, Shane E. Osteoporosis after solid organ transplantation. J Clin Endocrinol Metab. 2005;90(4):2456–65.
15. Chen Y, Dabbas W, Gangemi A, Benedetti E, Lash J, Finn PW, et al. Obesity management and chronic kidney disease. Semin Nephrol. 2021;41(4):392–402.
16. Naderi N, Kleine CE, Park C, Hsiung JT, Soohoo M, Tantisattamo E, et al. Obesity paradox in advanced kidney disease: from bedside to the bench. Prog Cardiovasc Dis. 2018;61(2):168–81.
17. Elsayed EF, Sarnak MJ, Tighiouart H, Griffith JL, Kurth T, Salem DN, et al. Waist-to-hip ratio, body mass index, and subsequent kidney disease and death. Am J Kidney Dis. 2008;52(1):29–38.
18. Kovesdy CP, Czira ME, Rudas A, Ujszaszi A, Rosivall L, Novak M, et al. Body mass index, waist circumference and mortality in kidney transplant recipients. Am J Transplant. 2010;10(12):2644–51.
19. Kim KM, Jang HC, Lim S. Differences among skeletal muscle mass indices derived from height-, weight-, and body mass index-adjusted models in assessing sarcopenia. Korean J Intern Med. 2016;31(4):643–50.
20. Kwan JM, Hajjiri Z, Metwally A, Finn PW, Perkins DL. Effect of the obesity epidemic on kidney transplantation: obesity is independent of diabetes as a risk factor for adverse renal transplant outcomes. PLoS One. 2016;11(11):e0165712.
21. Molnar MZ, Kovesdy CP, Mucsi I, Bunnapradist S, Streja E, Krishnan M, et al. Higher recipient body mass index is associated with post-transplant delayed kidney graft function. Kidney Int. 2011;80(2):218–24.

22. Lynch RJ, Ranney DN, Shijie C, Lee DS, Samala N, Englesbe MJ. Obesity, surgical site infection, and outcome following renal transplantation. Ann Surg. 2009;250(6):1014–20.
23. Goodpaster BH, Park SW, Harris TB, Kritchevsky SB, Nevitt M, Schwartz AV, et al. The loss of skeletal muscle strength, mass, and quality in older adults: the health, aging and body composition study. J Gerontol A Biol Sci Med Sci. 2006;61(10):1059–64.
24. Newman AB, Kupelian V, Visser M, Simonsick EM, Goodpaster BH, Kritchevsky SB, et al. Strength, but not muscle mass, is associated with mortality in the health, aging and body composition study cohort. J Gerontol A Biol Sci Med Sci. 2006;61(1):72–7.
25. Visser M, Goodpaster BH, Kritchevsky SB, Newman AB, Nevitt M, Rubin SM, et al. Muscle mass, muscle strength, and muscle fat infiltration as predictors of incident mobility limitations in well-functioning older persons. J Gerontol A Biol Sci Med Sci. 2005;60(3):324–33.
26. Fouque D, Kalantar-Zadeh K, Kopple J, Cano N, Chauveau P, Cuppari L, et al. A proposed nomenclature and diagnostic criteria for protein–energy wasting in acute and chronic kidney disease. Kidney Int. 2008;73(4):391–8.
27. Carrero JJ, Stenvinkel P, Cuppari L, Ikizler TA, Kalantar-Zadeh K, Kaysen G, et al. Etiology of the protein-energy wasting syndrome in chronic kidney disease: a consensus statement from the International Society of Renal Nutrition and Metabolism (ISRNM). J Ren Nutr. 2013;23(2):77–90.
28. Gracia-Iguacel C, Gonzalez-Parra E, Mahillo I, Ortiz A. Criteria for classification of protein-energy wasting in dialysis patients: impact on prevalence. Br J Nutr. 2019;121(11):1271–8.
29. Fu RG, Ge H, Yao GL, Wang L, Ren ST, Ma LQ, et al. Uremic anorexia and gastrointestinal motility dysfunction correlate with the changes of ghrelin system in hypothalamus. Nephrology (Carlton). 2013;18(2):111–6.
30. Fu RG, Xue RL, Wang J, Ma LQ, Lv JR, Wang L, et al. Uremic anorexia and ghrelin expression in the amygdala. Neurosci Lett. 2012;527(1):50–4.
31. Ikizler TA, Burrowes JD, Byham-Gray LD, Campbell KL, Carrero JJ, Chan W, et al. KDOQI clinical practice guideline for nutrition in CKD: 2020 update. Am J Kidney Dis. 2020;76(3):S1–07.
32. Mekki K, Bouzidi-bekada N, Kaddous A, Bouchenak M. Mediterranean diet improves dyslipidemia and biomarkers in chronic renal failure patients. Food Funct. 2010;1(1):110–5.
33. Hollingdale R, Sutton D, Hart K. Facilitating dietary change in renal disease: investigating patients'perspectives. J Ren Care. 2008;34(3):136–42.
34. MacLaughlin HL, Friedman AN, Ikizler TA. Nutrition in kidney disease: core curriculum 2022. Am J Kidney Dis. 2022;79(3):437–49.
35. Mc Causland FR, Brunelli SM, Waikar SS. Association of smoking with cardiovascular and infection-related morbidity and mortality in chronic hemodialysis. Clin J Am Soc Nephrol. 2012;7(11):1827–35.
36. Liebman SE, Lamontagne SP, Huang LS, Messing S, Bushinsky DA. Smoking in dialysis patients: a systematic review and meta-analysis of mortality and cardiovascular morbidity. Am J Kidney Dis. 2011;58(2):257–65.
37. Stack AG, Molony DA, Rives T, Tyson J, Murthy BV. Association of physical activity with mortality in the US dialysis population. Am J Kidney Dis. 2005;45(4):690–701.
38. Kutsuna T, Matsunaga A, Matsumoto T, Ishii A, Yamamoto K, Hotta K, et al. Physical activity is necessary to prevent deterioration of the walking ability of patients undergoing maintenance hemodialysis. Ther Apher Dial. 2010;14(2):193–200.
39. Chung YC, Yeh ML, Liu YM. Effects of intradialytic exercise on the physical function, depression and quality of life for haemodialysis patients: a systematic review and meta-analysis of randomised controlled trials. J Clin Nurs. 2017;26(13–14):1801–13.
40. Koh KP, Fassett RG, Sharman JE, Coombes JS, Williams AD. Effect of intradialytic versus home-based aerobic exercise training on physical function and vascular parameters in hemodialysis patients: a randomized pilot study. Am J Kidney Dis. 2010;55(1):88–99.

41. Castaneda C, Gordon PL, Parker RC, Uhlin KL, Roubenoff R, Levey AS. Resistance training to reduce the malnutrition-inflammation complex syndrome of chronic kidney disease. Am J Kidney Dis. 2004;43(4):607–16.
42. Afshar R, Shegarfy L, Shavandi N, Sanavi S. Effects of aerobic exercise and resistance training on lipid profiles and inflammation status in patients on maintenance hemodialysis. Indian J Nephrol. 2010;20(4):185–9.
43. Cheema B, Abas H, Smith B, O'Sullivan A, Chan M, Patwardhan A, et al. Progressive exercise for anabolism in kidney disease (PEAK): a randomized, controlled trial of resistance training during hemodialysis. J Am Soc Nephrol. 2007;18(5):1594–601.
44. Mori K. Maintenance of skeletal muscle to counteract sarcopenia in patients with advanced chronic kidney disease and especially those undergoing hemodialysis. Nutrients. 2021;13(5):1538.
45. Delgado C, Johansen KL. Barriers to exercise participation among dialysis patients. Nephrol Dial Transplant. 2012;27(3):1152–7.
46. Dobsak P, Homolka P, Svojanovsky J, Reichertova A, Soucek M, Novakova M, et al. Intradialytic electrostimulation of leg extensors may improve exercise tolerance and quality of life in hemodialyzed patients. Artif Organs. 2012;36(1):71–8.
47. Tsuruya K, Fukuma S, Wakita T, Ninomiya T, Nagata M, Yoshida H, et al. Dietary patterns and clinical outcomes in hemodialysis patients in Japan: a cohort study. PLoS One. 2015;10(1):e0116677.
48. Kistler BM, Benner D, Burrowes JD, Campbell KL, Fouque D, Garibotto G, et al. Eating during hemodialysis treatment: a consensus statement from the International Society of Renal Nutrition and Metabolism. J Ren Nutr. 2018;28(1):4–12.
49. Kelly JT, Palmer SC, Wai SN, Ruospo M, Carrero JJ, Campbell KL, et al. Healthy dietary patterns and risk of mortality and ESRD in CKD: a meta-analysis of cohort studies. Clin J Am Soc Nephrol. 2017;12(2):272–9.
50. March DS, Wilkinson TJ, Burnell T, Billany RE, Jackson K, Baker LA, et al. The effect of non-pharmacological and pharmacological interventions on measures associated with sarcopenia in end-stage kidney disease: a systematic review and meta-analysis. Nutrients. 2022;14(9):1817.
51. Gines P, Krag A, Abraldes JG, Sola E, Fabrellas N, Kamath PS. Liver cirrhosis. Lancet. 2021;398(10308):1359–76.
52. Haugen CE, McAdams-DeMarco M, Holscher CM, Ying H, Gurakar AO, Garonzik-Wang J, et al. Multicenter study of age, frailty, and waitlist mortality among liver transplant candidates. Ann Surg. 2020;271(6):1132–6.
53. Sinclair M, Poltavskiy E, Dodge JL, Lai JC. Frailty is independently associated with increased hospitalisation days in patients on the liver transplant waitlist. World J Gastroenterol. 2017;23(5):899–905.
54. Kardashian A, Ge J, McCulloch CE, Kappus MR, Dunn MA, Duarte-Rojo A, et al. Identifying an optimal liver frailty index cutoff to predict waitlist mortality in liver transplant candidates. Hepatology. 2021;73(3):1132–9.
55. Williams FR, Milliken D, Lai JC, Armstrong MJ. Assessment of the frail patient with end-stage liver disease: a practical overview of sarcopenia, physical function, and disability. Hepatol Commun. 2021;5(6):923–37.
56. Allen SL, Seabright AP, Quinlan JI, Dhaliwal A, Williams FR, Fine NHF, et al. The effect of ex vivo human serum from liver disease patients on cellular protein synthesis and growth. Cells. 2022;11(7):1098.
57. van Vugt JL, Levolger S, de Bruin RW, van Rosmalen J, Metselaar HJ, JN IJ. Systematic review and meta-analysis of the impact of computed tomography-assessed skeletal muscle mass on outcome in patients awaiting or undergoing liver transplantation. Am J Transplant. 2016;16(8):2277–92.

58. Lee CS, Cron DC, Terjimanian MN, Canvasser LD, Mazurek AA, Vonfoerster E, et al. Dorsal muscle group area and surgical outcomes in liver transplantation. Clin Transpl. 2014;28(10):1092–8.
59. Carey EJ, Lai JC, Wang CW, Dasarathy S, Lobach I, Montano-Loza AJ, et al. A multicenter study to define sarcopenia in patients with end-stage liver disease. Liver Transpl. 2017;23(5):625–33.
60. Tandon P, Montano-Loza AJ, Lai JC, Dasarathy S, Merli M. Sarcopenia and frailty in decompensated cirrhosis. J Hepatol. 2021;75(Suppl 1):S147–S62.
61. Sinclair M, Chapman B, Hoermann R, Angus PW, Testro A, Scodellaro T, et al. Handgrip strength adds more prognostic value to the model for end-stage liver disease score than imaging-based measures of muscle mass in men with cirrhosis. Liver Transpl. 2019;25(10):1480–7.
62. Qiu J, Thapaliya S, Runkana A, Yang Y, Tsien C, Mohan ML, et al. Hyperammonemia in cirrhosis induces transcriptional regulation of myostatin by an NF-kappaB-mediated mechanism. Proc Natl Acad Sci USA. 2013;110(45):18162–7.
63. Baczek J, Silkiewicz M, Wojszel ZB. Myostatin as a biomarker of muscle wasting and other pathologies-state of the art and knowledge gaps. Nutrients. 2020;12(8):2401.
64. Qiu J, Tsien C, Thapalaya S, Narayanan A, Weihl CC, Ching JK, et al. Hyperammonemia-mediated autophagy in skeletal muscle contributes to sarcopenia of cirrhosis. Am J Physiol Endocrinol Metab. 2012;303(8):E983–93.
65. Sinclair M, Grossmann M, Gow PJ, Angus PW. Testosterone in men with advanced liver disease: abnormalities and implications. J Gastroenterol Hepatol. 2015;30(2):244–51.
66. Kumar A, Davuluri G, Silva RNE, Engelen M, Ten Have GAM, Prayson R, et al. Ammonia lowering reverses sarcopenia of cirrhosis by restoring skeletal muscle proteostasis. Hepatology. 2017;65(6):2045–58.
67. Monegal A, Navasa M, Guanabens N, Peris P, Pons F, Martinez de Osaba MJ, et al. Osteoporosis and bone mineral metabolism disorders in cirrhotic patients referred for orthotopic liver transplantation. Calcif Tissue Int. 1997;60(2):148–54.
68. Abate EG, Vega MV, Rivas AM, Meek S, Yang L, Ball CT, et al. Evaluation of factors associated with fracture and loss of bone mineral density within 1 year after liver transplantation. Endocr Pract. 2021;27(5):426–32.
69. Jerman A, Lindic J, Skoberne A, Borstnar S, Martinuc Bergoc M, Godnov U, et al. Prevalence and risk factors for nonvertebral bone fractures in kidney transplant recipients—a single-center retrospective analysis. Clin Nephrol. 2017;88(13):101–8.
70. Kovvuru K, Kanduri SR, Vaitla P, Marathi R, Gosi S, Garcia Anton DF, et al. Risk factors and management of osteoporosis post-transplant. Medicina (Kaunas). 2020;56(6):302.
71. Kwong AJ, Kim WR, Lake JR, Smith JM, Schladt DP, Skeans MA, et al. OPTN/SRTR 2019 annual data report: liver. Am J Transplant. 2021;21(Suppl 2):208–315.
72. LaMattina JC, Foley DP, Fernandez LA, Pirsch JD, Musat AI, D'Alessandro AM, et al. Complications associated with liver transplantation in the obese recipient. Clin Transpl. 2012;26(6):910–8.
73. Engelmann C, Aehling NF, Schob S, Nonnenmacher I, Handmann L, Macnaughtan J, et al. Body fat composition determines outcomes before and after liver transplantation in patients with cirrhosis. Hepatol Commun. 2022;6(8):2198–209.
74. Dunn MA, Josbeno DA, Schmotzer AR, Tevar AD, DiMartini AF, Landsittel DP, et al. The gap between clinically assessed physical performance and objective physical activity in liver transplant candidates. Liver Transpl. 2016;22(10):1324–32.
75. Dharancy S, Lemyze M, Boleslawski E, Neviere R, Declerck N, Canva V, et al. Impact of impaired aerobic capacity on liver transplant candidates. Transplantation. 2008;86(8):1077–83.
76. Carey EJ, Steidley DE, Aqel BA, Byrne TJ, Mekeel KL, Rakela J, et al. Six-minute walk distance predicts mortality in liver transplant candidates. Liver Transpl. 2010;16(12):1373–8.
77. Grossmann M, Hoermann R, Gani L, Chan I, Cheung A, Gow PJ, et al. Low testosterone levels as an independent predictor of mortality in men with chronic liver disease. Clin Endocrinol (Oxf). 2012;77(2):323–8.

78. Kaplan DE, Serper M, John BV, Tessiatore KM, Lerer R, Mehta R, et al. Effects of metformin exposure on survival in a large national cohort of patients with diabetes and cirrhosis. Clin Gastroenterol Hepatol. 2021;19(10):2148–60 e14.
79. Vilar-Gomez E, Calzadilla-Bertot L, Wong VW, Castellanos M, Aller-de la Fuente R, Eslam M, et al. Type 2 diabetes and metformin use associate with outcomes of patients with nonalcoholic steatohepatitis-related, child-Pugh a cirrhosis. Clin Gastroenterol Hepatol. 2021;19(1):136–45.e6.
80. Cheung K, Lee SS, Raman M. Prevalence and mechanisms of malnutrition in patients with advanced liver disease, and nutrition management strategies. Clin Gastroenterol Hepatol. 2012;10(2):117–25.
81. Sam J, Nguyen GC. Protein-calorie malnutrition as a prognostic indicator of mortality among patients hospitalized with cirrhosis and portal hypertension. Liver Int. 2009;29(9):1396–402.
82. Ney M, Abraldes JG, Ma M, Belland D, Harvey A, Robbins S, et al. Insufficient protein intake is associated with increased mortality in 630 patients with cirrhosis awaiting liver transplantation. Nutr Clin Pract. 2015;30(4):530–6.
83. Nickkholgh A, Schneider H, Encke J, Buchler MW, Schmidt J, Schemmer P. PROUD: effects of preoperative long-term immunonutrition in patients listed for liver transplantation. Trials. 2007;8:20.
84. Booi AN, Menendez J, Norton HJ, Anderson WE, Ellis AC. Validation of a screening tool to identify undernutrition in ambulatory patients with liver cirrhosis. Nutr Clin Pract. 2015;30(5):683–9.
85. Bischoff SC, Bernal W, Dasarathy S, Merli M, Plank LD, Schutz T, et al. ESPEN practical guideline: clinical nutrition in liver disease. Nutr Hosp. 2022;39(2):434–72.
86. Mehta M, Louissaint J, Parikh NS, Long MT, Tapper EB. Cognitive function, sarcopenia, and inflammation are strongly associated with frailty: a Framingham cohort study. Am J Med. 2021;134(12):1530–8.
87. Murphy SL, Richardson JK, Blackwood J, Martinez B, Tapper EB. Neurocognitive and muscular capacities are associated with frailty in adults with cirrhosis. Dig Dis Sci. 2020;65(12):3734–43.
88. Bunce D, Batterham PJ, Mackinnon AJ. Long-term associations between physical frailty and performance in specific cognitive domains. J Gerontol B Psychol Sci Soc Sci. 2019;74(6):919–26.
89. Vilstrup H, Amodio P, Bajaj J, Cordoba J, Ferenci P, Mullen KD, et al. Hepatic encephalopathy in chronic liver disease: 2014 practice guideline by the American Association for the Study of Liver Diseases and the European Association for the Study of the Liver. Hepatology. 2014;60(2):715–35.
90. Das A, Dhiman RK, Saraswat VA, Verma M, Naik SR. Prevalence and natural history of subclinical hepatic encephalopathy in cirrhosis. J Gastroenterol Hepatol. 2001;16(5):531–5.
91. Ney M, Tangri N, Dobbs B, Bajaj J, Rolfson D, Ma M, et al. Predicting hepatic encephalopathy-related hospitalizations using a composite assessment of cognitive impairment and frailty in 355 patients with cirrhosis. Am J Gastroenterol. 2018;113(10):1506–15.
92. Felipo V. Hepatic encephalopathy: effects of liver failure on brain function. Nat Rev Neurosci. 2013;14(12):851–8.
93. Merli M, Giusto M, Lucidi C, Giannelli V, Pentassuglio I, Di Gregorio V, et al. Muscle depletion increases the risk of overt and minimal hepatic encephalopathy: results of a prospective study. Metab Brain Dis. 2013;28(2):281–4.
94. Bernardin F, Maheut-Bosser A, Paille F. Cognitive impairments in alcohol-dependent subjects. Front Psych. 2014;5:78.
95. Wijdicks EF. Hepatic encephalopathy. N Engl J Med. 2016;375(17):1660–70.
96. Bocarsly ME, Fasolino M, Kane GA, LaMarca EA, Kirschen GW, Karatsoreos IN, et al. Obesity diminishes synaptic markers, alters microglial morphology, and impairs cognitive function. Proc Natl Acad Sci USA. 2015;112(51):15731–6.
97. Miller AA, Spencer SJ. Obesity and neuroinflammation: a pathway to cognitive impairment. Brain Behav Immun. 2014;42:10–21.

98. Molteni R, Barnard RJ, Ying Z, Roberts CK, Gomez-Pinilla F. A high-fat, refined sugar diet reduces hippocampal brain-derived neurotrophic factor, neuronal plasticity, and learning. Neuroscience. 2002;112(4):803–14.
99. Cotter TG, Beresford T. Treatment of mental health in patients with chronic liver disease. Clin Liver Dis (Hoboken). 2022;20(2):57–60.
100. Mullish BH, Kabir MS, Thursz MR, Dhar A. Review article: depression and the use of antidepressants in patients with chronic liver disease or liver transplantation. Aliment Pharmacol Ther. 2014;40(8):880–92.
101. Singh N, Gayowski T, Wagener MM, Marino IR. Depression in patients with cirrhosis. Impact on outcome. Dig Dis Sci. 1997;42(7):1421–7.
102. Gedaly R, McHugh PP, Johnston TD, Jeon H, Koch A, Clifford TM, et al. Predictors of relapse to alcohol and illicit drugs after liver transplantation for alcoholic liver disease. Transplantation. 2008;86(8):1090–5.
103. Corruble E, Barry C, Varescon I, Durrbach A, Samuel D, Lang P, et al. Report of depressive symptoms on waiting list and mortality after liver and kidney transplantation: a prospective cohort study. BMC Psychiatry. 2011;11:182.
104. Al-Judaibi B, Alqalami I, Sey M, Qumosani K, Howes N, Sinclair L, et al. Exercise training for liver transplant candidates. Transplant Proc. 2019;51(10):3330–7.
105. Morkane CM, Kearney O, Bruce DA, Melikian CN, Martin DS. An outpatient hospital-based exercise training program for patients with cirrhotic liver disease awaiting transplantation: a feasibility trial. Transplantation. 2020;104(1):97–103.
106. Chen HW, Ferrando A, White MG, Dennis RA, Xie J, Pauly M, et al. Home-based physical activity and diet intervention to improve physical function in advanced liver disease: a randomized pilot trial. Dig Dis Sci. 2020;65(11):3350–9.
107. Wallen MP, Keating SE, Hall A, Hickman IJ, Pavey TG, Woodward AJ, et al. Exercise training is safe and feasible in patients awaiting liver transplantation: a pilot randomized controlled trial. Liver Transpl. 2019;25(10):1576–80.
108. Debette-Gratien M, Tabouret T, Antonini MT, Dalmay F, Carrier P, Legros R, et al. Personalized adapted physical activity before liver transplantation: acceptability and results. Transplantation. 2015;99(1):145–50.
109. Lin FP, Visina JM, Bloomer PM, Dunn MA, Josbeno DA, Zhang X, et al. Prehabilitation-driven changes in frailty metrics predict mortality in patients with advanced liver disease. Am J Gastroenterol. 2021;116(10):2105–17.
110. Zenith L, Meena N, Ramadi A, Yavari M, Harvey A, Carbonneau M, et al. Eight weeks of exercise training increases aerobic capacity and muscle mass and reduces fatigue in patients with cirrhosis. Clin Gastroenterol Hepatol. 2014;12(11):1920–6.e2.
111. Jetten WD, Hogenbirk RNM, Van Meeteren NLU, Cuperus FJC, Klaase JM, De Jong R. Physical effects, safety and feasibility of prehabilitation in patients awaiting orthotopic liver transplantation, a systematic review. Transpl Int. 2022;35:10330.
112. Garcia-Pagan JC, Santos C, Barbera JA, Luca A, Roca J, Rodriguez-Roisin R, et al. Physical exercise increases portal pressure in patients with cirrhosis and portal hypertension. Gastroenterology. 1996;111(5):1300–6.
113. Duarte-Rojo A, Bloomer PM, Rogers RJ, Hassan MA, Dunn MA, Tevar AD, et al. Introducing EL-FIT (exercise and liver FITness): a smartphone app to prehabilitate and monitor liver transplant candidates. Liver Transpl. 2021;27(4):502–12.
114. Meena BL, Taneja S, Tandon P, Sahni N, Soundararajan R, Gorsi U, et al. Home-based intensive nutrition therapy improves frailty and sarcopenia in patients with decompensated cirrhosis: a randomized clinical trial. J Gastroenterol Hepatol. 2023;38(2):210–8.
115. Park JG, Tak WY, Park SY, Kweon YO, Chung WJ, Jang BK, et al. Effects of branched-chain amino acid (BCAA) supplementation on the progression of advanced liver disease: a Korean nationwide, multicenter, prospective, observational, cohort study. Nutrients. 2020;12(5):1429.

116. Tsien C, Davuluri G, Singh D, Allawy A, Ten Have GA, Thapaliya S, et al. Metabolic and molecular responses to leucine-enriched branched chain amino acid supplementation in the skeletal muscle of alcoholic cirrhosis. Hepatology. 2015;61(6):2018–29.
117. Hume E, Ward L, Wilkinson M, Manifield J, Clark S, Vogiatzis I. Exercise training for lung transplant candidates and recipients: a systematic review. Eur Respir Rev. 2020;29(158):200053.
118. Wickerson L, Rozenberg D, Gottesman C, Helm D, Mathur S, Singer LG. Pre-transplant short physical performance battery: response to pre-habilitation and relationship to pre- and early post-lung-transplant outcomes. Clin Transpl. 2020;34(12):e14095.
119. Rozenberg D, Mathur S, Wickerson L, Chowdhury NA, Singer LG. Frailty and clinical benefits with lung transplantation. J Heart Lung Transplant. 2018;37(10):1245–53.
120. Koons B, Greenland JR, Diamond JM, Singer JP. Pathobiology of frailty in lung disease. Transl Res. 2020;221:1–22.
121. Schaenman JM, Diamond JM, Greenland JR, Gries C, Kennedy CC, Parulekar AD, et al. Frailty and aging-associated syndromes in lung transplant candidates and recipients. Am J Transplant. 2021;21(6):2018–24.
122. Martinu T, Babyak MA, O'Connell CF, Carney RM, Trulock EP, Davis RD, et al. Baseline 6-min walk distance predicts survival in lung transplant candidates. Am J Transplant. 2008;8(7):1498–505.
123. Singer JP, Diamond JM, Anderson MR, Katz PP, Covinsky K, Oyster M, et al. Frailty phenotypes and mortality after lung transplantation: a prospective cohort study. Am J Transplant. 2018;18(8):1995–2004.
124. Holeman TA, Peacock J, Beckstrom JL, Brooke BS. Patient-surgeon agreement in assessment of frailty, physical function, & social activity. J Surg Res. 2020;256:368–73.
125. Case AH, Hellkamp AS, Neely ML, Bender S, Dilling DF, Gulati M, et al. Associations between patient-reported outcomes and death or lung transplant in idiopathic pulmonary fibrosis. Data from the idiopathic pulmonary fibrosis prospective outcomes registry. Ann Am Thorac Soc. 2020;17(6):699–705.
126. Cruz-Jentoft AJ, Bahat G, Bauer J, Boirie Y, Bruyere O, Cederholm T, et al. Sarcopenia: revised European consensus on definition and diagnosis. Age Ageing. 2019;48(4):601.
127. Halpern AL, Boshier PR, White AM, Houk AK, Helmkamp L, Mitchell JD, et al. A comparison of frailty measures at listing to predict outcomes after lung transplantation. Ann Thorac Surg. 2020;109(1):233–40.
128. Rozenberg D, Wickerson L, Singer LG, Mathur S. Sarcopenia in lung transplantation: a systematic review. J Heart Lung Transplant. 2014;33(12):1203–12.
129. Agarwal A, Neujahr DC. Frailty in lung transplantation: candidate assessment and optimization. Transplantation. 2021;105(10):2201–12.
130. Rozenberg D, Orsso CE, Chohan K, Orchanian-Cheff A, Nourouzpour S, Nicholson JM, et al. Clinical outcomes associated with computed tomography-based body composition measures in lung transplantation: a systematic review. Transpl Int. 2020;33(12):1610–25.
131. Clausen ES, Frankel C, Palmer SM, Snyder LD, Smith PJ. Pre-transplant weight loss and clinical outcomes after lung transplantation. J Heart Lung Transplant. 2018;37(12):1443–7.
132. Singer JP, Peterson ER, Snyder ME, Katz PP, Golden JA, D'Ovidio F, et al. Body composition and mortality after adult lung transplantation in the United States. Am J Respir Crit Care Med. 2014;190(9):1012–21.
133. Bigelow B, Toci G, Etchill E, Krishnan A, Merlo C, Bush EL. Nutritional risk index: a predictive metric for mortality after lung transplant. Ann Thorac Surg. 2021;112(1):214–20.
134. Yamamoto H, Sugimoto S, Soh J, Shiotani T, Miyoshi K, Otani S, et al. The prognostic nutritional index is correlated negatively with the lung allocation score and predicts survival after both cadaveric and living-donor lobar lung transplantation. Surg Today. 2021;51(10):1610–8.
135. Upala S, Panichsillapakit T, Wijarnpreecha K, Jaruvongvanich V, Sanguankeo A. Underweight and obesity increase the risk of mortality after lung transplantation: a systematic review and meta-analysis. Transpl Int. 2016;29(3):285–96.

136. Soyseth TS, Lund MB, Bjortuft O, Heldal A, Soyseth V, Dew MA, et al. Psychiatric disorders and psychological distress in patients undergoing evaluation for lung transplantation: a national cohort study. Gen Hosp Psychiatry. 2016;42:67–73.
137. Vermeulen KM, Bosma OH, Bij W, Koeter GH, Tenvergert EM. Stress, psychological distress, and coping in patients on the waiting list for lung transplantation: an exploratory study. Transpl Int. 2005;18(8):954–9.
138. Pennington KM, Benzo RP, Schneekloth TD, Budev M, Chandrashekaran S, Erasmus DB, et al. Impact of affect on lung transplant candidate outcomes. Prog Transplant. 2020;30(1):13–21.
139. Courtwright AM, Salomon S, Lehmann LS, Wolfe DJ, Goldberg HJ. The effect of pretransplant depression and anxiety on survival following lung transplant: a meta-analysis. Psychosomatics. 2016;57(3):238–45.
140. Florian J, Watte G, Teixeira PJZ, Altmayer S, Schio SM, Sanchez LB, et al. Pulmonary rehabilitation improves survival in patients with idiopathic pulmonary fibrosis undergoing lung transplantation. Sci Rep. 2019;9(1):9347.
141. Hoffman M, Chaves G, Ribeiro-Samora GA, Britto RR, Parreira VF. Effects of pulmonary rehabilitation in lung transplant candidates: a systematic review. BMJ Open. 2017;7(2):e013445.
142. Maddocks M, Kon SS, Canavan JL, Jones SE, Nolan CM, Labey A, et al. Physical frailty and pulmonary rehabilitation in COPD: a prospective cohort study. Thorax. 2016;71(11):988–95.
143. Nyberg A, Martin M, Saey D, Milad N, Patoine D, Morissette MC, et al. Effects of low-load/high-repetition resistance training on exercise capacity, health status, and limb muscle adaptation in patients with severe COPD: a randomized controlled trial. Chest. 2021;159(5):1821–32.
144. Langer D. Rehabilitation in patients before and after lung transplantation. Respiration. 2015;89(5):353–62.
145. Jomphe V, Mailhot G, Damphousse V, Tahir MR, Receveur O, Poirier C, et al. The impact of waiting list BMI changes on the short-term outcomes of lung transplantation. Transplantation. 2018;102(2):318–25.
146. Denfeld QE, Winters-Stone K, Mudd JO, Gelow JM, Kurdi S, Lee CS. The prevalence of frailty in heart failure: a systematic review and meta-analysis. Int J Cardiol. 2017;236:283–9.
147. McDonagh J, Prichard R, Ferguson C, Phillips JL, Davidson PM, Macdonald PS, et al. Clinician estimates of frailty compared to formal frailty assessment in adults with heart failure: a cross-sectional analysis. Heart Lung Circ. 2022;31(9):1241–6.
148. Kobashigawa J, Dadhania D, Bhorade S, Adey D, Berger J, Bhat G, et al. Report from the American Society of Transplantation on frailty in solid organ transplantation. Am J Transplant. 2019;19(4):984–94.
149. Macdonald P. Frailty of the heart recipient. Transplantation. 2021;105(11):2352–61.
150. Drexler H, Riede U, Munzel T, Konig H, Funke E, Just H. Alterations of skeletal muscle in chronic heart failure. Circulation. 1992;85(5):1751–9.
151. Vescovo G, Volterrani M, Zennaro R, Sandri M, Ceconi C, Lorusso R, et al. Apoptosis in the skeletal muscle of patients with heart failure: investigation of clinical and biochemical changes. Heart. 2000;84(4):431–7.
152. Okoshi MP, Capalbo RV, Romeiro FG, Okoshi K. Cardiac cachexia: perspectives for prevention and treatment. Arq Bras Cardiol. 2017;108(1):74–80.
153. Evans WJ, Morley JE, Argiles J, Bales C, Baracos V, Guttridge D, et al. Cachexia: a new definition. Clin Nutr. 2008;27(6):793–9.
154. Anker SD, Ponikowski P, Varney S, Chua TP, Clark AL, Webb-Peploe KM, et al. Wasting as independent risk factor for mortality in chronic heart failure. Lancet. 1997;349(9058):1050–3.
155. Tsuji M, Kakuda N, Bujo C, Ishida J, Amiya E, Hatano M, et al. Sarcopenia and risk of infection in adult heart transplant recipients in Japan. ESC Heart Fail. 2022;9(2):1413–23.
156. Lopez-Sainz A, Barge-Caballero E, Barge-Caballero G, Couto-Mallon D, Paniagua-Martin MJ, Seoane-Quiroga L, et al. Late graft failure in heart transplant recipients: incidence, risk factors and clinical outcomes. Eur J Heart Fail. 2018;20(2):385–94.

157. Savage PA, Shaw AO, Miller MS, VanBuren P, LeWinter MM, Ades PA, et al. Effect of resistance training on physical disability in chronic heart failure. Med Sci Sports Exerc. 2011;43(8):1379–86.
158. Chung CJ, Wu C, Jones M, Kato TS, Dam TT, Givens RC, et al. Reduced handgrip strength as a marker of frailty predicts clinical outcomes in patients with heart failure undergoing ventricular assist device placement. J Card Fail. 2014;20(5):310–5.
159. Keller-Ross ML, Johnson BD, Carter RE, Joyner MJ, Eisenach JH, Curry TB, et al. Improved ventilatory efficiency with locomotor muscle afferent inhibition is strongly associated with leg composition in heart failure. Int J Cardiol. 2016;202:159–66.
160. Hulsmann M, Quittan M, Berger R, Crevenna R, Springer C, Nuhr M, et al. Muscle strength as a predictor of long-term survival in severe congestive heart failure. Eur J Heart Fail. 2004;6(1):101–7.
161. Kinugawa S, Takada S, Matsushima S, Okita K, Tsutsui H. Skeletal muscle abnormalities in heart failure. Int Heart J. 2015;56(5):475–84.
162. Koba S, Xing J, Sinoway LI, Li J. Sympathetic nerve responses to muscle contraction and stretch in ischemic heart failure. Am J Physiol Heart Circ Physiol. 2008;294(1):H311–21.
163. Arena R, Myers J, Williams MA, Gulati M, Kligfield P, Balady GJ, et al. Assessment of functional capacity in clinical and research settings: a scientific statement from the American Heart Association Committee on Exercise, Rehabilitation, and Prevention of the Council on Clinical Cardiology and the Council on Cardiovascular Nursing. Circulation. 2007;116(3):329–43.
164. Poty A, Krim F, Lopes P, Garaud Y, Lepretre PM. Benefits of a supervised ambulatory outpatient program in a cardiovascular rehabilitation unit prior to a heart transplant: a Case study. Front Cardiovasc Med. 2022;9:811458.
165. Mirza KK, Szymanski MK, Schmidt T, de Jonge N, Brahmbhatt DH, Billia F, et al. Prognostic value of peak oxygen uptake in patients supported with left ventricular assist devices (PRO-VAD). JACC Heart Fail. 2021;9(10):758–67.
166. Sato T, Yoshihisa A, Kanno Y, Suzuki S, Yamaki T, Sugimoto K, et al. Cardiopulmonary exercise testing as prognostic indicators: comparisons among heart failure patients with reduced, mid-range and preserved ejection fraction. Eur J Prev Cardiol. 2017;24(18):1979–87.
167. Josiak K, Jankowska EA, Piepoli MF, Banasiak W, Ponikowski P. Skeletal myopathy in patients with chronic heart failure: significance of anabolic-androgenic hormones. J Cachexia Sarcopenia Muscle. 2014;5(4):287–96.
168. Kerrigan DJ, Cowger JA, Keteyian SJ. Exercise in patients with left ventricular devices: the interaction between the device and the patient. Prog Cardiovasc Dis. 2022;70:33–9.
169. Tucker WJ, Beaudry RI, Samuel TJ, Nelson MD, Halle M, Baggish AL, et al. Performance limitations in heart transplant recipients. Exerc Sport Sci Rev. 2018;46(3):144–51.
170. Bussieres LM, Pflugfelder PW, Taylor AW, Noble EG, Kostuk WJ. Changes in skeletal muscle morphology and biochemistry after cardiac transplantation. Am J Cardiol. 1997;79(5):630–4.
171. Shimizu M, Hiraiwa H, Tanaka S, Tsuchikawa Y, Ito R, Kazama S, et al. Cardiac rehabilitation in severe heart failure patients with Impella 5.0 support via the subclavian artery approach prior to left ventricular assist device implantation. J Pers Med. 2023;13(4):630.
172. Gimeno-Santos E, Coca-Martinez M, Arguis MJ, Navarro R, Lopez-Hernandez A, Castel MA, et al. Multimodal prehabilitation as a promising strategy for preventing physical deconditioning on the heart transplant waiting list. Eur J Prev Cardiol. 2020;27(19):2367–70.
173. Nakaya Y, Akamatsu M, Ogimoto A, Kitaoka H. Early cardiac rehabilitation for acute decompensated heart failure safely improves physical function (PEARL study): a randomized controlled trial. Eur J Phys Rehabil Med. 2021;57(6):985–93.
174. Fisher S, Smart NA, Pearson MJ. Resistance training in heart failure patients: a systematic review and meta-analysis. Heart Fail Rev. 2022;27(5):1665–82.
175. Beckers PJ, Denollet J, Possemiers NM, Wuyts FL, Vrints CJ, Conraads VM. Combined endurance-resistance training vs. endurance training in patients with chronic heart failure: a prospective randomized study. Eur Heart J. 2008;29(15):1858–66.

176. Patti A, Merlo L, Ambrosetti M, Sarto P. Exercise-based cardiac rehabilitation programs in heart failure patients. Heart Fail Clin. 2021;17(2):263–71.
177. Toth MJ, Miller MS, VanBuren P, Bedrin NG, LeWinter MM, Ades PA, et al. Resistance training alters skeletal muscle structure and function in human heart failure: effects at the tissue, cellular and molecular levels. J Physiol. 2012;590(5):1243–59.
178. Nilsson BB, Westheim A, Risberg MA. Long-term effects of a group-based high-intensity aerobic interval-training program in patients with chronic heart failure. Am J Cardiol. 2008;102(9):1220–4.
179. McKelvie RS, Teo KK, Roberts R, McCartney N, Humen D, Montague T, et al. Effects of exercise training in patients with heart failure: the Exercise Rehabilitation Trial (EXERT). Am Heart J. 2002;144(1):23–30.
180. Belardinelli R, Georgiou D, Cianci G, Purcaro A. Randomized, controlled trial of long-term moderate exercise training in chronic heart failure: effects on functional capacity, quality of life, and clinical outcome. Circulation. 1999;99(9):1173–82.
181. Takada S, Sabe H, Kinugawa S. Treatments for skeletal muscle abnormalities in heart failure: sodium-glucose transporter 2 and ketone bodies. Am J Physiol Heart Circ Physiol. 2022;322(2):H117–H28.
182. Ferguson SK, Woessner MN, Holmes MJ, Belbis MD, Carlstrom M, Weitzberg E, et al. Effects of inorganic nitrate supplementation on cardiovascular function and exercise tolerance in heart failure. J Appl Physiol (1985). 2021;130(4):914–22.
183. Van Horn L, Carson JA, Appel LJ, Burke LE, Economos C, Karmally W, et al. Recommended dietary pattern to achieve adherence to the American Heart Association/American College of Cardiology (AHA/ACC) guidelines: a scientific statement from the American Heart Association. Circulation. 2016;134(22):e505–e29.
184. Sacks FM, Svetkey LP, Vollmer WM, Appel LJ, Bray GA, Harsha D, et al. Effects on blood pressure of reduced dietary sodium and the Dietary Approaches to Stop Hypertension (DASH) diet. DASH-Sodium Collaborative Research Group. N Engl J Med. 2001;344(1):3–10.
185. Chiavaroli L, Viguiliouk E, Nishi SK, Blanco Mejia S, Rahelic D, Kahleova H, et al. DASH dietary pattern and cardiometabolic outcomes: an umbrella review of systematic reviews and meta-analyses. Nutrients. 2019;11(2):338.
186. Appel LJ, Sacks FM, Carey VJ, Obarzanek E, Swain JF, Miller ER 3rd, et al. Effects of protein, monounsaturated fat, and carbohydrate intake on blood pressure and serum lipids: results of the OmniHeart randomized trial. JAMA. 2005;294(19):2455–64.

Prehabilitation for Infertility, Pregnancy, and the Postpartum Period

Sydney Diulus and Jaclyn Mirault

Pregnancy and the postpartum period are times of significant physical, psychological, and socioeconomic changes involving both the life of mother and baby. Prehabilitation may help to prepare for these changes and may even help them prepare to become pregnant. Because of the strong motivation for the healthiest pregnancy possible, it is also a time when patients can make lifestyle changes even though this can be difficult to do. This has the potential to lead to healthier families and hence healthier societies, so focusing on adopting healthier lifestyle changes surrounding pregnancy has both high stakes and high yield. Although this is an emerging field, available evidence shows significant benefits of prehabilitation for both mother and baby before pregnancy, while pregnant, and in the postpartum period.

1 Overview: The Continuum of Care in Pregnancy and the Postpartum Period

This is a general sequence of the steps that a patient can take while preparing for pregnancy, during pregnancy, and in the postpartum period to optimize their health and the health of the fetus.

- Preparing to become pregnant
- Lifestyle modifications during pregnancy
- Delivery
- Immediate postpartum period
- Long-term lifestyle changes

S. Diulus · J. Mirault (✉)
University of Pittsburgh Medical Center, Harrisburg, PA, USA
e-mail: diulussm2@upmc.edu; miraultj@upmc.edu

A. Watson, K. Barr (eds.), *A Prehabilitation Guide for All Providers*,
https://doi.org/10.1007/978-3-031-72862-4_10

2 Specialized Treatment Team

- Obstetrician & Gynecologist (OBGYN)—performs initial obstetric intake and evaluation, as well as subsequent prenatal care and delivery.
- Certified nurse midwife (CNM)—assists in care of pregnant patients during the prenatal period, intrapartum, and in the immediate postpartum period.
- Maternal & Fetal Medicine (MFM)—OBGYN specialists who care for pregnant patients who are categorized as high risk based on certain medical conditions including, but not limited to, preeclampsia, gestational diabetes, fetal congenital/developmental defects, multiple gestation pregnancy, and obesity.
- Physical therapist (PT)—experts in devising therapeutic exercise programs and increasing adherence to exercise.
- Pelvic floor physical therapists—these are PTs with additional training and expertise in rehabilitation of the pelvic floor musculature, which may be weakened during or after pregnancy.
- Physical trainers—can assist with the uptake and adherence of an exercise program but require additional education to have the expertise to understand changes to the musculoskeletal system and other aspects of exercising during this phase.
- Nutritionist/Dietician—specialists with added expertise in pregnancy who aid in the dietary needs of pregnant patients and help them to adhere to specific restrictive diets such as in patients with gestational diabetes.

Why Prehabilitation?

Although traditionally thought of in the setting of patients preparing for major surgeries, the principles of prehabilitation are applicable to pregnancy and childbirth. There are multiple lenses in which prehabilitation principles can be applied to this population:

1. Preparing the body and mind for the physiologic and psychological challenges of pregnancy.
2. Preventing or treating complications of pregnancy that can be mitigated through prehabilitation interventions such as low back pain and gestational diabetes.
3. Improving fetal outcomes through the promotion of healthy maternal habits.
4. Easing labor/improving recovery after cesarean section.
5. Hastening recovery to pre-pregnancy levels of physical performance after childbirth.

Pregnancy is an excellent time to make lifestyle changes to support health because of the high motivation that many patients feel and the frequent contact with healthcare professionals that can support behavioral change.

3 Preparing for Pregnancy: Preconception Prehabilitation

In the United States, only about half of pregnancies are planned [1]; although this percentage is rather low for a developed country, it still represents a significant number of patients who could benefit from applying prehabilitation principles in preparation for pregnancy. These modifications may help individuals to both achieve pregnancy and establish the foundation to maintain a healthy lifestyle throughout their pregnancy and into the postpartum period.

Exercise in Preparation for Pregnancy

Exercise and physical activity are important components in preparation for pregnancy. Recommendations for physical activity for healthy adults include at least 150 min (about 2½ h) of moderate-intensity exercise or 75 min of vigorous-intensity aerobic exercise/week [2]. When counseling patients regarding the effect of exercise on fertility, it is important to consider the patient's body mass index (BMI), current exercise routine, and underlying health conditions. One of the leading causes of female factor infertility is ovulatory dysfunction, with the most common form of anovulatory infertility being polycystic ovary syndrome (PCOS) [3]. PCOS is an endocrine disorder characterized by hyperandrogenism, oligomenorrhea or amenorrhea, and polycystic ovaries as identified by ultrasound. Two out of these three criteria must be met to establish a diagnosis [4]. Current research has shown that in patients diagnosed with PCOS, weight loss can lead not only to normal resumption of menses with lower levels of circulating androgens but also increased rates of spontaneous pregnancy [5, 6]. One study assessing the use of scheduled weekly exercise and dietary modifications in patients who were obese (BMI >30), showed that about 90% of patients who were previously anovulatory resumed normal ovulation cycles as compared to a control group [7]. A separate study concluded that in patients with diagnosed PCOS and morbid obesity (BMI >40) who underwent bariatric surgery, there was a significant decrease in health conditions like hypertension and type 2 diabetes mellitus as well as improvement in menstrual irregularities and fertility [8].

In a similar fashion, individuals who participate in intense physical activity, such as competitive athletes, can also have difficulty becoming pregnant. This effect is due to significant disruption in the hypothalamic-pituitary-ovarian (HPO) axis, leading to suppression of ovulation and low levels of estrogen [9]. This, in turn, leads to menstrual irregularities such as oligomenorrhea or amenorrhea. Menstrual irregularities tend to differ based on intensity, type, and frequency of exercise with the greatest effect noted to occur with athletes whose sport encourages a thin physique and low BMI [10]. Patients may counteract this effect by decreasing their exercise intensity or duration by at least 10% if possible and increasing caloric intake to promote weight gain.

When discussing exercise and fertility, patients should also be informed of exercise's effect on male factor infertility and sperm count. In one review of the literature, there was varying evidence and agreement on exercise's effect on male reproduction. The study concluded that there was evidence to prove that high-load exercise specifically, can influence the male reproductive system by means of physical stress exerting effects on the hypothalamic-pituitary-gonadal (HPG) axis, reproductive hormones, and testicular temperature [11]. In a separate study that assessed the effect of exercise on sperm concentration, volume, sperm motility, total motile sperm, and sperm morphology, it was found that none of these parameters were affected by regular exercise. However, the study did confirm previous research that suggests that using bicycling as the main form of exercise (>5 h/week) was associated with decreased sperm concentration and total motile sperm [12]. Given this information, moderate-intensity aerobic exercise for at least 30 min, 5 days/week should be recommended to male partners of patients wishing to conceive per the Physical Activities Guidelines for Americans [2].

Nutrition Recommendations Prior to Pregnancy

The diet in preparation for pregnancy is the same for all people. They should eat a diet that consists mainly of nutrient-dense foods that contain little to no added sugar or solid fats. This diet provides individuals with essential vitamins, minerals, fiber, and other important naturally occurring substances needed to support a healthy lifestyle. Special considerations are necessary for overweight and underweight patients. A prehabilitation plan before pregnancy should specifically outline a plan to address these issues. Obesity (BMI >30) is associated with infertility, miscarriage, stillbirth, birth defects, preterm birth, gestational diabetes, hypertensive disorders, and thromboembolic events during pregnancy [13]. However, weight loss should not come at the expense of meeting nutritional needs. It should therefore be approached with the goal of adopting lifelong healthy eating habits to achieve and maintain a normal BMI. Patients with an underweight BMI (<18.5) are at increased risk for delivering small for gestational age (SGA) and low birth weight infants [14]. In all women of reproductive age, it is recommended to take a prenatal vitamin containing at least 400 μg of folate daily at least 1 month prior to conception and to continue this well into the first trimester for prevention of neural tube defects (NTD) [15]. Patients with a history of a neonate with an NTD, or patients with a seizure disorder on certain medications, may require higher amounts of folate supplementation. In these cases, the increased recommendation is for 4 mg of folate for at least 3 months prior to conception. Similarly, patients who have certain gastrointestinal/malabsorptive disorders or those with a history of bariatric surgery may require further supplementation with specific vitamins and minerals to achieve an adequate nutritional status prior to pregnancy. Patients who follow a restrictive diet, such as a vegan diet, may benefit from consultation with a nutritionist with additional expertise in pregnancy to make sure nutritional needs are met prior to conception. Care should be taken to review all current medications, including prescription and over-the-counter supplements taken by the patient as many can be teratogenic, potentially causing harm to a fetus.

Other Healthy Behaviors to Adopt Prior to Pregnancy

Patients who use tobacco should be counseled regarding cessation. Desired pregnancy appears to be a strong motivator for smoking cessation according to CDC data, which shows that about 54% of patients will quit smoking directly prior to or during pregnancy [16]. Before attempting to achieve pregnancy, a discussion should be had with patients regarding alcohol cessation as there is no safe amount of alcohol use during pregnancy. Alcohol use may increase the risk of miscarriage and alcohol use while pregnant has been associated with fetal growth abnormalities, facial feature abnormalities, central nervous system, and behavioral disorders, including intellectual disability, with the most severe of these disorders being fetal alcohol syndrome (FAS) [17]. Because it may take several weeks between conception and a patient realizing they are pregnant, it makes sense to adopt healthy behaviors as soon as a patient desires pregnancy. For patients who believe they will have difficulty abstaining from alcohol use during pregnancy, this can be the time to make that change and obtain resources to help them abstain from alcohol prior to adding the stress of pregnancy.

Bariatric Surgery Prior to Pregnancy

Patients who are considering bariatric surgery for weight reduction should be counseled regarding its effects on future fertility and pregnancy outcomes. Significant and rapid weight reduction occurs after bariatric surgery, which leads to improvements in health outcomes such as decreased rates of hypertension and diabetes as well as improvements in menstrual irregularities and anovulatory cycles. However, bariatric surgery should not be considered as a treatment for infertility [18]. Patients should be informed that studies comparing maternal morbidity before and after bariatric surgery showed decreased rates of gestational hypertension, preeclampsia, and gestational diabetes [19, 20]. After undergoing bariatric surgery, patients should wait a minimum of 12–24 months before attempting to conceive due to the rapid weight changes and the possible nutritional deficiencies that occur immediately post-surgery which could potentially affect the fetus [21]. Common nutritional deficiencies for these patients include vitamin D, iron, vitamin B12, calcium, and folate, and should be replaced if a deficiency is found [22].

4 Pregnancy

Exercise During Pregnancy

The 2018 update to the U.S. Department of Health and Human Services Physical Activity Guidelines for Americans states that patients who are pregnant should follow the same guidelines as all other healthy people: perform at least 150 min of exercise/week with a typical exercise regimen of 30–60 min of moderate-intensity physical activity at least 3–4 days/week until time of delivery [2]. Patients who are already physically active and engage in vigorous aerobic exercise can continue to do so safely throughout their pregnancy. Patients who were less active or sedentary prior to pregnancy should begin exercise by gradually increasing their activity throughout the pregnancy, starting with low intensity, short periods of exercise. Extensive research demonstrates that walking, stationary cycling, aerobic exercises, dancing, resistance exercise (weights and elastic bands), stretching, and water aerobics are safe and beneficial for individuals during pregnancy [23]. Pregnant individuals should avoid contact sports and exercises that risk abdominal trauma. In patients who have uncomplicated pregnancies, studies have not shown any increased risk of miscarriage, poor fetal growth, musculoskeletal injury, or preterm delivery [24, 25] with regular exercise. In pregnant patients who exercise, there is higher incidence of vaginal birth and lower incidence of conditions such as gestational diabetes, excessive weight gain, hypertensive disorders, preterm birth, cesarean birth, and lower birth weight [23]. A 2017 systematic review showed that patients who performed aerobic exercise for 30–60 min about 2–7 times/week had significantly reduced risk of gestational hypertensive disorders, gestational diabetes, and cesarean birth compared with women who did not exercise [26, 27].

Patients must consider anatomic and physiologic changes associated with pregnancy when choosing an exercise routine. Breast volume and weight increase exponentially throughout pregnancy causing the shoulders to roll anteriorly, which may put some strain on the cervical spine and promote scapular dyskinesis [28]. Due to generalized weight gain and changes in the center of mass in the pregnant patient secondary to the gravid abdomen, a significant portion of patients develop lumbar lordosis and subsequently about 60% of patients report low back pain [28]. Performing strengthening and stretching exercises for abdominal and lower back musculature could help to minimize this risk. Aquatic-based exercise programs may be particularly beneficial for women who experience low back pain. One study measured a mean of 82.9% reduction of body weight during water immersion in pregnant patients in the third trimester, which lowered the maternal osteoarticular load due to buoyancy [29]. Patients may also benefit from referral to a licensed physical therapist (PT) for ongoing low back pain. PTs will not only be able to instruct patients on performing correct techniques for strengthening exercises but also provide patients with information regarding proper biomechanics while lifting relatively heavy objects, performing daily household activities, and remaining standing or seated for long periods of time [30].

Exercises that require a patient to lie supine for at least 20 min should be avoided after 20 weeks' gestation due to the risk of the gravid uterus compressing the inferior vena cava and leading to a decrease in venous return and potential hypotension [31]. It is recommended that pregnant patients follow common sense recommendations such as staying well hydrated, wearing loose-fitted clothing, and avoiding any added heat or humidity while exercising to avoid stress on the fetus [32]. For these reasons, aquatic therapies are especially beneficial as they improve heat dissipation. Although body temperatures increase secondary to hot tubs, saunas, and fever have been associated with NTDs, body temperature rise during exercise has not been shown to be associated with these conditions [33]. During exercise, there is a minimal to moderate increase in fetal heart rate (FHR) by about 10–30 beats/min [34]. Patients who continued to exercise during the third trimester delivered infants weighing 200–400 g less than comparable controls without any increased risk of intrauterine growth restriction (IUGR) [35]. One cohort study assessed fetal well-being before and after 30 min of strenuous exercise by measuring FHR, performing biophysical profiles (BPP), and assessing umbilical artery blood flow and found that exercise was well tolerated by fetuses [36]. In one RCT, patients who exercised with a birthing ball at least 3 times/week for 6–8 weeks during their pregnancy had a shorter length of the first stage of labor, decreased rates of epidural use, and decreased cesarean section rates [37]. The theory behind these benefits is that the birthing ball may help promote optimal fetal positioning within the pelvis due to gravity and the upright position while on the ball and it also may promote mobility of the pelvis [38].

When NOT to Recommend Exercise in Pregnancy

Exercise during pregnancy should be discontinued if patients develop any acute symptoms such as vaginal bleeding, leakage of fluid, abdominal pain, regular painful contractions, dyspnea before exertion, dizziness, headache, chest pain, muscle weakness affecting balance, and calf pain or swelling. Absolute contraindications to exercise include patients with preeclampsia, severe cardiovascular or pulmonary disease, patients with preterm prelabor rupture of membranes at risk for preterm labor, or patients with an incompetent cervix or cerclage in place. Relative contraindications include patients with poorly controlled seizure disorders, poorly controlled hypertension or diabetes, unevaluated maternal cardiac arrhythmias or those with orthopedic limitations [39].

Nutrition and Pregnancy

Broadly, pregnant patients should increase their nutritional intake by about 100–300 kcal/day [40]. During pregnancy, demand for protein increases due to the development of the growing fetus, uterus, placenta, breasts, and expansion of maternal blood volume, and patients should consume at *least* 1.1 g/kg/day of protein in their diet [39], preferably from animal sources such as meat, dairy, poultry, fish, and eggs as they contain additional nutrients and minerals necessary for fetal development. Almost all standard diets in the U.S. contain the proper amount of minerals to maintain adequate nutrition during pregnancy without supplementation except for iron. About 1000 mg of iron is required throughout a normal pregnancy. Of this total, 300 mg is transported to the fetus and placenta, 500 mg is used for the creation of erythrocytes for the expansion of maternal blood volume, and another 200 mg is lost through normal excretion by means of the gastrointestinal tract. Most of the iron is utilized in the second half of pregnancy, about 6–7 mg/day [39]. Most patients have neither sufficient iron reserves nor obtain enough iron through their diets to meet these requirements, so the American College of Obstetricians & Gynecologists

(ACOG) and American Academy of Pediatrics (AAP) recommend a prenatal vitamin that includes at least 27 mg of iron daily. In addition, iodine is important for fetal development but may not be in sufficient quantities in all diets. Individuals require the use of iodized salt and bread products to meet iodine intake requirements. Vitamin B12 levels should remain adequate in most pregnant patients who eat a diet consisting of animal proteins; however, pregnant individuals who consume a vegan or vegetarian diet may be insufficient without supplementation. Vitamin D deficiency is common in the general population and particularly in high-risk groups of pregnant patients such as vegetarians, individuals with darker complexions, and those with limited sun exposure [39] (Table 1).

When designing a nutritional strategy for pregnant patients, there are foods to avoid or to consume in limited amounts. Although the association between caffeine and fetal anomalies is unclear, pregnant patients should consume less than 200 mg/day of caffeine (approximately 2 cups of coffee) as research suggests the amount is likely safe with no association with increased rates of preterm labor or miscarriage [39]. Foodborne infections can have potentially life-threatening effects on the fetus and dictate many dietary recommendations in pregnancy. *Listeria monocytogenes* is a Gram-positive bacterium that can be found naturally throughout the environment but poses an increased risk of infection in pregnant patients, about 13 times that of the non-pregnant population [41]. Infection with this bacterium can lead to complications such as intrauterine fetal demise (IUFD), preterm labor, neonatal meningitis, and neonatal sepsis [42]. Foods that are easily contaminated with Listeria include deli/lunch meat, unwashed raw produce, raw (unpasteurized) soft cheeses and milk, and refrigerated smoked seafood. Patients should be instructed to avoid and properly prepare these foods to decrease their risk of infection. Patients should also avoid certain species of large fish and seafood that contain high levels of mercury, as it can cross the placenta and lead to a range of neurological disorders in the neonate. Examples of these types of fish include king mackerel, big eye tuna, orange roughie, and swordfish [39].

Table 1 Daily dietary recommendations for pregnant patients [39]

Vitamins/minerals	Daily dietary recommendations
Calcium	1000 mg/day
Iron	27 mg/day
Vitamin B6	6 mg/day
Vitamin B12	2.6 µg/day
Vitamin D	600 IU/day
Folate	600 µg/day
Carbohydrates	175 g/day (minimum)
Protein	1.1 g/kg/day (minimum)
Total fat	20–35% of total caloric intake

Other Healthy Behaviors

Patients who use tobacco, alcohol, or illicit substances should discontinue these prior to pregnancy; however, many will continue to use them throughout their pregnancy. Patients should understand that tobacco use during pregnancy increases their risk for conditions such as placenta previa, placental abruption, PPROM, orofacial clefts, IUGR, and low birth weight infants [43, 44]. Infants of mothers who have used tobacco during pregnancy also have increased rates of respiratory infections, asthma, bone fractures, and obesity [45, 46]. Motivational interviewing and cognitive behavioral therapy (CBT) are the two most efficacious non-pharmacologic strategies for promoting smoking cessation for pregnant patients. Patients should be informed that smoking cessation at any gestational age for any length of time will have positive effects on the outcome of the pregnancy but that the greatest benefit appears to occur with cessation prior to 15 weeks' gestation [47].

Prenatal Appointments

After the first prenatal visit, ideally completed within the first trimester between 8 and 13 weeks' gestation, follow-up appointments are recommended every 4 weeks until week 28. Appointments should then occur every 2 weeks until week 36 and finally once weekly until delivery unless complications arise, which would necessitate more frequent visits [39]. These are unique opportunities to promote improvement in lifestyle between a physician and their patient and may not occur again in the patient's lifetime. At each subsequent prenatal appointment, the well-being of the mother and fetus is evaluated. In addition to accepted medical practices such as obtaining a fetal heart rate, fundal height, maternal blood pressure and weight, determination of fetal activity, and any new or worsening symptoms, prehabilitation principles should be reinforced. In patients with no known risk factors, screening for gestational diabetes should occur between 24 and 28 weeks gestation.

Lifestyle Modification in Association with Gestational Diabetes Mellitus

Gestational diabetes mellitus (GDM) is a form of diabetes induced by physiologic changes to insulin sensitivity during pregnancy. Clinicians further classify GDM into categories of "diet-controlled," (also known as class A1GDM) and GDM in which medication is required to achieve euglycemia (also known as class A2GDM) [38]. About 6% of all pregnancies in 2016 were affected by some form of GDM [39]. Women with GDM have an increased risk of developing preeclampsia, undergoing cesarean section, and developing diabetes later in life [48, 49]. These patients also experience an increased risk of fetal macrosomia, shoulder dystocia, and birth trauma to the fetus like brachial plexus injuries or humeral fractures [50]. As this disorder is associated with many medical comorbidities for the mother and fetus, screening should be completed for all pregnant patients. Patients with GDM require referral to a registered dietician who can provide accurate counseling regarding diet and exercise to prevent ketosis, maintain proper blood glucose control, and ensure proper weight gain throughout pregnancy [51]. Regarding diet, about 33–40% of total calories throughout the day should come from carbohydrates, preferably complex carbohydrates as these are digested slower which helps to minimize postprandial hyperglycemia. About 20% of total calories should come from lean protein and the remaining 40% should come from healthy fats [52]. Exercise regimens for patients with GDM mirror those recommended for all pregnant patients, as there are currently only a few studies published with small sample sizes evaluating the role of exercise in GDM management.

Weight Gain During Pregnancy

The Institute of Medicine continues to update and publish recommendations by the World Health Organization (WHO) regarding weight gain during pregnancy using pre-pregnancy BMI [53]. If a patient's pre-pregnancy BMI is within the normal range (18.5–24.9), they are recommended to gain between 25 and 35 pounds throughout their pregnancy, with a rate of about 1 pound/week in the second and third trimesters. Patients with a pre-pregnancy BMI that is considered underweight (<18.5) should plan to gain between 28 and 40 pounds, again with an average of about 1 pound/week within the second and third trimesters. Patients with a BMI of 25–29.9 (overweight category) should plan to gain between 15 and 25 pounds, gaining an average of 0.6 pounds/week in the second and third trimesters. Lastly, patients who are considered obese (BMI >30) should plan to gain between 11 and 20 pounds, gaining an average of 0.5 pounds/week within the second and third trimesters [39]. These guidelines have met controversy specifically regarding guidelines for weight gain for patients who are overweight or obese. Several studies have shown that overweight women who gained an average of 6–14 pounds during their pregnancy had similar outcomes regarding fetal growth and neonatal health but with less difficulty with postpartum weight retention [54]. Recommendations for weight gain targets should be given based on the initial BMI obtained at the pregnant patient's first prenatal visit. Individualized discussion is needed, especially for patients with high BMIs who may wish to restrict weight gain.

Sleep During Pregnancy

Difficulty sleeping is common during pregnancy. Hormonal changes associated with pregnancy, including increased levels of estrogen and progesterone, can affect sleep patterns. Although length of sleep generally increases in the first trimester, it decreases by the third trimester with rising incidence of sleep disorders. In the first trimester, frequent waking due to urinary frequency, back pain, and nausea/vomiting can all contribute to poor sleep quality. Restless leg syndrome is more common during pregnancy and contributes to difficulty falling asleep and worse sleep quality. In addition, pregnant patients are at increased risk for obstructive sleep apnea in the third trimester due to weight gain and generalized edema, which itself increases the risk for preeclampsia and gestational hypertension. Insomnia generally worsens immediately before labor due to increased production of oxytocin, which promotes wakefulness. Poor sleep late in pregnancy is associated with increases in inflammatory markers. Women with sleep deprivation, defined as less than 5 h of sleep per night, are at increased risk for preterm birth. Commonly used medications for sleep, including benzodiazepines and hypnotic GABA receptor agonists (Zolpidem, Eszopiclone) are known to cross the placenta and are associated with adverse effects such as neonatal withdrawal syndrome and "floppy baby" syndrome, although studies to date have not shown an increased risk for congenital defects. Some studies have shown an increase in preterm labor, cesarean section, and SGA/low birth weight infants. Diphenhydramine is commonly used as a sleep aid and is generally considered safe in pregnancy with no known association with congenital effects [55].

5 Intrapartum Course

Labor Course and Vaginal Delivery

Before labor or induction of labor, patients should be counseled about their pain management options throughout the labor course. Pharmacologic options for pain control throughout labor include the use of inhaled nitrous oxide (NO) gas, intravenous or intramuscular opioids, or neuraxial analgesia by means of a spinal or epidural. Epidural anesthesia has been shown to have no effect on rates of cesarean section or operative deliveries although it may slightly lengthen the second stage of labor. Patients who wish to proceed through labor without medication should be encouraged to do so. Non-pharmacologic pain control strategies include massage, acupuncture, water immersion, use of heat/cold packs, maternal position changes, and continuous labor support by a trained labor support person (i.e., doula) [56].

There are many factors that influence the rate at which labor progresses. Patients may ask about adjunctive considerations studied regarding decreasing the total labor length. These include continuous one-to-one maternal support, peanut support ball usage, frequent position changes and ambulation, perineal massage, and water immersion. Throughout the labor course, a peanut support ball may be placed between the patient's knees while in the lateral recumbent position to widen the pelvis and promote fetal head descent to decrease the length of labor. However, a recent systematic review showed that there was no significant difference in the time of labor or incidence of vaginal or cesarean delivery with the use of a peanut support ball [57]. Ambulation and upright positions should be encouraged during the labor course, as this has been shown to decrease the length of the first stage of labor by over an hour and decrease rates of cesarean section. Studies concluded there was no significant difference in labor length with the use of perineal massage, water immersion, or acupuncture/acupressure [58].

When preparing for a vaginal delivery, many patients may have questions about how to prevent the risk of perineal laceration or trauma at the time of delivery. About 53–79% of patients will sustain some form of laceration at the time of delivery, with the most common being a second-degree perineal laceration [59]. There are multiple different methods that are currently used in practice and that have been studied regarding efficacy including perineal massage (antepartum and at time of delivery), warm compress use, perineal support at the time of delivery of the fetal head, delayed pushing and specific birthing positions. In one analysis of multiple randomized controlled trials, perineal massage after 34 weeks gestation and onward showed a modest reduction in perineal laceration and episiotomy rate in women who have had a prior vaginal delivery [60]. The most effective technique to decrease morbidity appears to be placing a warm compress at the perineum throughout the labor process, effectively decreasing rates of third and fourth-degree perineal lacerations [61] (Table 2).

Enhanced Recovery After Surgery (ERAS) Protocol for Cesarean Section

Cesarean section is one of the most common surgical procedures performed in the US. Indications for cesarean section include fetal malpresentation, arrest of the first or second stage of labor, failed operative vaginal delivery, non-reassuring fetal heart rate, cord prolapse, placenta previa, placenta accreta spectrum, and history of prior uterine surgery including prior cesarean section. With this procedure being so common, protocols to implement optimization using ERAS pathways have been put into place [63].

Prehabilitation for planned cesarean section is lacking in the literature. Patients undergoing a planned cesarean section should be encouraged to follow the lifestyle

Table 2 Defining degree of perineal lacerations and evidence to support prevention [62]

Degree of laceration	Definition	Evidence
First	Injury to perineal skin only	No evidence to support the prevention
Second	Injury to perineal skin and perineal muscles only	No evidence to support the prevention
Third	Injury to perineum that also involves anal sphincter complex 3a: Injury to <50% of external anal sphincter 3b: Injury to >50% of external anal sphincter 3c: Injury to both external and internal anal sphincters	Perineal massage in women with a history of prior vaginal delivery, warm compress use
Fourth	Injury through perineum, external and internal anal sphincter complex, and anal mucosa/epithelium	Perineal massage in women with a history of prior vaginal delivery, warm compress use

modifications for all pregnant patients listed above. ERAS protocol states that patients should be allowed to have a light meal about 6 h prior to their scheduled cesarean section and should be encouraged to drink clear liquids until about 2 h before the procedure [63]. Carbohydrate fluid supplementation may be offered 2 h prior to surgery for all non-diabetic patients, although a Cochrane Review found only a slight decrease in the length of hospital stay and a decrease in the time to flatus with the use of supplementation [64].

After the procedure, early mobilization should be encouraged although the evidence level for this is low as there are currently no studies evaluating early vs. delayed mobilization after cesarean section [65]. Still, it is theorized that encouragement of early mobilization promotes quicker return of bowel function, decreases the likelihood of developing a venous thromboembolism, and decreases the time to discharge. Barriers to early mobilization include indwelling Foley catheters and uncontrolled pain in the postoperative period, so these should be areas of focus when managing postoperative cesarean section patients. Regarding the postoperative diet, studies show that early versus delayed feeding (early feeding is defined as between 30 min to about 8 h postoperative [66, 67]) decreases patient length of stay without increasing readmission rates, improves maternal satisfaction, and promotes earlier ambulation [68]. A diet consisting of dairy, fruits, and vegetables should be encouraged for all patients, especially for those who are breastfeeding, along with a diet high in fiber to decrease rates of constipation [65].

6 Postpartum Period: Continuing Prehabilitation Lifestyle Changes and Postpartum Rehabilitation Strategies

Lifestyle Modification

Patients should be supported to achieve a healthy BMI, which may include returning to their pre-pregnancy weight and trying to achieve a normal BMI (18.5–24.9) before becoming pregnant again [13]. For patients desiring future pregnancies, studies have shown that a reduction in BMI improves perinatal outcomes while postpartum weight retention or weight gain has been associated with increased risk for gestational diabetes, hypertensive disorders, stillbirth, large-for-gestational age (LGA) neonates, cesarean section, and long-term obesity [69]. Patients with a BMI >40 or BMI >35 with at least one serious medical comorbidity who desire weight loss may reasonably consult with a bariatric surgeon in the postpartum period. Studies comparing pregnancies before and after bariatric surgery have shown decreased rates of gestational diabetes and hypertension and improved fertility in these patients [70, 71]. Continued support and encouragement to maintain smoking cessation is needed in the postpartum period as 50–60% of women who quit smoking prior to or during pregnancy will begin to smoke again within 1 year postpartum [72].

Exercise

Depending on the route of delivery (vaginal versus cesarean section) and the presence of medical or surgical complications, patients may gradually reintroduce exercise within days of delivery [73]. Reestablishing prior exercise routines is important for maintaining a healthy lifestyle after delivery. Patients may want to start increasing their activity by starting with easy-to-perform exercises like walking and can continue to increase the intensity and frequency of exercise as they progress through the postpartum period. In patients with an obstetrical laceration or who underwent cesarean section, water immersion exercises should be avoided for the first 6 weeks postpartum [74]. To decrease the risk of diastasis recti abdominis, patients may want to perform therapies like abdominal crunch exercises as well as the drawing-in exercise, which increases abdominal pressure by pulling in the abdominal wall musculature [75]. As encouraged during pregnancy, common sense recommendations when exercising in the postpartum period include gradually increasing exercise as able, increasing water intake for proper hydration, and wearing supportive bras due to the increase in the weight of the breasts secondary to lactation [74].

Breastfeeding

ACOG recommends exclusively breastfeeding for the first 6 months after birth (as able), then continuing to supplement with breast milk while foods are being introduced into a child's diet from 6 months to 1 year, or as long as a mother desires to breastfeed. Benefits of breastfeeding include ideal nutritional composition for developing infants, improved immunologic support in the early months of life, lower costs when compared to formula feeding, and lower rates of diabetes, hypertension, and certain cancers in breastfeeding mothers. However, breastfeeding can be challenging with only 25.4% of patients successfully breastfeeding at 6 months, with 45% of patients reporting early weaning despite a desire to continue breastfeeding [76]. Challenges to breastfeeding include difficulty latching, breast pain, mastitis, insufficient milk production, and societal barriers such as short maternity leave or inability to breastfeed while at work [77]. Negative experiences with breastfeeding increase the patient's risk for the development of postpartum depression.

Studies have shown that regular aerobic exercise does not affect milk production, composition or infant growth for patients who are breastfeeding. Regular exercise can be performed safely in breastfeeding patients who are consuming at least 1500 kcal/day and in those whose caloric intake does not fall more than 25% below caloric expenditure. In patients who wish to lose weight while breastfeeding, recommendations are to lose a maximum of 1 pound/week to ensure no changes to milk supply that could theoretically occur with more rapid weight loss [77]. Breastfeeding should also be encouraged immediately prior to exercise as this may help to decrease the size and weight of the breasts, therefore decreasing potential discomfort [74].

Postpartum Depression

Perinatal depression affects 1 in 7 patients, with about 40% of patients experiencing onset in the postpartum period [78]. Because of this, ACOG recommends that all patients be screened in the postpartum period for anxiety and depression. Risk factors for postpartum depression include a personal or family history of depression, lack of partner support, intimate partner violence, insomnia, incarceration, unemployment, or a history of other mental health disorders. Postpartum patients should be encouraged to take a holistic approach regarding their well-being by minimizing stressors when possible, getting adequate sleep, exercising regularly, and asking for support when needed [79]. Other options for management include cognitive behavioral therapy or pharmacotherapy with SSRIs or SNRIs.

References

1. Troutman M, Rafique S, Plowden TC. Are higher unintended pregnancy rates among minorities a result of disparate access to contraception? Contracept Reprod Med. 2020;5:1–6.
2. Elgaddal N, Kramarow EA, Reuben C. Physical activity among adults aged 18 and over: United States, 2020. NCHS Data Brief. 2022;443:1.
3. Hakimi O, Cameron L-C. Effect of exercise on ovulation: a systematic review. Sports Med. 2017;47:1555–67.
4. The Rotterdam ESHRE/ASRM-Sponsored PCOS Consensus Workshop Group. Revised 2003 consensus on diagnostic criteria and long-term health risks related to polycystic ovary syndrome. Fertil Steril. 2004;81(1):19–25.
5. Huber-Buchholz M-M, Carey D, Norman R. Restoration of reproductive potential by lifestyle modification in obese polycystic ovary syndrome: role of insulin sensitivity and luteinizing hormone. J Clin Endocrinol Metabol. 1999;84(4):1470–4.
6. Guzick DS, Wing R, Smith D, Berga SL, Winters SJ. Endocrine consequences of weight loss in obese, hyperandrogenic, anovulatory women. Fertil Steril. 1994;61(4):598–604.
7. Clark A, Thornley B, Tomlinson L, Galletley C, Norman R. Weight loss in obese infertile women results in improvement in reproductive outcome for all forms of fertility treatment. Hum Reprod (Oxford, England). 1998;13(6):1502–5.
8. Escobar-Morreale HF, Botella-Carretero JI, Alvarez-Blasco F, Sancho J, San Millán JL. The polycystic ovary syndrome associated with morbid obesity may resolve after weight loss induced by bariatric surgery. J Clin Endocrinol Metabol. 2005;90(12):6364–9.
9. Warren MP, Perlroth N. Hormones and sport-the effects of intense exercise on the female reproductive system. J Endocrinol. 2001;170(1):3–12.
10. Loucks AB. Physical health of the female athlete: observations, effects, and causes of reproductive disorders. Can J Appl Physiol. 2001;26(S1):S176–85.
11. du Plessis S, Kashou A, Vaamonde D, Agarwal A. Is there a link between exercise and male factor infertility? Open Reprod Sci J. 2011;3(1):105.
12. Wise LA, Cramer DW, Hornstein MD, Ashby RK, Missmer SA. Physical activity and semen quality among men attending an infertility clinic. Fertil Steril. 2011;95(3):1025–30.
13. ACOG Practice Bulletin No 156: obesity in pregnancy. Obstet Gynecol. 2015;126(6):e112–26.
14. Yu Z, Han S, Zhu J, Sun X, Ji C, Guo X. Pre-pregnancy body mass index in relation to infant birth weight and offspring overweight/obesity: a systematic review and meta-analysis. PLoS One. 2013;8(4):e61627.

15. Chitayat D, Matsui D, Amitai Y, Kennedy D, Vohra S, Rieder M, et al. Folic acid supplementation for pregnant women and those planning pregnancy: 2015 update. J Clin Pharmacol. 2016;56(2):170–5.
16. Tong VT, Dietz PM, Morrow B, D'Angelo DV, Farr SL, Rockhill KM, et al. Trends in smoking before, during, and after pregnancy—pregnancy risk assessment monitoring system, United States, 40 sites, 2000–2010. MMWR Surveill Summ. 2013;62(6):1–19.
17. American College of Obstetricians and Gynecologists. At-risk drinking and alcohol dependence: obstetric and gynecologic implications. Committee Opinion No. 496. Obstet Gynecol. 2011;118:383–8.
18. Merhi ZO. Weight loss by bariatric surgery and subsequent fertility. Fertil Steril. 2007;87(2):430–2.
19. Richards D, Miller D, Goodman G. Pregnancy after gastric bypass for morbid obesity. J Reprod Med. 1987;32(3):172–6.
20. Maggard MA, Yermilov I, Li Z, Maglione M, Newberry S, Suttorp M, et al. Pregnancy and fertility following bariatric surgery: a systematic review. JAMA. 2008;300(19):2286–96.
21. Apovian CM, Baker C, Ludwig DS, Hoppin AG, Hsu G, Lenders C, et al. Best practice guidelines in pediatric/adolescent weight loss surgery. Obes Res. 2005;13(2):274–82.
22. Wittgrove AC, Jester L, Wittgrove P, Clark GW. Pregnancy following gastric bypass for morbid obesity. Obes Surg. 1998;8(4):461–4.
23. Berghella V, Saccone G. Exercise in pregnancy! Am J Obstet Gynecol. 2017;216(4):335–7.
24. de Oliveria Melo AS, Silva JLP, Tavares JS, Barros VO, Leite DF, Amorim MM. Effect of a physical exercise program during pregnancy on uteroplacental and fetal blood flow and fetal growth: a randomized controlled trial. Obstet Gynecol. 2012;120(2 Part 1):302–10.
25. Barakat R, Pelaez M, Montejo R, Refoyo I, Coteron J. Exercise throughout pregnancy does not cause preterm delivery: a randomized, controlled trial. J Phys Act Health. 2014;11(5):1012–7.
26. Di Mascio D, Magro-Malosso ER, Saccone G, Marhefka GD, Berghella V. Exercise during pregnancy in normal-weight women and risk of preterm birth: a systematic review and meta-analysis of randomized controlled trials. Am J Obstet Gynecol. 2016;215(5):561–71.
27. Magro-Malosso ER, Saccone G, Di Tommaso M, Roman A, Berghella V. Exercise during pregnancy and risk of gestational hypertensive disorders: a systematic review and meta-analysis. Acta Obstet Gynecol Scand. 2017;96(8):921–31.
28. Harrison KD, Mancinelli C, Thomas K, Meszaros P, McCrory JL. The relationship between lower extremity alignment and low back, hip, and foot pain during pregnancy: a longitudinal study of primigravid women versus nulliparous controls. J Womens Pelvic Health Phys Ther. 2016;40(3):139–46.
29. Alberton CL, Bgeginski R, Pinto SS, Nunes GN, Andrade LS, Brasil B, et al. Water-based exercises in pregnancy: apparent weight in immersion and ground reaction force at third trimester. Clin Biomech. 2019;67:148–52.
30. Pain CP. ACOG practice bulletin number 218. Obstet Gynecol. 2020;3:e98–109.
31. Clark SL, Cotton DB, Pivarnik JM, Lee W, Hankins GD, Benedetti TJ, et al. Position change and central hemodynamic profile during normal third-trimester pregnancy and post partum. Am J Obstet Gynecol. 1991;164(3):883–7.
32. Liguori G, Medicine ACoS. ACSM's guidelines for exercise testing and prescription. Lippincott Williams & Wilkins; 2020.
33. Milunsky A, Ulcickas M, Rothman KJ, Willett W, Jick SS, Jick H. Maternal heat exposure and neural tube defects. JAMA. 1992;268(7):882–5.
34. Carpenter MW, Sady SP, Hoegsberg B, Sady MA, Haydon B, Cullinane EM, et al. Fetal heart rate response to maternal exertion. JAMA. 1988;259(20):3006–9.
35. Leet T, Flick L. Effect of exercise on birthweight. Clin Obstet Gynecol. 2003;46(2):423–31.
36. Szymanski LM, Satin AJ. Exercise during pregnancy: fetal responses to current public health guidelines. Obstet Gynecol. 2012;119(3):603–10.
37. Gau M-L, Chang C-Y, Tian S-H, Lin K-C. Effects of birth ball exercise on pain and self-efficacy during childbirth: a randomised controlled trial in Taiwan. Midwifery. 2011;27(6):e293–300.
38. Perez P. Birth balls: use of physical therapy balls in maternity care. Cutting Edge Press; 2000.

39. Cunningham FG, Leveno KJ, Bloom SL, Spong CY, Dashe JS, Hoffman BL, et al. Williams obstetrics. New York: McGraw-Hill Medical; 2014.
40. Williamson C. Nutrition in pregnancy. Nutr Bull. 2006;31(1):28–59.
41. Silk BJ, Date KA, Jackson KA, Pouillot R, Holt KG, Graves LM, et al. Invasive listeriosis in the Foodborne Diseases Active Surveillance Network (FoodNet), 2004–2009: further targeted prevention needed for higher-risk groups. Clin Infect Dis. 2012;54(Suppl_5):S396–404.
42. Mylonakis E, Paliou M, Hohmann EL, Calderwood SB, Wing EJ. Listeriosis during pregnancy: a case series and review of 222 cases. Medicine. 2002;81(4):260–9.
43. Castles A, Adams EK, Melvin CL, Kelsch C, Boulton ML. Effects of smoking during pregnancy: five meta-analyses. Am J Prev Med. 1999;16(3):208–15.
44. Spinillo A, Nicola S, Piazzi G, Ghazal K, Colonna L, Baltaro F. Epidemiological correlates of preterm premature rupture of membranes. Int J Gynecol Obstet. 1994;47(1):7–15.
45. Li Y-F, Langholz B, Salam MT, Gilliland FD. Maternal and grandmaternal smoking patterns are associated with early childhood asthma. Chest. 2005;127(4):1232–41.
46. Ayubi E, Safiri S, Mansori K. Association between maternal smoking during pregnancy and risk of bone fractures in offspring: a systematic review and meta-analysis. Clin Exp Pediatr. 2021;64(3):96.
47. Siu AL, U.S. Preventive Services Task Force. Behavioral and pharmacotherapy interventions for tobacco smoking cessation in adults, including pregnant women: US Preventive Services Task Force recommendation statement. Ann Intern Med. 2015;163(8):622–34.
48. Yogev Y, Xenakis EM, Langer O. The association between preeclampsia and the severity of gestational diabetes: the impact of glycemic control. Am J Obstet Gynecol. 2004;191(5):1655–60.
49. England LJ, Dietz PM, Njoroge T, Callaghan WM, Bruce C, Buus RM, et al. Preventing type 2 diabetes: public health implications for women with a history of gestational diabetes mellitus. Am J Obstet Gynecol. 2009;200(4):365.e1–8.
50. Rosenstein MG, Cheng YW, Snowden JM, Nicholson JM, Caughey AB. Risk of stillbirth and infant death stratified by gestational age. Obstet Gynecol. 2012;120(1):76–82.
51. Mellitus GD. ACOG practice bulletin summary.
52. Mulford MI, Jovanovic-Peterson L, Peterson CM. Alternative therapies for the management of gestational diabetes. Clin Perinatol. 1993;20(3):619–34.
53. Yaktine AL, Rasmussen KM. Weight gain during pregnancy: reexamining the guidelines. Washington, DC: National Academies Press; 2010.
54. Update I. ACOG practice bulletin. 2021.
55. Reichner CA. Insomnia and sleep deficiency in pregnancy. Obstet Med. 2015;8(4):168–71.
56. Smith A, LaFlamme E, Komanecky C. Pain management in labor. Am Fam Physician. 2021;103(6):355–64.
57. Grenvik JM, Rosenthal E, Saccone G, Della Corte L, Quist-Nelson J, Gerkin RD, et al. Peanut ball for decreasing length of labor: a systematic review and meta-analysis of randomized controlled trials. Eur J Obstet Gynecol Reprod Biol. 2019;242:159–65.
58. Myers ER, Sanders GD, Coeytaux RR, McElligott KA, Moorman PG, Hicklin K, et al. Labor dystocia. Rockville, MD: Agency for Healthcare Research and Quality; 2020.
59. Smith LA, Price N, Simonite V, Burns EE. Incidence of and risk factors for perineal trauma: a prospective observational study. BMC Pregnancy Childbirth. 2013;13:1–9.
60. Beckmann MM, Garrett AJ. Antenatal perineal massage for reducing perineal trauma. Cochrane Database Syst Rev. 2006;1:CD005123.
61. Aasheim V, Nilsen ABV, Reinar LM, Lukasse M. Perineal techniques during the second stage of labour for reducing perineal trauma. Cochrane Database Syst Rev. 2017;6:CD006672.
62. Waldman R. ACOG Practice Bulletin No. 198: prevention and management of obstetric lacerations at vaginal delivery. Obstet Gynecol. 2019;133(1):185.
63. Wilson RD, Caughey AB, Wood SL, Macones GA, Wrench IJ, Huang J, et al. Guidelines for antenatal and preoperative care in cesarean delivery: enhanced recovery after surgery society recommendations (part 1). Am J Obstet Gynecol. 2018;219(6):523.e1–e15.

64. Smith MD, McCall J, Plank L, Herbison GP, Soop M, Nygren J. Preoperative carbohydrate treatment for enhancing recovery after elective surgery. Cochrane Database Syst Rev. 2014;8:CD009161.
65. Macones GA, Caughey AB, Wood SL, Wrench IJ, Huang J, Norman M, et al. Guidelines for postoperative care in cesarean delivery: Enhanced Recovery After Surgery (ERAS) Society recommendations (part 3). Am J Obstet Gynecol. 2019;221(3):247.e1–9.
66. Teoh W, Shah M, Mah C. A randomised controlled trial on beneficial effects of early feeding post-caesarean delivery under regional anaesthesia. Singapore Med J. 2007;48(2):152.
67. Izbizky G, Minig L, Sebastiani M, Otano L. The effect of early versus delayed postcaesarean feeding on women's satisfaction: a randomised controlled trial. BJOG Int J Obstet Gynaecol. 2008;115(3):332–8.
68. Jalilian N, Ghadami MR. Randomized clinical trial comparing postoperative outcomes of early versus late oral feeding after cesarean section. J Obstet Gynaecol Res. 2014;40(6):1649–52.
69. Villamor E, Cnattingius S. Interpregnancy weight change and risk of adverse pregnancy outcomes: a population-based study. Lancet. 2006;368(9542):1164–70.
70. Johansson K, Cnattingius S, Näslund I, Roos N, Trolle Lagerros Y, Granath F, et al. Outcomes of pregnancy after bariatric surgery. N Engl J Med. 2015;372(9):814–24.
71. Mechanick JI, Youdim A, Jones DB, Garvey WT, Hurley DL, McMahon MM, et al. Clinical practice guidelines for the perioperative nutritional, metabolic, and nonsurgical support of the bariatric surgery patient—2013 update: cosponsored by American Association of Clinical Endocrinologists, the Obesity Society, and American Society for Metabolic & Bariatric Surgery. Surg Obes Relat Dis. 2013;9(2):159–91.
72. Colman GJ, Joyce T. Trends in smoking before, during, and after pregnancy in ten states. Am J Prev Med. 2003;24(1):29–35.
73. Syed H, Slayman T, Thoma KD. ACOG committee opinion no. 804: physical activity and exercise during pregnancy and the postpartum period. Obstet Gynecol. 2021;137(2):375–6.
74. Bane SM. Postpartum exercise and lactation. Clin Obstet Gynecol. 2015;58(4):885–92.
75. Mota P, Pascoal AG, Carita AI, Bø K. The immediate effects on inter-rectus distance of abdominal crunch and drawing-in exercises during pregnancy and the postpartum period. J Orthop Sports Phys Ther. 2015;45(10):781–8.
76. Rupnicki S. Breastfeeding report card United States, 2020. Atlanta, GA: CDC; 2020.
77. Tomori C. Overcoming barriers to breastfeeding. Best Pract Res Clin Obstet Gynaecol. 2022;83:60–71.
78. Wisner KL, Sit DK, McShea MC, Rizzo DM, Zoretich RA, Hughes CL, et al. Onset timing, thoughts of self-harm, and diagnoses in postpartum women with screen-positive depression findings. JAMA Psychiatry. 2013;70(5):490–8.
79. Leboffe EN, Pietragallo HC, Liu G, Ba D, Leslie D, Chuang CH. The impact of the 2015 ACOG screening guidelines on the diagnosis of postpartum depression among privately insured women. J Affect Disord. 2023;328:103–7.

Index

A. Watson, K. Barr (eds.), *Prehabilitation Guide for All Providers*, https://doi.org/10.1007/978-3-031-72862-4

MIX
Papier aus verantwortungsvollen Quellen
Paper from responsible sources
FSC® C105338

If you have any concerns about our products,
you can contact us on
ProductSafety@springernature.com

In case Publisher is established outside the EU,
the EU authorized representative is:
Springer Nature Customer Service Center GmbH
Europaplatz 3, 69115 Heidelberg, Germany

Printed by Libri Plureos GmbH
in Hamburg, Germany